Pediatric and Adolescent Knee Injuries: Evaluation, Treatment and Rehabilitation

Editor

MATTHEW D. MILEWSKI

CLINICS IN SPORTS MEDICINE

www.sportsmed.theclinics.com

Consulting Editor
MARK D. MILLER

October 2022 • Volume 41 • Number 4

ELSEVIER

1600 John F. Kennedy Boulevard • Suite 1800 • Philadelphia, Pennsylvania, 19103-2899

http://www.theclinics.com

CLINICS IN SPORTS MEDICINE Volume 41, Number 4
October 2022 ISSN 0278-5919, ISBN-13: 978-0-323-84957-9

Editor: Megan Ashdown
Developmental Editor: Diana Grace Ang

Clinics in Sports Medicine (ISSN 0278-5919) is published quarterly by Elsevier Inc., 360 Park Avenue South, New York, NY 10010-1710. Months of issue are January, April, July, and October. Business and Editorial Offices: 1600 John F. Kennedy Blvd., Ste. 1800, Philadelphia, PA 19103-2899. Customer Service Office: 3251 Riverport Lane, Maryland Heights, MO 63043. Periodicals postage paid at New York, NY and additional mailing offices. Subscription prices are $368.00 per year (US individuals), $959.00 per year (US institutions), $100.00 per year (US students), $409.00 per year (Canadian individuals), $988.00 per year (Canadian institutions), $100.00 (Canadian students), $480.00 per year (foreign individuals), $988.00 per year (foreign institutions), and $235.00 per year (foreign students). Foreign air speed delivery is included in all *Clinics* subscription prices. All prices are subject to change without notice. **POSTMASTER:** Send address changes to *Clinics in Sports Medicine*, Elsevier Health Sciences Division, Subscription Customer Service, 3251 Riverport Lane, Maryland Heights, MO 63043. Customer Service (orders, claims, online, change of address): Elsevier Health Sciences Division, Subscription Customer Service, 3251 Riverport Lane, Maryland Heights, MO 63043. **Tel: 1-800-654-2452 (U.S. and Canada); 314-447-8871 (outside U.S. and Canada). Fax: 314-447-8029. E-mail: journalscustomerservice-usa@elsevier.com (for print support); journalsonlinesupport-usa@elsevier.com (for online support).**

Reprints. For copies of 100 or more of articles in this publication, please contact the Commercial Reprints Department, Elsevier Inc., 360 Park Avenue South, New York, NY 10010-1710. Tel.: 212-633-3874; Fax: 212-633-3820; E-mail: reprints@elsevier.com.

Clinics in Sports Medicine is covered in *MEDLINE/PubMed (Index Medicus) Current Contents/Clinical Medicine, Excerpta Medica,* and *ISI/Biomed.*

Contributors

CONSULTING EDITOR

MARK D. MILLER, MD
S. Ward Casscells Professor, Head, Department of Orthopaedic Surgery, Division of Sports Medicine, University of Virginia, Charlottesville, Virginia, USA; Team Physician, Miller Review Course, Harrisonburg, Virginia, USA

EDITOR

MATTHEW D. MILEWSKI, MD
Past President, Pediatric Research in Sports Medicine Society (PRiSM), Associate Professor, Division of Sports Medicine, Department of Orthopaedic Surgery, Boston Children's Hospital, Harvard Medical School, Boston, Massachusetts, USA

AUTHORS

SOROUSH BAGHDADI, MD
Children's Hospital of Philadelphia, Philadelphia, Pennsylvania, USA

TARA BAXTER, MD, MSc
Boston, Massachusetts, USA

DAVID BAZETT-JONES, PhD, AT, ATC, CSCS
Associate Professor, Program Director, School of Exercise and Rehabilitation Sciences, University of Toledo, School of Exercise and Rehabilitation Sciences, Toledo, Ohio, USA

SAMUEL CLIFTON WILLIMON, MD
Children's Orthopedics and Sports Medicine, Children's Healthcare of Atlanta, Atlanta, Georgia, USA

JENNIFER BECK, MD
Associate Professor, Orthopaedic Institute for Children/UCLA Department of Orthopaedic Surgery

JENNIFER BREY, MD
Assistant Professor, Department of Orthopaedic Surgery, University of Louisville

NAOMI BROWN, MD
Department of Orthopedics, Sports Medicine and Performance Center, Children's Hospital of Philadelphia, Philadelphia, Pennsylvania, USA

LAUREN S. BUTLER, PT, DPT, SCS
Nicklaus Children's Hospital, Miami, Florida, USA

CORDELIA W. CARTER, MD
Attending Physician, Associate Professor, Orthopedic Surgery, NYU Langone Orthopedic Hospital, NYU Langone Health, NYU Grossman School of Medicine, New York, New York, USA

ROSS CHAFETZ, PT, DPT, PhD, MPH
Corporate Director, Motion Analysis Centers at Shriners Childrens, Department of Orthopedics, Shriners Hospital for Children, Department of Orthopedics, Hahnemann University Hospital, Philadelphia, Pennsylvania, USA

MICHAEL M. CHAU, MD, PhD
Department of Orthopedic Surgery, University of Minnesota, Minneapolis, Minnesota, USA

DANIELLE E. CHIPMAN, BS
Division of Pediatric Orthopedic Surgery, Hospital for Special Surgery, New York, New York, USA

MELISSA A. CHRISTINO, MD
Division of Sports Medicine, Department of Orthopaedic Surgery, Boston Children's Hospital, Boston, Massachusetts, USA

FRANK A. CORDASCO, MD, MS
Sports Medicine Institute, Hospital for Special Surgery, New York, New York, USA; Professor of Orthopaedic Surgery, Weill Cornell Medical College, Attending Surgeon, Sports Medicine Institute, Senior Scientist, Research Division

ARISTIDES I. CRUZ Jr, MD, MBA
Assistant Professor, Department of Orthopedics, Warren Alpert Medical School of Brown University, Hasbro Children's Hospital, Providence, Rhode Island, USA

BIANCA R. EDISON, MD, MS
Attending Physician, Assistant Professor, Orthopaedics, Children's Hospital Los Angeles, University of Southern California, Los Angeles, California, USA

HENRY B. ELLIS Jr, MD
Department of Orthopaedic Surgery, Associate Professor, UT Southwestern Medical Center, Texas Scottish Rite Hospital for Children, Dallas, Texas, USA

CRAIG J. FINLAYSON, MD
Assistant Professor of Orthopaedic Surgery, Northwestern University Feinberg School of Medicine, Ann & Robert H. Lurie Children's Hospital of Chicago, Chicago, Illinois, USA

CORINNA FRANKLIN, MD
Associate Professor, Chief, Pediatric Orthopaedic Surgery, Department of Orthopedics, Shriners Hospital for Children, Philadelphia, Pennsylvania, USA

NICOLE FRIEL, MD
Shriners Hospital for Children, Northern California, Sacramento, California, USA

THEODORE J. GANLEY, MD
Associate Professor of Orthopaedic Surgery, Perelman School of Medicine, University of Pennsylvania, Children's Hospital of Philadelphia, Philadelphia, Pennsylvania, USA

JAYDEN GLOVER, BS
Lake Erie College of Osteopathic Medicine, Bradenton, Florida, USA

DANIEL W. GREEN, MD, MS, FACS
Division of Pediatric Orthopedic Surgery, Hospital for Special Surgery, Director, Pediatric Orthopedic Surgery Fellowship, Associate Director, HSS Orthopedic Surgery Residency Program, Professor of Clinical Orthopedic Surgery, Weill Cornell Medical College New York, New York, USA

ELLIOT M. GREENBERG, PT, DPT, PhD
Clinical Specialist/Research Scientist, Children's Hospital of Philadelphia Sports Medicine and Performance Center, Philadelphia, Pennsylvania, USA

BENTON E. HEYWORTH, MD
Associate Program Director, Orthopedic Sports Medicine Fellowship, Associate Professor of Orthopedic Surgery, Harvard Medical School, Boston Children's Hospital, Boston, Boston, Massachusetts, USA

JOSEPH J. JANOSKY, DrPHc, MSc, PT, ATC
Sports Medicine Institute, Hospital for Special Surgery, New York, New York, USA

ELAINE JOUGHIN, MD
Clinical Assistant Professor of Orthopaedic Surgery, Alberta Children's Hospital, Calgary, Alberta, Canada

JAPSIMRAN KAUR, BS
University of Rochester School of Medicine and Dentistry, Rochester, New York, USA

EMILY KRAUS, MD
Division of Physical Medicine and Rehabilitation, Department of Orthopedic Surgery, Stanford University, Center for Academic Medicine, Pediatric Orthopaedic Surgery, Stanford, California, USA

INDRANIL KUSHARE, MD
Associate Professor, Department of Orthopedic Surgery, Texas Children's Hospital, Houston, Texas, USA

RUSHYUAN JAY LEE, MD
Director, Pediatric Orthopaedic Fellowship, Associate Professor of Orthopaedic Surgery, The Johns Hopkins School of Medicine, Baltimore, Maryland, USA

LISE LEVEILLE, MD
Clinical Assistant Professor & Director, Undergraduate Medical Education, Department of Orthopaedics, BC Children's Hospital, Vancouver, British Columbia, Canada

DANIELLE MAGRINI, DO
Division of Pediatric Sports Medicine, Swedish Medical Center, Seattle, Washington, USA

ADITI MAJUMDAR, MD, MSc
Sports Medicine Division, Orthopedic Sports Medicine Attending, Children's Hospital Orange County, Orange, California, USA

ANDREW MCCOY, MD
Department of Physical Medicine and Rehabilitation, Children's Hospital Colorado, Aurora, Colorado, USA

DONNA MERKEL, PT, DPT, SCS, CSCS
Physical Therapist, Mainline Health System, Collegeville, Pennsylvania, USA

MATTHEW D. MILEWSKI, MD
Past President, Pediatric Research in Sports Medicine Society (PRiSM), Associate Professor, Division of Sports Medicine, Department of Orthopaedic Surgery, Boston Children's Hospital, Harvard Medical School, Boston, Massachusetts, USA

RONALD JUSTIN MISTOVICH, MD, MBA
Associate Professor, Case Western Reserve University School of Medicine, Rainbow Babies & Children's Hospital, Cleveland, Ohio, USA

JOSEPH T. MOLONY Jr, PT, MS. SCS, CSCS
Manager, Young Athlete Program, Department of Pediatric Rehabilitation, Hospital for Special Surgery, New York, New York, USA

MARIE LYNE NAULT, MD
Associate Professor, Pediatric Orthopaedic Surgery, University of Montreal

EMILY L. NIU, MD
Assistant Professor of Orthopaedic Surgery, George Washington University School of Medicine, Children's National Hospital, Washington, DC, USA

ERIC NUSSBAUM, ATC
Division of Orthopaedic Surgery, Rutgers, Robert Wood Johnson Medical School, New Brunswick, New Jersey, USA

NIRAV K. PANDYA, MD
Attending Physician, Associate Professor, Orthopaedic Surgery, UCSF Benioff Children's Hospital, Oakland, California, USA; University California, San Francisco, San Francisco, California, USA

SHITAL N. PARIKH, MD, FACS
Professor of Orthopedic Surgery, Cincinnati Children's Hospital Medical Center, Cincinnati, Ohio, USA

NICOLAS PASCUAL-LEONE, BA
Division of Pediatric Orthopedic Surgery, Hospital for Special Surgery, New York, New York, USA

ANEESH G. PATANKAR, BS
Rutgers Robert Wood Johnson Medical School, New Brunswick, New Jersey, USA

NEERAJ M. PATEL, MD, MPH, MBS
Attending Physician, Assistant Professor, Orthopaedic Surgery, Ann & Robert H. Lurie Children's Hospital of Chicago, Northwestern University Feinberg School of Medicine, Chicago, Illinois, USA

SOFIA HIDALGO PEREA, BS
Hospital for Special Surgery, New York, New York, USA

CRYSTAL A. PERKINS, MD
Children's Orthopedics and Sports Medicine, Children's Healthcare of Atlanta, Atlanta, Georgia, USA

MIMI RACICOT, PT, DPT, SCS
Manager, Rehabilitation and Sports, Department of Rehabilitation, Seattle Children's Hospital, Seattle, Washington, USA

LAUREN REDLER, MD
Columbia University, New York, New York, USA

JASON RHODES, MD
Associate Professor, Clinical Director Center for Gait and Movement Analysis, Department of Orthopedics, Children's Hospital Colorado, Aurora, Colorado, USA

KATHERINE RIZZONE, MD, MPH
Division of Orthopaedics and Pediatrics, University of Rochester Medical Center, Rochester, New York, USA

JOHN SCHLECHTER, DO
Children's Hospital of Orange County, Orange, California, USA

SARA ROSE SHANNON
Hospital for Special Surgery, New York, New York, USA

BRENDAN SHI, MD
Resident Physician, UCLA Department of Orthopaedic Surgery

AUSTIN SKINNER, BS
Department of Orthopedics, Children's Hospital Colorado, Musculoskeletal Research Center, Aurora, Colorado, USA

ZACHARY STINSON, MD
Attending Surgeon, Nemours Children's Health

DAI SUGIMOTO, PhD, ATC
The Micheli Center for Sports Injury Prevention, Waltham, Massachusetts, USA; Faculty of Sport Sciences, Waseda University, Nishi-Tokyo City, Tokyo, Japan

ALEX TAGAWA, BS
Department of Orthopedics, Children's Hospital Colorado, Musculoskeletal Research Center, Aurora, Colorado, USA

MARC A. TOMPKINS, MD
Department of Orthopedic Surgery, University of Minnesota, Minneapolis, Minnesota, USA; TRIA Orthopedic Center, Bloomington, Minnesota, USA; Gillette Children's Specialty Healthcare, St Paul, Minnesota, USA

KIRSTEN TULCHIN-FRANCIS, PhD
Director, Orthopedic Research & Director, Honda Center for Gait Analysis and Mobility Enhancement, Department of Orthopedic Surgery, Nationwide Children's Hospital, Columbus, Ohio, USA

MATTHEW VEERKAMP, BA
Cincinnati Children's Hospital Medical Center, Cincinnati, Ohio, USA

MAHALA WALKER, BS
University of Kentucky College of Medicine, Lexington, Kentucky, USA

ADAM P. WEAVER, PT, DPT
Sports Physical Therapist, Connecticut Children's, Farmington, Connecticut, USA

BRENDAN A. WILLIAMS, MD
Children's Hospital of Philadelphia, Philadelphia, Pennsylvania, USA

MOSHE YANIV, MD
Dana-Dwek Children's Hospital - Tel Aviv Sourasky Medical Center. Tel Aviv, Israel

CHRISTIN ZWOLSKI, PT, DPT, PhD
Division of Occupational Therapy and Physical Therapy, Cincinnati Children's Hospital Medical Center, Cincinnati, Ohio, USA

Contents

The Micheli anterior cruciate ligament reconstruction (ACLR) procedure is a combined intra-articular and extra-articular knee stabilization technique that combines lateral augmentation with ACL reconstruction using iliotibial band autograft for both aspects of the technique. Its primary indication is for ACL reconstruction in skeletally immature patients with more than 2 years of growth remaining. Studies have shown it to be effective at restoring knee biomechanics, to have minimal risk of complications, including those associated with growth disturbances, and to have a relatively low ACL graft rupture rate. Additional studies are needed to better understand the potential utilization of this technique and related modifications in the marginally skeletally immature patient, skeletally mature adolescent, adult, and in revision ACL reconstruction settings.

All-epiphyseal anterior cruciate ligament reconstruction (AE ACLR) has become an alternative technique for skeletally immature patients with a significant amount of growth remaining. This technique involves graft fixation within the epiphysis without crossing the physis. Either quadriceps tendon or hamstring autograft can be used when performing this procedure. Previous studies have shown that the complication rate is not higher in AE techniques versus previously developed techniques. Additionally, in our hands, the revision rate was found to be significantly lower in an AE ACLR compared with patients who had a transphyseal ACLR.

Osteochondritis dissecans of the knee is a relatively rare disorder in young athletes that can lead to premature osteoarthritis. It may be caused by multiple factors, including repetitive stress, local ischemia, aberrant endochondral ossification of the subarticular physis, and hereditary disposition. Nonoperative treatment is typically attempted for patients with open physes, stable lesions, and minimal symptoms. Operative treatment is offered to patients with closed physes, unstable lesions, mechanical symptoms, and failure of nonoperative treatment. Customized rehabilitation and return to sport programs are important for successful outcomes regardless of treatment type.

Knee injuries are prevalent in pediatric and adolescent athletes, leading to both physical and psychological disturbances following injury. Various preoperative psychological measures of maladaptive beliefs—including kinesiophobia, fear avoidance, and pain catastrophizing—can predict responses to recovery, such as knee function, knee-related quality of life, and return-to-sport. Treatment recommendations for the psychological aspect of adolescent knee injuries can include screening patients to identify those at high risk for poor recovery. These patients can be targeted with psychologically informed media or cognitive-behavioral therapy models aimed at reducing maladaptive beliefs and supporting individualized motivations and recovery goals.

Evaluation and management of multiligament knee injuries (MLKI) require a comprehensive understanding of anatomy and biomechanics. In addition to a thorough history and physical examination, stress radiographs provide a reliable method to assess knee stability. Single-stage anatomic reconstruction techniques should be performed, as they restore native knee kinematics and enable early knee range of motion and superior outcomes.

This article summarizes the latest research related to pediatric patellar instability. The epidemiology, patterns of patellar instability, and underlying pathoanatomy are unique in children and adolescents. Information related to the natural history and predictive factors of patellar instability in young patients would allow for better patient counseling and management decisions. The components of nonoperative treatment for first patellar dislocation are outlined. Physeal-respecting surgical techniques, including medial patellofemoral ligament reconstruction in skeletally immature patients, are discussed. The indications and outcomes for quadricepsplasty to address more complex instability patterns are presented. Evaluation and management strategies for specific anatomic risk factors is provided.

> Tibial spine fractures are a relatively rare injury in the young athlete. Previously thought to be the equivalent of a "pediatric anterior cruciate ligament (ACL) tear," contemporary understanding of these injuries classifies them as distinct from ACL injuries in this patient population. Successful treatment hinges on accurate diagnosis paying special attention to fracture displacement and the presence of concomitant intraarticular injury. Surgery can be performed using open or arthroscopic techniques and a variety of fixation options. The most common complication after surgical treatment is arthrofibrosis and, therefore, stable fixation is necessary to allow for early, unimpeded knee motion postoperatively.

> Three-dimensional motion capture systems may improve evaluation, treatment, and rehabilitation of knee injuries, because quantitative assessment of the knee improves understanding of biomechanical mechanisms. The benefit of using motion analysis in pediatric sports medicine is that it allows closer and more focused evaluation of sports injuries using kinematics, kinetics, and electromyogram with physical and imaging to determine what is happening dynamically during sports. Future research investigating knee injuries should focus on identifying risk factors, assessing the effectiveness of surgical and nonsurgical interventions, and developing return to sport/rehabilitation protocols. The literature is focused on motion capture in adults with knee injuries.

> According to epidemiology studies, the majority of youth sports injuries presenting to primary care, athletic trainers, and emergency departments impact the musculoskeletal system. Both acute and overuse knee injuries can contribute to sports attrition before high school. Effective rehabilitation of knee injuries ensures a timely return to sports participation and minimizes the negative physical, psychological, and social consequences of becoming injured. The following article provides rehabilitation and return to play strategies for postsurgical and nonsurgical injuries of the young athlete's knee.

> Stress injuries to the bone and physis of the knee are common in the active adolescent patient and can be broken down into bone stress injuries (BSIs)

and chronic physeal stress injuries. BSIs result from prolonged, repetitive bone loading, whereas chronic physeal stress injuries develop from repetitive loading to the apophysis or epiphysis. Most stress injuries of the knee resolve with relative rest but will occasionally need surgical intervention in more severe cases. Early and accurate identification is paramount for optimal management and to avoid long-term consequences.

Discoid meniscus is the most common congenital variant of the meniscus. Its variability in pathology leads to a spectrum of clinical presentations in patients. Treatment must be tailored to the specific pathology of the discoid meniscus. Imaging studies such as radiographs and magnetic resonance imaging can be useful in confirming the diagnosis, but may not be the most accurate in determining specific pathology. Thorough intraoperative evaluation of the discoid is critical to appropriate surgical management. Rim preservation and repair is preferred to prevent degenerative changes in the knee.

Meniscus tears are common in the pediatric population, typically occur after noncontact injuries, and can be diagnosed clinically with MRI confirmation. Surgery should be offered to patients with loss of range of motion, persistent symptoms, or displaced/complex tears. Given poor long-term outcomes reported after meniscectomy, repair should be attempted when possible as pediatric menisci are well vascularized and have better outcomes after repair than their adult counterparts. The location of the tear is an important determining factor when deciding on the type of repair to use. Pediatric meniscus repair techniques will be discussed noting differences between pediatric and adult procedures. Further studies are needed to explore the role of biologics and define postoperative protocols.

The participation of females in sports has increased significantly since the passage of Title IX. Sports participation may place young athletes at risk for knee injuries, including patellofemoral pain syndrome (PFPS), osteochondritis dissecans (OCD), and anterior cruciate ligament (ACL) rupture. Differences in anatomy, hormone production, and neuromuscular patterns between female and male athletes can contribute to disparities in knee injury rates with female athletes more vulnerable to PFPS and ACL injury. Biological differences between sexes alone cannot fully explain worldwide differences in musculoskeletal health outcomes. Social, cultural and societal attitudes toward gender and the participation of girls and women in sports may result in a lack of accessible training for both injury prevention and performance optimization; one must recognize the effects of gender disparities on injury risk. More nuanced approaches to assess the complex interplay among biological, physiologic, and social influences are needed to inform best practices for intervention and sports injury prevention.

Disparities persist in pediatric sports medicine along the lines of race, ethnicity, insurance status, and other demographic factors. In the context of knee injuries such as anterior cruciate ligament (ACL) ruptures, meniscus tears, and tibial spine fractures, these inequalities affect evaluation, treatment, and outcomes. The long-term effects can be far-reaching, including sports and physical activity participation, comorbid chronic disease, and socio-emotional health. Further research is needed to more concretely identify the etiology of these disparities so that effective, equitable care is provided for all children.

 Video content accompanies this article at http://www.sportsmed. theclinics.com.

It is estimated that approximately 2.5 million sports-related knee injuries occur in the pediatric population annually in the United States. Thus, identifying appropriate screening tools and injury prevention strategies is imperative. To develop successful injury prevention strategies, risk factor identification is the first step. There are two types of risk factors: non-modifiable (age, gender, injury history, and anatomical alignment) and modifiable risk factors (biomechanical and neuromuscular control, training loads, and body mass index). These risk factors can be addressed by three types of preventive interventions: primary, secondary, and tertiary. To translate study evidence to clinical practices and routine trainings, awareness of injury prevention and health promotion needs to be further strengthened.

CLINICS IN SPORTS MEDICINE

FORTHCOMING ISSUES

January 2023
Advances in the Treatment of Rotator Cuff Tears
Brian Werner, *Editor*

April 2023
Equality, Diversity, and Inclusion in Sports Medicine
Joel Boyd, Constance Chu, Erica Taylor, *Editors*

July 2023
On the Field Emergencies
Eric McCarty, Sourav K. Poddar and Alex Ebinger, *Editors*

RECENT ISSUES

July 2022
Sports Cardiology
Peter Nelson Dean, *Editor*

April 2022
Sports Anesthesia
Ashley Matthews Shilling, *Editor*

January 2022
Patellofemoral Instability Decision Making and Techniques
David Diduch, *Editor*

SERIES OF RELATED INTERESTED

Orthopedic Clinics
https://www.orthopedic.theclinics.com/
Foot and Ankle Clinics
https://www.foot.theclinics.com/
Hand Clinics
https://www.hand.theclinics.com/
Physical Medicine and Rehabilitation Clinics
https://www.pmr.theclinics.com/

Foreword

Pediatric and Adolescent Knee Injuries: The PRiSM Vision

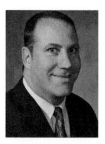

Mark D. Miller, MD
Consulting Editor

It has been a while since we had an issue of *Clinics in Sports Medicine* focusing on the Pediatric Knee. Therefore, I asked my former Fellow, now an associate professor at Boston's Children Hospital at Harvard and past president of the Pediatric Research in Sports Medicine Society (PRiSM) (Yes, we are proud of him), to serve as guest editor for this issue. Not surprisingly, he put together an excellent compilation that gives us important updates for the management of pediatric and adolescent knee injuries. He has included the entire gambit of injuries, including ACL, MLI, OCD, patellar instability, meniscal pathology, and a wide variety of associated problems. Thank you to Dr Milewski for putting this together and thank you to all the PRiSM members who contributed. I encourage all readers to analyze and reflect the light from this important society.

Mark D. Miller, MD
Division of Sports Medicine
Department of Orthopaedic Surgery
University of Virginia
400 Ray C. Hunt Drive
Suite 330
Charlottesville, VA 22908-0159, USA

E-mail address:
MDM3P@hscmail.mcc.virginia.edu

https://doi.org/10.1016/j.csm.2022.07.003
0278-5919/22/© 2022 Published by Elsevier Inc.
sportsmed.theclinics.com

Preface

Pediatric and Adolescent Knee Injuries: Evaluation, Treatment, and Rehabilitation

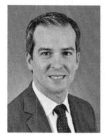

Matthew D. Milewski, MD
Editor

It is my extreme privilege to serve as guest editor for this issue of *Clinics in Sports Medicine* entitled Pediatric and Adolescent Knee Injuries: Evaluation, Treatment, and Rehabilitation. This issue was produced collaboratively from the Pediatric Research in Sports Medicine Society (PRiSM), and I had the honor of serving as president of this society in 2021.

PRiSM is a multidisciplinary group of sports medicine clinicians and researchers, including athletic trainers, physical therapists, nurse practitioners, physician assistants/associates, PhDs, radiologists, primary care sports medicine physicians, and orthopedic surgeons. The purpose of PRiSM is to lead interdisciplinary research, education, and advancement in pediatric and adolescent sports medicine. Our society is devoted to improving not only injury diagnosis and treatment but also injury prevention and sports performance optimization.

PRiSM was founded in 2012 by our founding board of directors to improve collaboration and education in pediatric and adolescent sports medicine. We strive to foster the growth of an incredibly diverse membership, representative of all aspects of sports medicine. Many pediatric sports injuries, conditions, and such are unique to young athletes and do not occur in other age groups. By combining research across multiple centers and different practitioners, PRiSM members are uniquely positioned to

Clin Sports Med 41 (2022) xvii–xviii
https://doi.org/10.1016/j.csm.2022.07.002
0278-5919/22/© 2022 Published by Elsevier Inc.

sportsmed.theclinics.com

increase the impact of research. We intend to move beyond research-based retrospective case series and expand our ability to conduct prospective research on outcomes, optimal treatment, injury prevention, and so forth. By developing processes and systems to allow sharing of data, we can answer research questions with greater power, confidence, and generalizability.

PRiSM's research endeavors are centered within research interest groups that study 16 different pediatric adolescent sports conditions that cover concussions, overuse injuries, and fractures and ligament/structural injuries in a multidisciplinary team approach.

As you will see in the subsequent articles for this issue, the collaborative multidisciplinary teamwork is showcased by our members and research interest groups for this amazing issue of *Clinics in Sports Medicine*.

We hope that you enjoy and learn from the collective knowledge of our collaborations for the evaluation, treatment, and rehabilitation of pediatric and adolescent knee injuries and pathologic conditions. If you have like-minded interest in the treatment or research of pediatric and adolescent athletes and their injuries, please check out our Web site (prismsports.org) and consider membership!

Thanks again.

Matthew D. Milewski, MD
Division of Sports Medicine
Department of Orthopaedic Surgery
Boston Children's Hospital
Harvard Medical School
300 Longwood Avenue
Boston, MA 02115, USA

E-mail address:
matthew.milewski@childrens.harvard.edu

Erratum

In the article, "Differentiating Physiology from Pathology," by Alfred Danielian and Ankit B. Shah., published in the July 2022 issue (Volume 41, number 3, pages 426), Figure 1 should be:

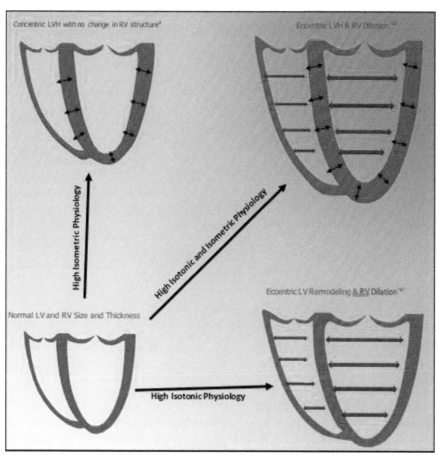

Anterior Cruciate Ligament Reconstruction Procedures Using the Iliotibial Band Autograft

Aditi Majumdar, MD, MSc[a], Tara Baxter, MD, MSc[b],
Benton Heyworth, MD[b],*

KEYWORDS

- ACL • ITB • Anterior cruciate ligament • Iliotibial band • Pediatric • Knee instability
- Reconstruction • Graft

KEY POINTS

- The Micheli anterior cruciate ligament (ACL) reconstruction procedure is a combined intra-articular and extra-articular procedure that adds anterolateral augmentation to an ACL reconstruction, using an extended central portion of the native iliotibial band as a single autograft for both components of the reconstruction.
- The Micheli procedure is primarily indicated for skeletally immature patients with ACL tears and more than 2 years of growth remaining, but its indications and uses may be expanding, with some having explored modified applications of the technique in skeletally mature patients.
- The Micheli procedure has demonstrated excellent postoperative functional and patient-reported outcomes and favorable ACL re-tear/graft rupture rates in several studies.
- There has been growing interest in using a shorter central or posterior portion of the iliotibial band as a graft in lateral extra-articular augmentation procedures, which are often combined with ACL reconstruction using other autograft options, such as hamstring, quadriceps, or patellar tendon.

INTRODUCTION/BACKGROUND

Anterior cruciate ligament (ACL) injuries in skeletally immature patients were once a rare occurrence, but have become increasingly common secondary to increased athletic participation, intensity, and sheer numbers of potential exposures in youth sports today. Most of these injuries benefit from surgery to stabilize the knee, facilitate return

[a] Sports Medicine, Children's Hospital Orange County, 1310 W Stewart Drive, Suite 508, Orange, CA 92868, USA; [b] Sports Medicine, Children's Hospital Orange County, 1310 W Stewart Drive, Suite 508, Orange, CA 92868, USA
* Corresponding author.
E-mail address: benton.heyworth@childrens.harvard.edu

Clin Sports Med 41 (2022) 549–567
https://doi.org/10.1016/j.csm.2022.05.001
0278-5919/22/© 2022 Published by Elsevier Inc.

to cutting and pivoting sports and recreational activities, and minimize secondary intra-articular injuries, such as meniscal and chondral injuries. A recent national database study of ACL injuries in pediatric patients found that the rate of ACL reconstructions (ACLRs) in this population increased 5.7 fold between 2004 and 2014.[1] The risk of physeal injury associated with traditional techniques performed in younger patients has driven the emergence of several physeal-sparing techniques, the earliest and best studied of which is the combined intra-articular and extra-articular physeal-sparing technique with autologous iliotibial band (ITB) graft. The current review aims to describe the specific considerations inherent to the technique and provide insight into its emerging role in lateral augmentation, revision ACLR and primary ACLR in other populations and settings, such as in skeletally mature adolescents.

The use of the ITB as a graft in surgical stabilization procedures of the knee is not a novel concept. Its use as a graft was initially popularized in the 1970s and 1980s for lateral extra-articular stabilization procedures,[2] which were used in ACL-deficient knees as an isolated procedure in an attempt to address anterolateral rotational laxity. Many such extra-articular procedures were described during this time period, including the Lemaire,[3] Ellison,[4] MacIntosh,[5,6] and Andrews[7] techniques. However, these techniques were later abandoned in favor of intra-articular ACLR, coinciding with the advent and popularization of arthroscopic-assisted ACLR, which seemed to produce better results. Interestingly, in cyclical fashion, this concept has recently experienced an explosion of renewed interest as an *adjunctive* procedure to ACLR, first in selective clinical scenarios or specific patient populations,[8–11] but may be increasingly paired with more routine primary ACLR in broader populations of young patients.

After the original MacIntosh procedure described in 1976, MacIntosh also described a modification of his technique which included both an extra-articular component and an intra-articular component to address ACL deficiency.[12] In this modification, a long segment of intact ITB was routed posteriorly over the top of the lateral femoral condyle into the knee joint and secured on the tibial side through a tibial bone tunnel,[6] thus combining a lateral extra-articular augmentation procedure with an ACLR. This technique was later modified by Micheli to an exclusively physeal-sparing technique, devoid of bone tunnels, for use in pediatric patients with open growth plates, with the first report in 1999.[13] In this physeal-sparing ACLR, in addition to avoiding a tunnel in the distal femoral physis, the proximal tibial physis is avoided by using a bony trough in the epiphysis in place of a tunnel and using suture fixation of the distal extent of the ITB graft to the anterior tibial metaphyseal periosteum[14] (**Fig. 1**). Kocher and Micheli have since popularized the technique with longer term patient-based outcomes reported in 2006 and 2018, and it has remained a preferred ACLR procedure in prepubescent patients with substantial growth remaining.[14,15]

ANATOMY

The ITB is a tendinous band of dense fibrous connective tissue in the lateral thigh. It takes its origin from the tensor fascia lata and gluteus maximus muscles proximally and has a broad distal insertion into Gerdy's tubercle after crossing the knee joint. The posterior portion of the ITB is confluent with the lateral intermuscular septum, whereas the anterior portion is confluent with the superficial fascia of the vastus lateralis. These features can make its margins challenging to define surgically.[16] The ITB acts as a knee extensor when the knee is at 0 to 30° of flexion, and as a knee flexor when the knee is flexed beyond 30°. The tension in the distal ITB shifts from anterior to posterior as the loaded knee goes from extension to flexion.[16] The ITB has a role in restricting both anterior tibial translation and internal rotation of the tibia.[17] The distal

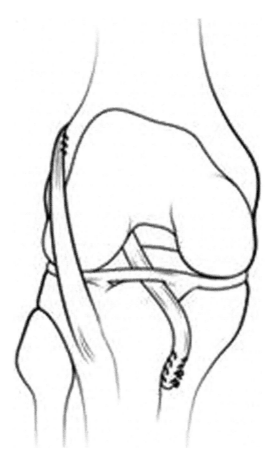

Fig. 1. An illustration of the Micheli physeal-sparing, ACL reconstruction technique, which combines extra-articular and intra-articular reconstruction. A long segment of ITB autograft is harvested proximally and preserved distally at the tibial insertion. The graft is then routed posteriorly over the top of the lateral femoral condyle, intra-articularly and under the intermeniscal ligament, and secured distally within a bony trough and anterior tibial metaphyseal periosteum using suture fixation.

portion of the ITB overlies the lateral epicondyle of the distal femur, the lateral collateral ligament, and the anterolateral ligament (ALL).

The recent surge in orthopedic research related to the ALL, spurred by trending anatomic descriptions of the ligament and attention to anterolateral rotatory instability,[18–21] has generated renewed interest in lateral extra-articular augmentation procedures to complement, and reinforce, ACLRs.[18] Several anatomic studies have identified the ALL as a distinct ligament presenting as a thickening of the lateral side of the knee joint capsule, with a prominent attachment to the lateral meniscus.[18,19,21,22] The femoral footprint of the ALL is described to be just posterior and proximal to the lateral epicondyle with the tibial footprint located on the anterolateral proximal tibia between the fibular head and Gerdy's tubercle.[18,22–24] The ALL functions in resisting anterolateral rotatory instability in the knee.[25] Currently, most lateral extra-articular augmentation procedures attempt to either anatomically reconstruct the ALL with a separate graft, or approximate its function with a portion of the ITB in a "nonanatomic" reconstruction, such as the lateral extra-articular tenodesis

(LET) and many of the previously mentioned isolated extra-articular techniques developed in the 1970s and 1980s.[26]

LATERAL EXTRA-ARTICULAR AUGMENTATION AND ANTEROLATERAL LIGAMENT RECONSTRUCTION PROCEDURES

Among the most well-cited investigations of ACLR combined with either ALL reconstruction or LET are the research efforts of the Scientific ACL NeTwork International (SANTI) (502 patients) and STABILITY (618 patients) study groups, respectively. Proponents for ALL reconstruction may contend that an anatomic technique is less likely to result in iatrogenic overconstraint of the knee or alter knee kinematics or biomechanics. Although some biomechanical studies have indicated potential overconstraint of the lateral compartment with LET, this has not been shown to have an adverse clinical effect in larger patient-based follow-up studies.[27] Regardless of the precise technique selected, biomechanical investigations and clinical outcomes have indicated that lateral extra-articular augmentation with ITB decreases forces on the ACL graft through load sharing and results in a lower incidence of ACL graft failure in young, pivoting athletes.[11,27,28]

In a 2-year follow-up of one of the original SANTI cohort studies, a prospective comparison of primary ACLR with a hamstring tendon (HT) autograft with anterolateral ligament reconstruction (ALLR) (HT + ALLR) had a significantly lower rate of graft failure in comparison to isolated bone–patellar tendon–bone (BTB) and quadrupled HT ACLR, respectively. In addition, HT + ALLR patients were more likely to return to pre-injury level of sport than hamstring graft alone.[11] Longer term results of this cohort (mean, 104.3 months) show combined ACL + ALLR patients had significantly better ACL graft survivorship (96.5%) and lower overall rates of reoperation in comparison to ACLR alone, with no increase in complications.[29] Independent of preinjury activity level, patients undergoing isolated ACLR had a greater than 5-fold increased risk in ACL graft rupture and need for revision surgery.[29]

Two year outcomes from the STABILITY study, a randomized control trial of ACLR in patients less than 25 years of age with hamstring autograft with or without LET, showed similar patient-reported outcomes between groups, but the LET group had significantly lower ACL graft rupture rates (4% vs 11%).[26,30] Another meta-analysis study found that patients having undergone a lateral extra-articular procedure in addition to an ACLR had a 3-fold reduction in ACL graft rupture and slightly improved International Knee Documentation Committee (IKDC) scores.[31] This study showed that although the LET addition yielded no significant effect on anterior (Lachman) translation, it decreased residual pivot shift significantly.

The Micheli technique of physeal-sparing ACLR, comparable to the techniques explored in the SANTI and STABILITY study groups, combines a lateral extra-articular augmentation procedure with an ACLR. The biomechanics of the Micheli ACLR technique have been compared with those of an all-epiphyseal ACLR with ALL reconstruction, demonstrating superior ability to control tibial internal rotation compared with the all-epiphyseal reconstruction with ALL reconstruction, which was less successful in restoring rotational control between 60° and 90° of knee flexion.[32] Importantly, to investigate concerns about the "nonanatomic" nature of the Micheli ACLR and the potential for lateral compartment overconstraint or altered knee kinematics,[33,34] Sugimoto and colleagues performed a 3-dimensional motion analysis study on patients ranging from 1 to 20 years following the procedure and found no differences between reconstructed and non-reconstructed knees in any kinematic parameter at any postoperative time point.[35]

Specific indications for the addition of a lateral extra-articular augmentation procedure remain incompletely delineated in the literature, but the risk factors of ligamentous laxity, revision surgery, high grade pivot shift, young age (<25 year-old), female sex, and involvement in competitive cutting and pivoting sports seem to be at least relative indications for consideration of extra-articular stabilization techniques.[2,9–11,25,26]

PATIENT EVALUATION
History

Evaluation of the pediatric patient with a suspected ACL injury begins with a thorough history. Acute ACL injuries are typically associated with significant knee swelling, and the patient may report feeling or hearing a "pop" at the time of injury. It is especially important to understand the mechanism of injury, the patient's desired activity and level of participation and competition, symptoms and frequency of instability episodes, and interval treatment since the time of injury. Specific locations of pain and mechanical symptoms should be noted. Knowledge of prior knee injuries or surgeries is helpful for the treating surgeon to potentially predict altered or more challenging surgical anatomy. Patients or parents should be asked about recent growth spurts and onset of menarche for girls.

Physical Examination

The ability to perform a thorough physical examination may be limited in the immediate post-injury period, secondary to a large knee effusion and associated discomfort. It is, however, imperative to obtain a good physical examination of the injured knee, either at the time of initial presentation or at a future planned follow-up, once inflammation and pain subsides.

The examination begins with inspection of effusion, muscle atrophy, obvious deformity, gait asymmetry, and standing alignment of the lower extremities. Specific to the young patient, a general assessment of physical appearance and visible signs of puberty should be made to help inform the physician regarding the patient's state of skeletal maturity. This may include signs such as facial hair growth, deepening of voice, acne, height, weight, body build, and a comparison to accompanying family members. Formal designation of Tanner staging is generally not appropriate in the orthopedic clinic in the modern era, but a bone age radiograph of the left hand can be obtained and provide relatively accurate estimates of the number of years of growth remaining of an adolescent or preadolescent child. A neurologic and vascular examination of the extremity should be performed and documented, although no deficits are generally anticipated with an isolated ACL injury. Range of motion should be assessed and carefully documented. The Beighton score should be determined for all patients, which can help identify patients with generalized ligamentous laxity. Palpation of all bony and soft tissue structures around the knee should proceed systematically, with an identification of areas of tenderness. Ligamentous stability of the knee is then assessed in the anteroposterior plane with the anterior and posterior drawer tests to assess the ACL and posterior cruciate ligament (PCL) and in the medial and lateral planes using varus and valgus stress to assess the lateral collateral ligament (LCL) and medial collateral ligament (MCL), respectively. The pivot shift is the most specific physical examination maneuver for ACL injury in both the acute and chronic settings. However, patient guarding and apprehension present a challenge and may contribute to a low sensitivity for this test if not appreciated and addressed. The Lachman test is another essential maneuver in the assessment for an ACL tear. It has good sensitivity and specificity and is relatively simple to perform. Grades or millimeters of translation should be documented for all stability tests, always relative to the normal, unaffected side.

Patients should be reexamined, as needed, before undergoing surgery to ensure return of near full range of motion, resolution of effusion, and return of quadriceps function and reasonable quadriceps strength and a normal gait without ambulatory aids.

Imaging

All patients presenting to a sports clinician for initial evaluation of a knee injury should undergo radiographs of the affected knee with AP and lateral views. If surgical intervention is being considered, skeletally immature patients should additionally undergo full-length standing alignment (hips to ankles or EOS scanner) views and a left-hand radiograph for bone age. Bone age determination from the hand radiograph can be undertaken by the treating clinician via the Greulich and Pyle atlas,[36] Tanner–Whitehouse method,[37] or shorthand bone age method[38] or is often reported by the radiology department if requested at the time the x-ray is ordered. Recent studies demonstrating the utility of knee radiographs or knee MRI to determine bone age have also emerged, potentially obviate a left-hand radiograph in the future.[39–43] Preoperative knee and long-leg alignment x-rays may be used, most importantly, as a baseline against which to compare future postoperative radiographs to monitor for growth disturbances, most commonly in the form of leg length discrepancy or valgus distal femoral deformity. Suspicion of ligamentous injury or positive clinical examination for ligamentous or meniscal injury in the clinical setting should prompt evaluation with an MRI. In the case of suspected ACL injury, it is important to assess for continuity of the ACL fibers on both the coronal and sagittal MRI cuts, and for the presence of pathognomonic pivot shift bone bruise patterns, which are best seen on sagittal sequences at the sulcus terminalis and posterolateral tibia and highly indicates ACL injury (**Fig. 2**). The radiographic finding of a Segond fracture is consistent with avulsion of the anterolateral complex, which includes the ALL, and is pathognomonic for an ACL injury.[44,45] All imaging should be thoroughly reviewed to determine the nature

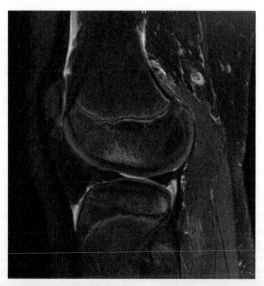

Fig. 2. A sagittal T2-weighted MRI of the knee demonstrating a pivot shift bone bruise pattern at the lateral femoral sulcus terminalis and posterolateral tibia, highly indicates an ACL injury.

and extent of any additional injuries. Physes should be carefully assessed on all knee imaging to determine if they are open, closing, or closed (**Fig. 3**).

Assessment of Skeletal Maturity and Growth Remaining

For adolescent and preadolescent patients with open physes, it is critical to make a determination of skeletal maturity and the number of years of growth remaining. This assessment is made by combining the data gathered during the history, examination, and imaging to assess the patient's skeletal maturity status.

Taken together, the following factors will help the clinician categorize patients into one of the three categories:

1. Greater than 2 years of growth remaining: Generally, prepubertal appearance, premenarchal, bone age less than 14 years for boys and less than 12 years for girls.
2. One to two years of growth remaining: Beginning to show signs of physical and sexual maturation, have started or are actively experiencing a growth spurt, onset of menarche took place less than 2 years prior, bone age 14 to 15 years for boys and 12 to 13 years for girls.
3. Skeletally mature/approaching skeletal maturity: Have the physical maturity and appearance of an adult, minimal change in height in the last year, onset of menarche greater than 2 years prior, physes closing or nearly closed, bone age of 15+ years for boys and 14+ years for girls.

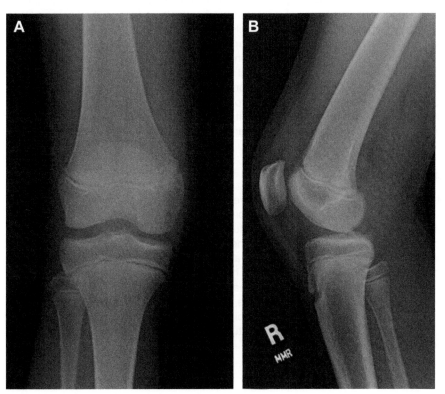

Fig. 3. Anteroposterior (A) and lateral (B) radiographs of the knee demonstrating open distal femoral and proximal tibial physes, indicates skeletal immaturity.

If a patient falls between categories, it may be advisable to err conservatively and assume that the patient has additional growth remaining.

NONOPERATIVE CARE

With a suspected acute ACL injury, all pediatric patients should be provided with crutches, allowed to pursue weight bearing as tolerated, assuming no significant meniscal or chondral pathology is suspected, and placed in a knee brace or immobilizer for support or stability until the diagnosis can be confirmed by a sports clinician. A hinged knee brace (eg, Bledsoe) is generally preferable to a knee immobilizer for its advantages in the prevention of stiffness and deep vein thrombosis, though these are rare in the pediatric population. Patients should begin working with a physical therapist as soon as possible to improve range of motion, initiate gentle strengthening and quadriceps recruitment, minimize gait asymmetry, and maintain compliance with cryotherapy and strategies to decrease edema and effusion. Such strategies may require 4 to 6 weeks post-injury before the knee, and the pediatric patient is optimized for surgery; therefore, scheduling a procedure before 3 to 4 weeks post-injury may risk stiffness. The presence of concomitant injuries, such as a displaced bucket-handle meniscus tears, osteochondral shear injuries, or loose bodies, may inhibit restoration of full motion and may benefit from restricted weight bearing until the time of surgery, the timeline for which may be expedited, compared with normal circumstances.

Nonsurgical care as definitive management in a pediatric patient with a complete ACL tear and unstable knee, by physical examination, remains a controversial concept at this stage and has been advocated more frequently in Europe than among North American investigators.[46] Although children who do not participate in competitive sports are much less likely to suffer symptomatic and recurrent instability episodes, the risk of concomitant meniscal or chondral injury remains during free play in recess, physical education classes, recreational activities, and even activities of daily life for a child or preadolescent.[47–50] As such, nonoperative management is generally reserved for low-demand patients without symptomatic instability, those anticipated to comply with aggressive strength-based rehabilitation and ongoing restrictions and modifications, and those with parents who clearly understand the ongoing risks of potential instability and future injury.

SURGICAL DECISION-MAKING

It is generally recommended that active pediatric and adolescent patients undergo ACLR if they wish to partake in future competitive or recreational sports and activities. In younger children, the spectrum of return to sports and unrestricted activity may be extended to include simple free play and gym class. The Micheli technique of ACLR with an autologous ITB graft has generally been used for pediatric patients with 2 or more years of growth remaining, but it has also been used successfully in skeletally immature children with less than 2 years of growth remaining, older adolescents, and even adults.[51] Modifications of the Micheli technique may include the passage of the ITB graft through femoral and tibial ACL tunnels in older children or skeletally mature patients, and preliminary literature suggests results comparable to modern adult techniques.[51–53]

SURGICAL TECHNIQUE

The Micheli surgical technique has been previously described.[14] The patient is placed supine on the operating room table. General anesthesia is induced. A regional block is administered, if desired. A thorough examination of the knee under anesthesia is performed and documented. If a tourniquet is used, it should be placed as high as possible on the patient's thigh so as not to interfere with ITB harvest. A sterile tourniquet can also be considered for shorter lower extremities to potentially allow for slightly more proximal access on the thigh. A standard arthroscopy setup with a lateral knee post is used at the mid-thigh level. A circumferential leg holder may also be used, particularly if a known posterior horn tear of the medial meniscus warrants optimal posterior medial compartment access for safe repair.

A 3 to 5 cm longitudinal or slightly oblique incision is made centered over the lateral epicondyle or just proximal. When choosing the placement of this incision, keep in mind that it will later be used to access the over-the-top position on the lateral femoral condyle. Dissection proceeds through skin and subcutaneous tissue, until the ITB is identified. Care must be taken to make the skin incision just through the level of the dermis in knees with minimal subcutaneous tissue to avoid injury to the ITB. A Cobb elevator is used to thoroughly separate the subcutaneous tissue from the ITB for ~20 cm proximally and far enough anterior and posterior to identify its borders. At the posterior border of the ITB, the surgeon may encounter the biceps femoris, and the ITB in this region is typically confluent with the lateral intermuscular septum. Anteriorly, the border is identified as a change in thickness of the tissue, transitioning from the robust ITB to the thinner retinaculum and vastus lateralis fascia. A ruler is used to mark the anticipated harvest of approximately 70% to 85% of the anteroposterior width of the ITB, with care to leave some posterior fibers intact, as these contribute to the stabilizing function of the knee. Two 2 to 4 cm longitudinal cuts are created in the ITB with a knife in line with the fibers to establish the anterior and posterior borders of the graft intended for harvest. Care should also be taken to avoid violation of the LCL posteriorly and knee joint capsule deep to the ITB, given the risk of fluid extravasation once arthroscopy is commenced. Meniscotomes are inserted into the anterior and posterior graft incisions, respectively, and slid proximally 18 to 20 cm, although an assistant retracts the overlying lateral thigh subcutaneous tissue laterally and proximally with a long retractor. Ensure the meniscotome blades are facing in divergent directions from the graft to avoid converging proximally or amputating the graft prematurely. Free the ITB from its underlying fascial tissue and attachment to the lateral epicondyle. Release the proximal end of the ITB graft using the curved meniscotome. This step requires countertraction on the graft distally and may require alternating a lever force posteriorly from the anterior aspect and anteriorly from the posterior aspect of the graft. Alternatively, the utilization of closed tendon strippers in smaller patients versus a secondary proximal 2 to 3 cm incision for graft harvest under direct visualization are effective methods for safe proximal transection of the ITB graft.

An extended whip stitch is placed on the free end of the graft for ~3 to 5 cm with heavy nonabsorbable suture (we use #5 ethibond) to tubularize the distal third of the graft. Further dissection of the anterior and posterior edges of the ITB graft is then carried distally for several centimeters toward Gerdy's tubercle, separating the graft from the capsule until the lateral margin of the lateral femoral condyle cartilage is palpated, ensuring preservation of the distal attachment of the graft to Gerdy's tubercle. The graft is provisionally tucked into the posterior aspect of the open wound during the next portion of the operation.

Attention is turned to preparation of the tibia. A 5 cm incision is made 1 cm medial to the tibial tuberosity just proximal to the pes anserinus, which is preserved. The deep incision is carried proximally to the level just distal to the proximal tibial physis, taking care to preserve the underlying physeal cartilage. Electrocautery is used to make a longitudinal 2.5 to 3.0 cm cut through the periosteum overlying the proximal tibial metaphysis. To ensure deep dissection proceeds sufficiently distal to the proximal tibial physis, the level of the physis may be approximated clinically by the proximal extent of the patellar tendon insertion on the tibial tuberosity and intraoperatively by a leash of subcutaneous pretibial vessels encountered on skin incision. A subperiosteal elevator is used to separate the medial and lateral edges of the periosteum, with care to avoid excessive elevation laterally so as not to violate the tibial tubercle apophysis, clearing an 8 to 10 mm tract of cortical bone on the metaphysis. A small burr or the sharp edge of the periosteal elevator is used to decorticate the bone 3 to 4 mm deep to establish a metaphyseal trough for later graft placement and periosteal suture fixation.

Arthroscopy is commenced. Consider placing the medial portal slightly more medial than a standard anteromedial portal to facilitate inserting a long curved clamp through this portal into the over-the-top position. Perform the diagnostic arthroscopy and address non-ACL pathology, if present. Thoroughly debride the anterior fat pad and clearly identify the intermeniscal ligament (IML). When debriding the notch, it is critical to maintain a cuff of femoral ACL footprint tissue posterolaterally, so as to serve as a sling of soft tissue which will hold the new graft proximally on the posterolateral corner of the lateral condyle within the notch. Debride the tibial stump, taking care to maintain a cuff of native tibial ACL footprint within which the graft will be situated (**Fig. 4**).

A Schnidt forceps or long curved Kelly clamp is placed through the medial portal into the intercondylar notch. Under arthroscopic guidance, gently wiggle the tip of the clamp through the posterolateral soft tissue sling that was left intact in the previous step. Be sure to advance the tip along the posterolateral margin of the lateral femoral condyle toward the over-the-top position. The surgeon should be able to palpate, with a forefinger, the tip of the clamp posterolateral to the lateral femoral condyle through the lateral incision that was used for the ITB harvest, taking care to maintain the clamp's position deep to the lateral gastrocnemius tendon. The tip of the clamp is slowly advanced through the posterolateral capsule of the knee until it is visualized. The clamp is then opened to establish an aperture for graft passage. The free limbs of the heavy nonabsorbable suture on the ITB graft are then fed, with a second curved clamp, into the opened tips of the clamp previously placed through the capsule. The

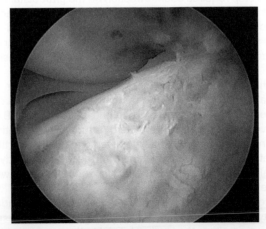

Fig. 4. Arthroscopic image of the remnant ACL following debridement, demonstrating a preserved cuff of tissue at the native tibial footprint, within which the graft will be situated.

free sutures on the ITB graft are then pulled through the intercondylar notch and out the anteromedial to advance the graft into the over-the-top position, with the free end of the graft left provisionally hanging freely out the anteromedial portal.

Under arthroscopic guidance, a Schnidt clamp or long curved Kelly clamp is then introduced into the tibial incision and advanced proximally from the proximal end of the previously established metaphyseal trough. The tip of the clamp should be advanced in extra-periosteal fashion into the knee joint under arthroscopic visualization, taking care to stay under the IML when entering the joint. After the clamp tips are spread several times to maintain a tract for graft passage, the clamp is removed and a rat-tailed rasp is passed along the same tract. The rasp is then oscillated back and forth to create a trough from the posterior aspect of the center of the tibial ACL footprint to the anterior epiphysis under the IML. Care is taken to line up the vector of the epiphyseal trough with the vector of the tibial metaphyseal trough more distally. After removing the rat-tailed rasp, a small straight or curved shaver is then introduced from the anterior tibial incision into the joint along the same tract, maintaining its position under the IML. The shaver is used to clear the epiphyseal trough of rasped ACL tissue and bony debris, ensuring an adequate 5 to 6 mm deep trough for graft placement, which will allow for eventual tendon-to-bone healing between the graft and the underlying bony epiphyseal trough.

The ITB graft is pulled backwards from the posterolateral incision until the free tagging sutures are visible in the intercondylar notch and pulled down into the anterior tibial incision with a reintroduced curved clamp. The free end of the ITB graft is then pulled out into the medial tibial incision.

Attention is turned to fixation of the graft to the posterolateral aspect of the lateral femoral condyle, which is performed with the knee positioned in 75 to 90° of flexion off of the lateral side of the operating table and leg maintained in neutral (0°) rotation. Although keeping maximal tension on the graft distally out the anteromedial incision, two to three figure-of-8 sutures with high-strength braided #2 suture material are placed between the graft and the capsular tissue of the posterolateral femoral condyle, just before the graft turns medially toward the posterolateral capsular aperture. The sutures are tied down in sequence while maintaining distal graft tension. These steps allow for fixation between the graft remaining attached distally to Gerdy's tubercle and the native ALL femoral footprint just posterior and proximal to the lateral epicondyle, thereby completing the lateral extra-articular augmentation portion of the procedure.

Attention is then turned to distal fixation of the intra-articular portion of the reconstruction, which represents the ACLR. For this step, the knee is placed in full extension. With the graft tensioned distal to the anteromedial wound and the graft sitting in the metaphyseal trough, three-to-four figure-of-8 sutures with high-strength braided #2 suture material are placed between the graft and the previously elevated periosteum on either side of the trough. This is achieved by passing the graft through the lateral trough periosteum, then looped twice through the graft approximately 1 cm proximal to the level of the periosteal entry point, and then back to the medial periosteal tissue 1 cm distally, such that the two periosteal suture passes line up side-by-side. This technique allows for additional distal tension on the graft when the sutures are hand-tied. A Lachman test should reveal optimal knee stability, and arthroscopic confirmation of adequate intra-articular ACL graft tension is performed (**Fig. 5**). After copious irrigation of all wounds, the subcutaneous wound edges are approximated with an absorbable 2.0 suture, followed by subcuticular skin closure with an absorbable 3.0 suture. A sterile dressing, cryotherapy sleeve, and hinged knee brace are applied in the operating room.

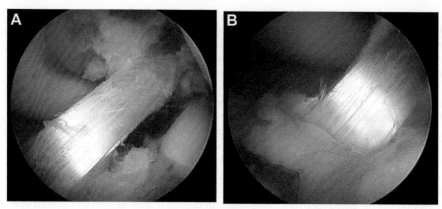

Fig. 5. Arthroscopic images of a completed Micheli technique physeal-sparing ACL reconstruction with an ITB autograft, demonstrating (*A*) an intact sling of soft tissue holding the graft proximally at the posterolateral corner of the lateral femoral condyle and (*B*) graft under an intact intermeniscal ligament distally.

POSTOPERATIVE PROTOCOL

Postoperatively, the patient is made touch-down weight bearing for the first 6 weeks, with a rapid increase to weight bearing as tolerated thereafter. Physical therapy is commenced within the first 1 to 2 weeks. Early on, the hinged knee brace is maintained locked in full extension for mobilization pending restoration of protective quadriceps control. Range of motion from 0 to 30° is allowed for the first 2 weeks, increased to 0 to 90° for weeks 3 to 6, and unlimited thereafter. In the younger population with inherent challenges adhering to activity precautions, this extended period of restricted weight bearing and bracing is imperative to elicit early graft protection, soft tissue healing and gradual return of motion, particularly in the setting of extraosseous, suture-graft-periosteal fixation. The rationale for conservative early rehabilitation progression may be less crucial in older adolescents or adults undergoing isolated ACLR, given overall differences in graft integration, physiologic healing, emotional maturity, strength development, and arthrofibrosis. Once full motion, symmetric gait, and protective strength are achieved, patients may return to straight line jogging at 3 to 4 months and initiate agility training and sport-specific exercises at 4 to 5 months. Return to full sporting activity is expected at 6 to 9 months, depending on the results of return-to-sport strength, balance, and functional hop testing. For this age group, it is recommended that patients wear a custom-fitted ACL sports brace during cutting and pivoting sport activity for 1 year following sports clearance postoperatively. Knee radiographs and lower limb standing alignment views are taken at 6 months and 12 months post-procedure, followed by annually until skeletal maturity to monitor for potential growth disturbance (**Fig. 6**).

OUTCOMES

Studies evaluating the outcomes of the Micheli technique in children have shown excellent results. The most rigorous follow-up study of 240 knees in children found the retear rate to be 6.6% at a mean of over 6 years postoperatively,[15] though other studies have reported retear rates as high as 14%.[54] By comparison, the reported retear rate for other pediatric ACLRs may be 9% to 22%[55,56] and the rate for all-epiphyseal reconstructions is 5% to 18%.[56–59] At our institution, the return to sport

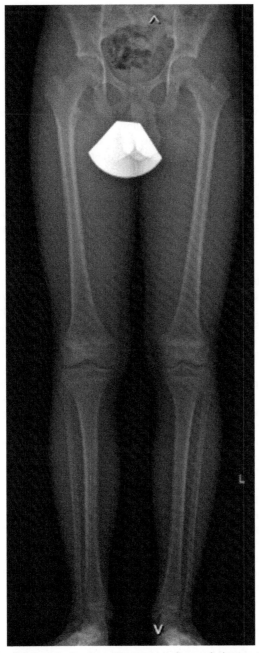

Fig. 6. Postoperative full-length standing alignment radiograph demonstrating neutral limb alignment and closed physes of the distal femur and proximal tibia. A standing alignment radiograph is obtained annually until skeletal maturity to monitor for potential growth disturbance or malalignment.

following the Micheli procedure is near 97%,[15] which is higher than that reported for all-epiphyseal reconstruction (93%)[57] and all pediatric ACLR patients (92%).[60] Patient-reported outcome measures have also shown excellent results, with the mean Lysholm scores of 93 to 95, Pedi-IKDC of 93 to 96.5, and Tegner score of 8.[15,54] The Pediatric ACL: Understanding Treatment Options (PLUTO) study is a large scale multicenter observational study that is currently underway and investigating the outcomes of all pediatric ACLR options.[a] This study will likely help to further delineate the safety and effectiveness of the various treatment options in comparative, prospective fashion in this age-based subpopulation.

As previously described above, knee kinematics were assessed between 1 and 20 years postoperatively in patients having undergone ACLR with the Micheli technique, demonstrating no significant difference in any kinematic metrics, when compared with the non-operated side.[35] Patients have also shown to have significantly less hamstring weakness at 6 months postoperatively compared with those having undergone ACLR with a transphyseal hamstring technique, which is a commonly used technique in patients with less than 2 years of growth remaining.[61]

COMPLICATIONS

In skeletally immature patients, the greatest concern with ACLR is the potential risk of growth disturbance, which may manifest as limb length discrepancy or angular deformity. In general, surgeries near a growing physis inherently carry the risk of physeal injury. Two studies specifically reporting on the outcomes of the Micheli ACLR technique did not identify any cases of angular deformity or leg length discrepancy on long-term follow-up.[15,54] Furthermore, both studies reported relatively low postoperative complication rates with this particular technique. Other studies investigating all extra-physeal, epiphyseal, and trans-physeal reconstruction techniques in skeletally immature patients have identified sporadic cases of growth disturbance.[57–59,62] Strategies to limit the occurrence of growth disturbance include using extra-physeal or all-epiphyseal techniques and minimizing aggressive dissection near the perichondral ring, particularly in establishing the over the top position. By comparison, with techniques that involve epiphyseal tunnel creation, additional technical demands include balancing tunnel size, optimizing tunnel placement between the articular surface and physes with use of intraoperative fluoroscopic guidance, and navigating optimal placement of implants, all of which are irrelevant to the Micheli technique free of bone tunnels and intraosseous fixation.

Owing to the residual deficit of the ITB on the lateral thigh in the Micheli technique, cosmetic asymmetry of the thigh is a common postoperative finding, but reported in less than half of patients, with only 1.6% of patients reporting discomfort at the donor site.[15] Although one cadaveric biomechanical study simulating the Micheli ACLR technique suggested a risk of lateral compartment overconstraint at certain knee flexion angles, such concerns have not been replicated in clinical studies.[33]

NEW DEVELOPMENTS

Given the success of the Micheli ACLR procedure in pediatric patients, some investigators have sought to apply the same technique and principles to adults. One systematic review looked at the outcomes of the Macintosh intra- and extra-physeal ACLR

[a] PLUTO Study Group. Pediatric ACL: Understanding Treatment Options. Published 2016. Accessed December 15, 2021. Available at: https://www.plutoacl.org/pediatric-acl-acl-injury-treatments.html.

technique in adult patients and found similar graft failure and patient-reported outcomes compared with numbers reported in the literature for other graft types in this age group.[63] Stensbirk and colleagues randomized 60 adult patients to either receive an ACLR using BTB autograft or an ACLR using ITB autograft with drilled tunnels on both the femur and tibial side.[51] The investigators found no significant differences between the two groups at long-term follow-up in terms of graft rupture, patient-reported outcomes measures (KOOS, Tegner, Lysholm), and objective outcomes measures (heel height, single hop for distance, and crossover hop for distance). The institution at which the Micheli technique was developed is currently investigating a novel modification of the technique using ITB autograft with tibial and femoral bone tunnels in skeletally mature adolescent and adult patients.

Ellis and colleagues investigated the use of a trans-physeal ACLR using hamstring autograft with the addition of an extra-osseous femoral ITB technique in young patients.[53] The intra-articular combined hamstring and ITB grafts were fixed together within the tibial bone tunnel. This approach resulted in a 2% rerupture rate, good patient outcomes, and a low complication rate.

The ITB can also be considered as a graft in the revision setting, but additional research is needed before widespread adoption.

SUMMARY

The Micheli technique is a combined extra-articular and intra-articular stabilization procedure that combines lateral augmentation with ACLR, using ITB autograft. Its primary indication is for ACLR in skeletally immature patients with more than 2 years of growth remaining. Studies have shown it to be effective at restoring knee biomechanics have minimal risk of complications, including those associated with growth disturbances, with a relatively low graft rupture rate. There may be benefits to performing this surgery in older children, adults, and revision cases, but the precise indications warrant continued investigation.

DISCLOSURE

The authors have nothing to disclose.

REFERENCES

1. Tepolt FA, Feldman L, Kocher MS. Trends in Pediatric ACL Reconstruction From the PHIS Database. J Pediatr Orthop 2018;38(9):e490–4.
2. Lording TD, Lustig S, Servien E, et al. Lateral reinforcement in anterior cruciate ligament reconstruction. Asia Pacific J Sports Med Arthrosc Rehabil Technol 2014;1(1):3–10.
3. Lemaire M. [Chronic knee instability. Technics and results of ligament plasty in sports injuries]. J Chir (Paris) 1975;110(4):281–94.
4. Ellison AE. Distal iliotibial-band transfer for anterolateral rotatory instability of the knee. J Bone Joint Surg Am 1979;61(3):330–7.
5. Ireland J, Trickey EL. Macintosh tenodesis for anterolateral instability of the knee. J Bone Joint Surg Br 1980;62(3):340–5.
6. Amirault JD, Cameron JC, Macintosh DL, et al. Chronic anterior cruciate ligament deficiency: long-term results of MacIntosh's lateral substitution reconstruction. J Bone Joint Surg Br 1988;70B(4):622–4.
7. Andrews JR, Sanders R. A "mini-reconstruction" technique in treating anterolateral rotatory instability (ALRI). Clin Orthop Relat Res 1983;172(172):93–6.

8. Lee DW, Kim JG, Cho SI, et al. Clinical Outcomes of Isolated Revision Anterior Cruciate Ligament Reconstruction or in Combination With Anatomic Anterolateral Ligament Reconstruction. Am J Sports Med 2019;47(2):324–33.

9. Helito CP, Sobrado MF, Giglio PN, et al. Combined Reconstruction of the Anterolateral Ligament in Patients With Anterior Cruciate Ligament Injury and Ligamentous Hyperlaxity Leads to Better Clinical Stability and a Lower Failure Rate Than Isolated Anterior Cruciate Ligament Reconstruction. Arthroscopy 2019;35(9): 2648–54.

10. Helito CP, Camargo DB, Sobrado MF, et al. Combined reconstruction of the anterolateral ligament in chronic ACL injuries leads to better clinical outcomes than isolated ACL reconstruction. Knee Surg Sports Traumatol Arthrosc 2018;26(12): 3652–9.

11. Sonnery-Cottet B, Saithna A, Cavalier M, et al. Anterolateral Ligament Reconstruction Is Associated With Significantly Reduced ACL Graft Rupture Rates at a Minimum Follow-up of 2 Years: A Prospective Comparative Study of 502 Patients From the SANTI Study Group. Am J Sports Med 2017;45(7):1547–57.

12. Bertoia JT, Urovitz EP, Richards RR, et al. Anterior cruciate reconstruction using the MacIntosh lateral-substitution over-the-top repair. J Bone Joint Surg Am 1985;67(8):1183–8.

13. Micheli LJ, Rask B, Gerberg L. Anterior cruciate ligament reconstruction in patients who are prepubescent. Clin Orthop Relat Res 1999;364(364):40–7.

14. Kocher MS, Garg S, Micheli LJ. Physeal Sparing Reconstruction of the Anterior Cruciate Ligament in Skeletally Immature Prepubescent Children and Adolescents: Surgical Technique. J Bone Joint Surg Am 2006;88(1_suppl_2 Suppl 1): 283–93.

15. Kocher MS, Heyworth BE, Fabricant PD, et al. Outcomes of Physeal-Sparing ACL Reconstruction with Iliotibial Band Autograft in Skeletally Immature Prepubescent Children. J Bone Joint Surg Am 2018;100(13):1087–94.

16. Fairclough J, Hayashi K, Toumi H, et al. The functional anatomy of the iliotibial band during flexion and extension of the knee: implications for understanding iliotibial band syndrome. J Anat 2006;208(3):309–16.

17. Kittl C, El-Daou H, Athwal KK, et al. The Role of the Anterolateral Structures and the ACL in Controlling Laxity of the Intact and ACL-Deficient Knee. Am J Sports Med 2016;44(2):345–54.

18. Claes S, Vereecke E, Maes M, et al. Anatomy of the anterolateral ligament of the knee. J Anat 2013;223(4):321–8.

19. Caterine S, Litchfield R, Johnson M, et al. A cadaveric study of the anterolateral ligament: re-introducing the lateral capsular ligament. Knee Surg Sports Traumatol Arthrosc 2015;23(11):3186–95.

20. Vincent JP, Magnussen RA, Gezmez F, et al. The anterolateral ligament of the human knee: an anatomic and histologic study. Knee Surg Sports Traumatol Arthrosc 2011;20(1):147–52.

21. Cruells Vieira EL, Vieira EÁ, Teixeira da Silva R, et al. An Anatomic Study of the Iliotibial Tract. Arthroscopy 2007;23(3):269–74.

22. Kennedy MI, Claes S, Fuso FAF, et al. The Anterolateral Ligament: An Anatomic, Radiographic, and Biomechanical Analysis. Am J Sports Med 2015;43(7): 1606–15.

23. Daggett M, Busch K, Sonnery-Cottet B. Surgical Dissection of the Anterolateral Ligament. Arthrosc Tech (Amsterdam) 2016;5(1):e185–8.

24. Helito CP, Demange MK, Bonadio MB, et al. Anatomy and Histology of the Knee Anterolateral Ligament. Orthop J Sports Med 2013;1(7). 2325967113513546.

25. Weber AE, Zuke W, Mayer EN, et al. Lateral Augmentation Procedures in Anterior Cruciate Ligament Reconstruction: Anatomic, Biomechanical, Imaging, and Clinical Evidence. Am J Sports Med 2019;47(3):740–52.

26. Getgood AM, Bryant DM, Litchfield R, et al. Lateral Extra-articular Tenodesis Reduces Failure of Hamstring Tendon Autograft Anterior Cruciate Ligament Reconstruction: 2-Year Outcomes From the STABILITY Study Randomized Clinical Trial. Am J Sports Med 2020;48(2):285–97.

27. Slette EL, Mikula JD, Schon JM, et al. Biomechanical Results of Lateral Extra-articular Tenodesis Procedures of the Knee: A Systematic Review. Arthroscopy 2016;32(12):2592–611.

28. Engebretsen L, Lew WD, Lewis JL, et al. The effect of an iliotibial tenodesis on intraarticular graft forces and knee joint motion. Am J Sports Med 1990;18(2):169–76.

29. Sonnery-Cottet B, Haidar I, Rayes J, et al. Long-term Graft Rupture Rates After Combined ACL and Anterolateral Ligament Reconstruction Versus Isolated ACL Reconstruction: A Matched-Pair Analysis From the SANTI Study Group. Am J Sports Med 2021;49(11):2889–97.

30. Getgood A, Hewison C, Bryant D, et al. No Difference in Functional Outcomes When Lateral Extra-Articular Tenodesis Is Added to Anterior Cruciate Ligament Reconstruction in Young Active Patients: The Stability Study. Arthroscopy 2020;36(6):1690–701.

31. Onggo JR, Rasaratnam HK, Nambiar M, et al. Anterior Cruciate Ligament Reconstruction Alone Versus With Lateral Extra-articular Tenodesis With Minimum 2-Year Follow-up: A Meta-analysis and Systematic Review of Randomized Controlled Trials. Am J Sports Med 2021. https://doi.org/10.1177/03635465211004946. 3635465211004946.

32. Trentacosta N, Pace JL, Metzger M, et al. Biomechanical Evaluation of Pediatric Anterior Cruciate Ligament (ACL) Reconstruction Techniques With and Without the Anterolateral Ligament (ALL). J Pediatr Orthop 2020;40(1):8–16.

33. Kennedy A, Coughlin DG, Metzger MF, et al. Biomechanical Evaluation of Pediatric Anterior Cruciate Ligament Reconstruction Techniques. Am J Sports Med 2011;39(5):964–71.

34. Sena M, Chen J, Dellamaggioria R, et al. Dynamic Evaluation of Pivot-Shift Kinematics in Physeal-Sparing Pediatric Anterior Cruciate Ligament Reconstruction Techniques. Am J Sports Med 2013;41(4):826–34.

35. Sugimoto D, Whited AJ, Brodeur JJ, et al. Long-Term Follow-up of Skeletally Immature Patients With Physeal-Sparing Combined Extra-/Intra-articular Iliotibial Band Anterior Cruciate Ligament Reconstruction: A 3-Dimensional Motion Analysis. Am J Sports Med 2020;48(8):1900–6.

36. Greulich WW, Pyle SI, Todd TW. Radiographic atlas of skeletal development of the hand and Wrist. University Press; 1950.

37. Tanner JM. Assessment of skeletal maturity and prediction of adult height (TW3 method). 3rd edition. WBSaunders; 2001.

38. Heyworth BE, Osei DA, Fabricant PD, et al. The Shorthand Bone Age Assessment: A Simpler Alternative to Current Methods. J Pediatr Orthop 2013;33(5):569–74.

39. Politzer CS, Bomar JD, Pehlivan HC, et al. Creation and Validation of a Shorthand Magnetic Resonance Imaging Bone Age Assessment Tool of the Knee as an Alternative Skeletal Maturity Assessment. Am J Sports Med 2021;49(11):2955–9.

40. Yu KE, Coghill GA, Vernik D, et al. Combining Lower Extremity Radiographic Markers Begets More Accurate Predictions of Remaining Skeletal Growth. J Pediatr Orthop 2021;41(6):362–7.
41. Benedick AJ, Hogue B, Furdock RJ, et al. Estimating Skeletal Maturity Using Knee Radiographs During Preadolescence: The Epiphyseal Metaphyseal Ratio. J Pediatr Orthop 2021;41(9):566–70.
42. O'Connor JE, Coyle J, Bogue C, et al. Age prediction formulae from radiographic assessment of skeletal maturation at the knee in an Irish population. Forensic Sci Int 2013;234:188.e1-8.
43. Dekhne MS, Kocher ID, Hussain ZB, et al. Tibial Tubercle Apophyseal Stage to Determine Skeletal Age in Pediatric Patients Undergoing ACL Reconstruction: A Validation and Reliability Study. Orthop J Sports Med 2021;9(9). 232596712110368-23259671211036896.
44. Claes S, Luyckx T, Vereecke E, et al. The Segond Fracture: A Bony Injury of the Anterolateral Ligament of the Knee. Arthroscopy 2014;30(11):1475–82.
45. Albers M, Shaikh H, Herbst E, et al. The iliotibial band and anterolateral capsule have a combined attachment to the Segond fracture. Knee Surg Sports Traumatol Arthrosc 2017;26(5):1305–10.
46. Moksnes H, Engebretsen L, Eitzen I, et al. Functional outcomes following a non-operative treatment algorithm for anterior cruciate ligament injuries in skeletally immature children 12 years and younger. A prospective cohort with 2 years follow-up. Br J Sports Med 2013;47(8):488–94.
47. Moksnes H, Engebretsen L, Risberg MA. Prevalence and Incidence of New Meniscus and Cartilage Injuries After a Nonoperative Treatment Algorithm for ACL Tears in Skeletally Immature Children: A Prospective MRI Study. Am J Sports Med 2013;41(8):1771–9.
48. Funahashi KM, Moksnes H, Maletis GB, et al. Anterior Cruciate Ligament Injuries in Adolescents With Open Physis: Effect of Recurrent Injury and Surgical Delay on Meniscal and Cartilage Injuries. Am J Sports Med 2014;42(5):1068–73.
49. Henry J, Chotel F, Chouteau J, et al. Rupture of the anterior cruciate ligament in children: early reconstruction with open physes or delayed reconstruction to skeletal maturity? Knee Surg Sports Traumatol Arthrosc 2009;17(7):748–55.
50. Millett PJ, Willis AA, Warren RF. Associated injuries in pediatric and adolescent anterior cruciate ligament tears: Does a delay in treatment increase the risk of meniscal tear? Arthroscopy 2002;18(9):955–9.
51. Stensbirk F, Thorborg K, Konradsen L, et al. Iliotibial band autograft versus bone-patella-tendon-bone autograft, a possible alternative for ACL reconstruction: a 15-year prospective randomized controlled trial. Knee Surg Sports Traumatol Arthrosc 2014;22(9):2094–101.
52. Abreu FG, Pioger C, Franck F, et al. Femoral Physeal-Sparing Anterior Cruciate Ligament Reconstruction Using the Iliotibial Band: Over-The-Top Technique. Arthrosc Tech (Amsterdam) 2020;9(6):e691–5.
53. Ellis HB, Boes N, Mitchell P, et al. Can Combined Trans-physeal and Lateral Extra-Articular Pediatric ACL Reconstruction Techniques Be Employed to Reduce ACL Re-Injury While Allowing for Growth? Orthop J Sports Med 2019; 7(7_suppl5):2325967119.
54. Willimon SC, Jones CR, Herzog MM, et al. Micheli Anterior Cruciate Ligament Reconstruction in Skeletally Immature Youths: A Retrospective Case Series With a Mean 3-Year Follow-up. Am J Sports Med 2015;43(12):2974–81.
55. Wong SE, Feeley BT, Pandya NK. Complications After Pediatric ACL Reconstruction: A Meta-analysis. J Pediatr Orthop 2019;39(8):E566–71.

56. DeFrancesco CJ, Striano BM, Bram JT, et al. An In-Depth Analysis of Graft Rupture and Contralateral Anterior Cruciate Ligament Rupture Rates After Pediatric Anterior Cruciate Ligament Reconstruction. Am J Sports Med 2020;48(10): 2395–400.

57. Knapik DM, Voos JE. Anterior Cruciate Ligament Injuries in Skeletally Immature Patients: A Meta-analysis Comparing Repair Versus Reconstruction Techniques. J Pediatr Orthop 2020;40(9):492–502.

58. Gupta A, Tejpal T, Shanmugaraj A, et al. All-epiphyseal anterior cruciate ligament reconstruction produces good functional outcomes and low complication rates in pediatric patients: a systematic review. Knee Surg Sports Traumatol Arthrosc 2020;28(8):2444–52.

59. Wall EJ, Ghattas PJ, Eismann EA, et al. Outcomes and Complications After All-Epiphyseal Anterior Cruciate Ligament Reconstruction in Skeletally Immature Patients. Orthop J Sports Med 2017;5(3). 2325967117693604.

60. Kay J, Memon M, Marx RG, et al. Over 90 % of children and adolescents return to sport after anterior cruciate ligament reconstruction: a systematic review and meta-analysis. Knee Surg Sports Traumatol Arthrosc 2018;26(4):1019–36.

61. Sugimoto D, Heyworth BE, Collins SE, et al. Comparison of Lower Extremity Recovery After Anterior Cruciate Ligament Reconstruction With Transphyseal Hamstring Versus Extraphyseal Iliotibial Band Techniques in Skeletally Immature Athletes. Orthop J Sports Med 2018;6(4). 2325967118768044.

62. Wong SE, Feeley BT, Pandya NK. Comparing Outcomes Between the Over-the-Top and All-Epiphyseal Techniques for Physeal-Sparing ACL Reconstruction: A Narrative Review. Orthop J Sports Med 2019;7(3). 2325967119833689.

63. Sarraj M, de Sa D, Shanmugaraj A, et al. Over-the-top ACL reconstruction yields comparable outcomes to traditional ACL reconstruction in primary and revision settings: a systematic review. Knee Surg Sports Traumatol Arthrosc 2019;27(2): 427–44.

Anterior Cruciate Ligament Reconstruction in Skeletally Immature Athletes Using All-Epiphyseal Techniques

Check for updates

Danielle E. Chipman, BS[a], Nicolas Pascual-Leone, BA[a],
Frank A. Cordasco, MD, MS[b], Daniel W. Green, MD, MS[a],*

KEYWORDS

- Anterior cruciate ligament reconstruction • Pediatric ACL • All-epiphyseal technique
- Quadriceps tendon autograft

KEY POINTS

- All-epiphyseal anterior cruciate ligament reconstruction (AE ACLR) in pediatrics is a suitable technique for skeletally immature patients with a significant amount of growth remaining.
- To align the trajectory of the tunnel correctly, the posterolateral femoral condyle is palpated with respect to the distal femoral physis; the insertion of the popliteus tendon can be a useful landmark for the placement of the guide pin.
- Previous studies have shown the rates of revision and the return-to-sport to be equal or lower in AE ACLR compared with a partial transphyseal and complete transphyseal hamstring autograft technique.

HISTORY

There have been various surgical techniques developed for skeletally immature anterior cruciate ligament reconstructions (ACLRs) but recent focus has turned toward all-epiphyseal (AE) techniques.

In 2003, Anderson described an epiphyseal technique for skeletally immature patients.[1] This technique described an ACLR without the need to drill across the physis (**Fig. 1**). AE ACLRs involve graft fixation within the epiphysis without crossing the physis.[1] In 2010, Ganley further modified this technique to include a tibial socket instead of a complete through-and-through tibial tunnel.[2] In 2012, Cordasco and

[a] Division of Pediatric Orthopedic Surgery, Hospital for Special Surgery, 535 East 70th Street, New York, NY, 10021, USA; [b] Sports Medicine Institute, Hospital for Special Surgery, 525 East 71st Street, New York, NY, 10021, USA
* Corresponding author.
E-mail address: greendw@hss.edu

Clin Sports Med 41 (2022) 569–577
https://doi.org/10.1016/j.csm.2022.05.002
0278-5919/22/Published by Elsevier Inc.
sportsmed.theclinics.com

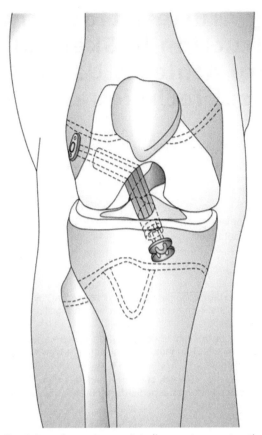

Fig. 1. All-inside, all-epiphyseal anterior cruciate ligament reconstruction technique.

Green modified the Anderson technique to include an all-inside, AE technique using retrograde sockets instead of tunnels at both the femur and tibia.[3,4]

The technique for an AE all-inside ACLR using a quadriceps tendon autograft is outlined below.

TECHNIQUE
Preoperative Technique

All children are assessed by physical examination including Beighton score for ligamentous laxity. Preoperative imaging is obtained and includes knee X-rays (anterior-posterior (AP), lateral, merchant), MRI, standing hip-to-ankle leg length to evaluate for preoperative leg length discrepancy or genu valgum, and hand X-ray for bone age.

A full examination under anesthesia is performed in the operating room.

Landmarks Identified

The subcutaneous landmarks of interest are identified: the tibial tubercle, the distal femoral physis, the tibiofemoral joint line, the inferior pole of the patella, and the proximal tibia physis. These landmarks are marked to aid in anatomic orientation.

Graft Harvest

A soft tissue autograft, either hamstring or quadriceps tendon, is the graft of choice. An Esmarch band is used to exsanguinate the lower extremity and then a tourniquet is inflated. A 5-cm incision is made over the quadriceps tendon extending proximally from the superior pole of the patella. When performing the procedure with a quadriceps tendon autograft, the quadriceps tendon is localized, and a surgical marker is used to mark the proximal and central aspect of the tendon. A double-bladed scalpel is used to cut the quadriceps tendon from the superior pole of the patella to the proximal end of the central part of the tendon. The graft is then released from the superior pole of the patella to the proximal end of the quadriceps tendon. The quadriceps tendon autograft typically has a length of 60 to 65 mm. A full-thickness graft is preferred, including the rectus femoris and the rectus intermedius, while leaving the synovial capsular layer of the quadriceps tendon intact.[3] The quadriceps tendon defect is then repaired with #1 absorbable sutures.

Graft Preparation

Using a graft preparation board, the graft is constructed. We prefer the quadriceps graft because it is a robust, all-soft tissue graft with a solid piece of collagen. If a hamstring autograft is performed, the tendons are looped together to increase the graft's diameter, which results in a shorter and thicker graft. On both the femoral and tibial ends of the graft, a TightRope RT suture is used (Arthrex Inc., Naples, FL, USA). Additional sutures are used at each end to augment the suspensory fixation. Ideally, the graft is symmetric in diameter throughout (about 9–10 mm). The graft is covered in a moist gauze and stored in a sealed plastic bag.

Diagnostic Knee Arthroscopy and Site Preparation

A standard diagnostic knee arthroscopy is performed using anteromedial and anterolateral portals. The anterolateral portal is used to assess the femoral footprint with a 70° lens for optimal visualization, and all intact portions of the ACL are left in place. Rubberized cannulas are placed through the portal sites to facilitate graft passage and prevent suture soft tissue bridges (**Fig. 2**). We recommend using a large enough diameter of the portal cannula to allow graft passage. For example, for a 10 mm graft, we use 10 mm cannula.

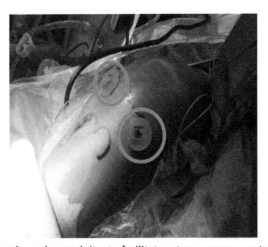

Fig. 2. Cannulas are through portal sites to facilitate suture management and graft passage.

Femoral Socket Preparation

The femoral socket is prepared under visualization through the anteromedial portal with a 30° lens. The optimal angle for the distal femur pediatric guide is between 90° and 95° onto the center of the femoral footprint and about 2 to 3 mm from the back wall. The femoral marking hook (Arthrex) side is first placed through the antero-lateral portal. To align the trajectory of the tunnel correctly, the posterolateral femoral condyle is palpated with respect to the distal femoral physis. The insertion of the pop-liteus tendon can be a useful landmark for the placement of the guide pin.[5] Then, a less than 1 cm incision is made just anterior to the lateral epicondyle, and the guide is seated onto the lateral cortex of the lateral femoral condyle. Next, a small guide pin is inserted under fluoroscopic guidance (we prefer using a Ziehm device (Nuremberg, Germany) for three-dimensional [3D] evaluation to precisely assess the

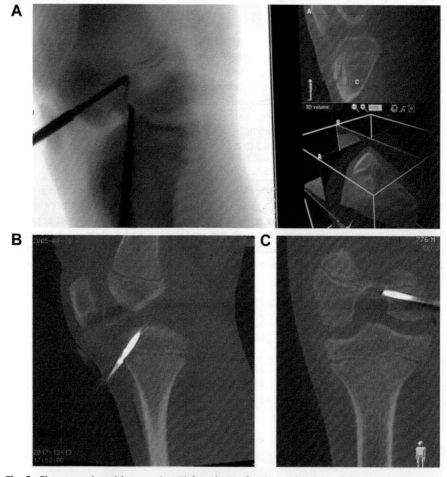

Fig. 3. Fluoroscopic guidance using Ziehm device for 3D evaluation of the proximity to the physis after flip cutter placement but before reeming of the epiphyseal sockets. (A) Plain fluoroscopic images next to 3D reconstructions. (B) Sagittal reconstruction demonstrating the flipcutter within the proximal tibial epiphysis. (C) Coronal reconstruction demonstrating the flipcutter withing the femoral epiphysis.

proximity to the physis) to assess its position relative to the physis and articular surfaces (**Fig. 3**). A FlipCutter (Arthrex) of the appropriate diameter is drilled through the stepped drill sleeve to reach the ACL footprint in the notch, and the position of the FlipCutter is again confirmed by fluoroscopy. The stepped drill sleeve is gently placed through the lateral cortex using a mallet to ensure a bone bridge of at least 7 mm between the end of the tunnel and the lateral cortex of the lateral femoral condyle. The FlipCutter is deployed, and the femoral socket is reamed retrograde to approximately 25 mm. Finally, the FlipCutter is removed and a FiberStick (Arthrex) is inserted through the drill sleeve and exits via the anteromedial portal for later graft passage.

Tibial Socket Preparation

The arthroscope is now placed back in the anterolateral portal using a 70° lens. The tibial footprint of ACL is debrided. The tibial ACL guide is inserted through the anteromedial portal and correct placement is confirmed by palpation of the physis. The tibial marking hook (Arthrex) is inserted and placed onto the tibial footprint, and a guide pin is used to confirm correct placement fluoroscopically (once again, using the Ziehm device for 3D precision) (**Fig. 4**). The stepped drill sleeve is gently placed through the tibial cortex using a mallet; then, the FlipCutter is drilled through the guide and exits through the tibial footprint. A FiberStick is advanced through the guide, traversing the socket, and retrieved intra-articularly to exit through the anterolateral portal for later graft passage.

All-Inside Graft Passage

The graft is passed through the anteromedial portal into the femoral socket, and the RT button is passed through the lateral femoral epiphyseal cortex, flipped, and secured onto the lateral epiphyseal cortex. The slack is removed from the suture and is partially tensioned. The tibial end of the graft is then passed through the anteromedial portal using the previously placed FiberStick that has been shuttled from the anterolateral to anteromedial portals. The TightRope suture is shuttled into the suture in the FiberStick, and that stitch is passed through the tibial drill hole, pulling the tibial end of the graft into the tibial socket. The whipstitch sutures are loaded onto the button and secured for backup fixation. The graft is finally tensioned with the knee in 0° of

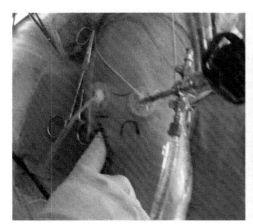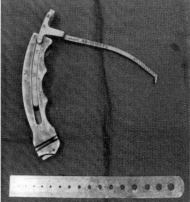

Fig. 4. Tibial Socket Preparation, the zone of the physis between the convex epiphysis and the flatter metaphysis can often be palpated thru the anterior medial incision.

flexion, first on the femoral side and then on the tibial side. The knots are tied over the self-tensioning buttons for back-up fixation.

The graft is then evaluated throughout a full range of motion, the pivot shift and Lachman tests are performed. A hinged knee brace locked in extension is placed on the patient in the operating room.

Postoperative Rehabilitation

Typically, patients are evaluated at 10 days, and 1, 2, 3, 4.5, 6, 9, 12, 18, and 24 months postoperative, and then are followed annually until they reach skeletal maturity. At 10 days postoperative, routine AP and lateral radiographs are evaluated to check the hardware and sockets. Standing hip-to-ankle X-rays and physeal-specific MRI scans are obtained at 6 months, 1 year, and 2 years postoperative. Standing radiographs were assessed for alignment and leg length discrepancy.

Implants used

1. ACL TightRope RT x2

Instruments used

1. Arthrex RetroConstruction Drill Guide Set
2. Pin Tip Tibial Marking Hook ACL Guide, small angle
3. Epiphyseal Femoral ACL Guide, small angle (Right and Left)
4. FlipCutter III
5. Drill Sleeve for RetroConstruction Drill Guide
6. PassPort Cannulas
7. Epiphyseal ACL guide (Arthrex Inc., Naples, FL)
8. 3D Intraoperative Fluoroscopy
9. Double blade 10 or 11 blade for quad harvest
10. 30° and 70° scopes

LITERATURE REVIEW

AE ACLR has been shown to be an effective technique for treating skeletally immature patients with a significant degree of growth remaining.[6] In Cruz and colleagues'[7] review of 103 AE ACLR patients treated at Children's Hospital of Pennsylvania, the average age was 12.1 with a range of 6.3 to 15.7 years. In Cordasco and colleagues'[8] prospective evaluation of 49 AE ACLR athletes treated at Hospital for Special Surgery (HSS), the average skeletal age was 12.0 ± 1.5 years.

Previous studies have cited numerous theoretic and practical advantages to the AE ACLR technique. Compared with over-the-top reconstructions, AE ACLR is an anatomic ACLR technique that does not involve transphyseal drilling.[9]

The AE ACLR technique has been shown in biomechanical studies to have favorable kinematics and contact stress in cadaveric knees.[9] The rates of revision and the return-to-sport rate have also been demonstrated to be significantly lower in AE ACLR compared with a partial transphyseal and complete transphyseal hamstring autograft technique.[8] Patient reported outcomes have also shown favorable results of the AE ACLR technique in the pediatric population with consistently high mean Pedi-International Knee Documentation Committee (IKDC), Pedi-Funtional Activity Brief Scale (FABS), and Pedi-Patient-Reported Outcomes Measurement Information System (PROMIS) scores.[10] Similarly, AE ACLR has shown good functional outcomes, low failure rates, at over 2-year follow-up.[11] In a systematic review of 3798 skeletally immature patients performed by Fury and colleagues[12] in 2021, the incidence of postoperative leg-length discrepancy greater than 10 mm was 2.1%, and the incidence of angular deformity greater than 5° was 1.3%.

A 2017 study by Wall and colleagues[13] of Cincinnati Children's Hospital Medical Center retrospectively reviewed 27 patients with a mean age of 11.4 ± 1.9 years (85% men). There was a 48% complication rate, including ACL retear (11%), lax ACL graft (4%), leg-length discrepancy greater than or equal to 2 cm (11%), lateral meniscus tear (11%), medial meniscus tear (7%), notch impingement (7%), hardware displaced/prominent (7%), postoperative skin infection (7%), patellar dislocation (4%), lateral femoral condyle fracture (4%), and genu valgum (4%).[13]

Moreover, in 2017, a retrospective study by Cruz and colleagues[7] reviewed 103 patients at Children's Hospital of Philadelphia that underwent AE ACLR with a mean follow-up of 21 months. The mean age of the patients was 12.1 years (range 6.3–15.7; 23.3% women).[7] Nineteen patients used allograft, 81 autograft, and 3 hybrid.[7] Overall, the complication rate was 16.5%, including rerupture (10.7%), arthrofibrosis (1.9%), growth disturbance (<1%), superficial infection (<1%), prominent hardware (<1%), and persistent instability (<1%).[7]

A study at Hospital for Special Surgery by Cordasco and colleagues[8] in 2019, prospectively, evaluated 49 patients with a mean skeletal age of 12 years ± 1.5 (82% men). Of the patients, 3 (6%) underwent a revision ACL surgery and 7 (14%) patients had a second surgery to the same knee excluding revision surgery.[8] Additionally, 5 (10%) patients had a contralateral ACL surgery.[8] The return to sport rate was 100% and 92% of patients returned to their sport as the same level as before surgery.[8]

In a study from 2020 by Ranade and colleagues,[10] 83 subjects were retrospectively reviewed with an average age of 12.3 years at initial surgery. Eleven patients (13%) had a reinjury to the ipsilateral ACL at an average of 2.7 years postoperative.[10]

Recently, DeFrancesco and colleagues[14] reported that 161 patients with a mean age of 12.1 ± 1.78 that underwent AE ACLR (78.3% men) were retrospectively reviewed. A total of 145 (90.1%) patients used hamstring autografts, 12 (7.45%) used tendon allografts, and 4 (2.48%) used hamstring autografts with allograft supplementation.[14] The cumulative graft rupture rate was 18.2% by 4 years postoperative and the cumulative contralateral ACL rupture rate was 6.63% by 4 years postoperative.[14]

Complications after AE ACLR can occur, including growth arrest, angular deformity, limb-length discrepancy, rerupture, contralateral rerupture, other injuries, arthrofibrosis, and infection (**Figs. 5** and **6**). A previous study in 2017 has shown a small physeal violation (<5% of the surface area of the respective physis) by either the femoral or

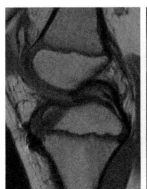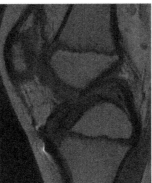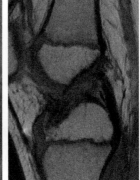

Fig. 5. Consecutive sagittal slices of 10-year-old boy 11 month postoperative displaying the tibial socket.

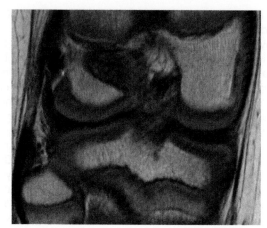

Fig. 6. MRI image at 6 months postoperative displaying the femoral socket.

tibial tunnel was seen in 52.2% of patients. In a recent follow-up study on 3D imaging, we found that 11.1% of sockets touched the distal femoral physis and 16.6% of sockets reamed into the proximal tibial physis during the placement of the AE ACLR socket.[15] Longer term follow-up of a large prospective cohort of AE ACLR is needed to determine the exact rate of significant growth disturbance and angular deformity.

SUMMARY

AE ACL reconstruction techniques have been developed to treat skeletally immature patients undergoing ACLR without crossing the physis. The surgical technique was first published in 2003 and has been slightly modified to date. Numerous studies have shown the effectiveness of this technique; however, future studies with longer term follow-up are needed.

DISCLOSURES

D W. Green is a paid consultant and has intellectual property (IP) royalties in Arthrex, Inc. F.A. Cordasco is a paid consultant and has IP royalties in Arthrex, Inc.

REFERENCES

1. Anderson AF. Transepiphyseal replacement of the anterior cruciate ligament in skeletally immature patients A preliminary report. J Bone Joint Surg 2003;85(7): 1255–63.

2. Lawrence JTR, Bowers AL, Belding J, et al. All-epiphyseal anterior cruciate ligament reconstruction in skeletally immature patients. Clin Orthop Relat Res 2010; 468(7):1971.

3. Aitchison AH, Schlichte LM, Green DW, et al. Open full-thickness quadriceps tendon autograft harvest with repair for anterior cruciate ligament reconstruction. Arthrosc Tech 2020;9(10):e1459–65.

4. McCarthy MM, Graziano J, Green DW, et al. All-epiphyseal, all-inside anterior cruciate ligament reconstruction technique for skeletally immature patients. Arthrosc Tech 2012;1(2):e231-9.

5. Xerogeanes JW, Hammond KE, Todd DC. Anatomic landmarks utilized for physeal-sparing, anatomic anterior cruciate ligament reconstruction: an MRI-based study. J Bone Joint Surg Ser A 2012;94(3):268–76.
6. Gausden EB, Green DW, Cordasco FA. Technique: anterior cruciate ligament reconstruction: all-epiphyseal sockets. In: Pediatric and adolescent knee injury. Wolters Kluwer; 2015. p. 53–60.
7. Cruz AI, Fabricant PD, McGraw M, et al. All-Epiphyseal ACL reconstruction in children: review of safety and early complications. J Pediatr Orthop 2017;37(3): 204–9.
8. Cordasco FA, Black SR, Price M, et al. Return to sport and reoperation rates in patients under the age of 20 after primary anterior cruciate ligament reconstruction: risk profile comparing 3 patient groups predicated upon skeletal age. Am J Sports Med 2019;47(3):628–39.
9. McCarthy MM, Tucker S, Nguyen JT, et al. Contact stress and kinematic analysis of all-epiphyseal and over-the-top pediatric reconstruction techniques for the anterior cruciate ligament. Am J Sports Med 2013;41(6):1330–9.
10. Ranade SC, Refakis CA, Cruz Cruz AI, et al. Validated pediatric functional outcomes of all-epiphyseal ACL reconstructions: does reinjury affect outcomes? J Pediatr Orthop 2018. https://doi.org/10.1097/BPO.0000000000001217.
11. Pennock AT, Chambers HG, Turk RD, et al. Use of a modified all-epiphyseal technique for anterior cruciate ligament reconstruction in the skeletally immature patient. Orthopaedic J Sports Med 2018;6(7). https://doi.org/10.1177/2325967118781769.
12. Fury MS, Paschos NK, Fabricant PD, et al. Assessment of skeletal maturity and postoperative growth disturbance after anterior cruciate ligament reconstruction in skeletally immature patients: a systematic review. Am J Sports Med 2021. https://doi.org/10.1177/03635465211008656. 3635465211008656.
13. Wall EJ, Ghattas PJ, Eismann EA, et al. Outcomes and complications after all-epiphyseal anterior cruciate ligament reconstruction in skeletally immature patients. Orthopaedic J Sports Med 2017;5(3). https://doi.org/10.1177/2325967117693604.
14. DeFrancesco CJ, Striano BM, Bram JT, et al. An in-depth analysis of graft rupture and contralateral anterior cruciate ligament rupture rates after pediatric anterior cruciate ligament reconstruction. Am J Sports Med 2020;48(10):2395–400.
15. Aitchison AH, Perea SH, Cordasco FA, et al. Improved epiphyseal socket placement with intraoperative 3D fluoroscopy: a consecutive series of pediatric all-epiphyseal anterior cruciate ligament reconstruction. Knee Surg Sports Traumatol Arthrosc 2022. https://doi.org/10.1007/S00167-021-06809-Z.

Osteochondritis Dissecans of the Knee in Young Athletes

Michael M. Chau, MD, PhD[a], Marc A. Tompkins, MD[a,b,c,*]

KEYWORDS

- Osteochondritis dissecans • Young athletes • Local ischemia
- Endochondral ossification • Subarticular physis • Premature osteoarthritis

KEY POINTS

- Osteochondritis dissecans of the knee is a relatively rare disorder in young athletes that can lead to premature osteoarthritis.
- The causes may be multifactorial, involving repetitive stress or microtrauma, local ischemia, disruption of the endochondral ossification program in the subarticular physis, and hereditary predisposition.
- Nonoperative treatment is typically attempted for patients with open physes, stable lesions, and minimal symptoms.
- Operative treatment is typically offered to patients with closed physes, unstable lesions, mechanical symptoms, and failure of 3 to 6 months of nonoperative treatment.
- Individualized rehabilitation is critical for both nonoperative and postoperative management to maximize function by enhancing strength and flexibility while protecting the lesion against further degeneration.

INTRODUCTION

The occurrence of loose osteochondral bodies within a joint was initially described and hypothesized to be caused by "quiet necrosis" by James Paget in 1870.[1] Franz König coined the term "osteochondritis dissecans" in 1887.[2] More recently, in 2013, members of an international study group dedicated to Research in OsteoChondritis dissecans of the Knee (ROCK) published a working definition to aid research

The authors declare no commercial or financial conflicts of interest and no funding sources were associated with this work.

[a] Department of Orthopedic Surgery, University of Minnesota, 2450 Riverside Avenue South Suite R200, Minneapolis, MN 55454, USA; [b] TRIA Orthopedic Center, 8100 Northland Drive, Bloomington, MN 55431, USA; [c] Gillette Children's Specialty Healthcare, 200 University Avenue East, St Paul, MN 55101, USA

* Corresponding author. Department of Orthopedic Surgery, University of Minnesota, 2450 Riverside Avenue South Suite R200, Minneapolis, MN 55454.

E-mail address: marc.tompkins@tria.com

collaborations: "Osteochondritis dissecans (OCD) is a focal idiopathic alteration of subchondral bone with risk of instability and disruption of adjacent articular cartilage that may result in premature osteoarthritis."[3] Knee OCD is a relatively rare disorder in young athletes that is typically managed by sports medicine specialists.

OCD is divided into juvenile and adult forms based on skeletal maturity at the time of diagnosis.[4] The distinction between juvenile and adult OCD is important for management and prognosis because younger patients with open physes usually require less invasive treatment and have more favorable outcomes.[4] Knee OCD has a reported incidence of up to 29/100,000 in young patients and is rarely found in those who are less than 10 or greater than 50 years old.[4–7] Boys have a 4 times higher risk compared with girls.[6] Involvement in high-level athletics, such as soccer, football, and basketball, has been correlated with knee OCD in the majority of cases in some studies.[4,8,9] Earlier sports participation or single sport specialization is speculated to be related to an observed trend of younger disease onset.[10]

The exact etiology of OCD has not been fully elucidated. It has been particularly challenging to study early stages of the disease as patients often do not present until later when they develop persistent pain or mechanical symptoms. Nevertheless, the underlying cause has been postulated to be multifactorial, involving repetitive stress or microtrauma, local ischemia, disruption of the endochondral ossification program in the subarticular physis, and hereditary predisposition.[11] The nomenclature implying an inflammatory process (osteochondritis) is a misnomer with minimal supporting histologic evidence. Current literature instead suggests local ischemic necrosis of epiphyseal cartilage to be a common pathologic pathway (**Fig. 1**).[12–14]

Modern advanced imaging protocols have permitted more in-depth investigation into the epiphyseal cartilage origin of OCD. Using a 3T MRI protocol called T2* (T2

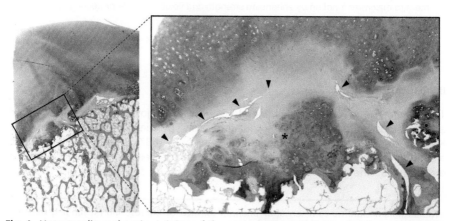

Fig. 1. Hematoxylin and eosin staining of the central aspect of the medial femoral condyle from an 8-year-old male human cadaveric donor. The high magnification inset image on the right demonstrates early cleft formation in the epiphyseal cartilage along a necrotic vascular profile (*arrowheads*). Failure of endochondral ossification of the secondary subarticular physis will result in an island of necrotic epiphyseal cartilage (*asterisks*) retained within subchondral bone, which provides poor mechanical support for overlying articular cartilage. This defect will either heal or subsequently be exposed to biomechanical trauma in a single event or multiple events to generate an osteochondritis dissecans lesion. (*Courtesy of* Alexandra Armstrong, DVM; Ferenc Tóth, DVM, PhD, DACVS; and Cathy Carlson, DVM, PhD, DACVP; Department of Veterinary Clinical Sciences, College of Veterinary Medicine, University of Minnesota, St. Paul, MN.)

"star") mapping, which allows differentiation of otherwise hypointense and indistinguishable tissues, the natural history of juvenile OCD was shown to progress in a step-wise fashion from necrotic epiphyseal cartilage to lesions that either heal or fail to heal.[15] Histologic studies of pediatric cadaveric knees with juvenile OCD have similarly revealed epiphyseal cartilage necrosis associated with failed endochondral ossification at predilection sites.[16] Furthermore, animal models in which ischemic necrosis was induced in the epiphyseal cartilage demonstrated aberrant endochondral ossification and corresponding areas of weak articular cartilage supported only by underlying necrotic tissue reminiscent of OCD lesions.[17]

The classic site for an OCD lesion in the knee is the posterior-central aspect of the medial femoral condyle (63.6%–85%).[6] Lesions occur less commonly in the inferior-central aspect of the lateral condyle (15%–32.5%), inferomedial aspect of the patella (1.5%–10%), the trochlea (2%), and the tibial plateau (0.5%).[6] These predilection sites have been shown to be associated with vascular watershed areas in the subchondral epiphysis, repetitive stress on the corresponding subchondral bone produced by the patella or tibial spine at varying degrees of knee flexion, and mechanical axis deviation into the respective knee compartment.[18,19] Lesions are often isolated but can occur at multiple sites in different disease stages and can be bilateral with the contralateral knee either being symptomatic or having no symptoms.[20,21]

The "stability" of an OCD lesion is defined by the presence or absence of an articular cartilage fracture and subchondral bone separation.[22] Lesion stability is typically inferred by history and physical examination, deduced by MRI, and verified by diagnostic arthroscopy. Lesion stability, lesion size, adjacent cyst, subchondral bone status, and patient age are important factors for clinical decision-making when deciding between nonoperative versus operative treatment and the specific type of surgical intervention. Other factors that may need to be addressed concomitantly include mechanical malalignment (genu varum, genu valgum, and torsional deformities), patellofemoral maltracking, and meniscal pathology.[23–25] The relationship between lateral femoral condyle OCD and discoid lateral meniscus has been reported to have a concurrence rate up to 14.5%. The specific location of the lateral femoral condyle OCD lesion may be related to the discoid meniscus morphology or injury pattern.[25,26]

EVALUATION
Differential Diagnoses

Knee OCD can be diagnosed by integrating information from the history, physical examination, and imaging findings. However, there are normal variations and similar but distinct pathologies that should be ruled out. Normal irregular distal femoral epiphyseal ossification and accessory epiphyseal ossification nuclei have been described.[10] These ordinary variations can be differentiated by recognizing the common appearance and predilection sites of OCD lesions on standard imaging. Osteochondral stress or impaction fractures are not uncommon in athletes but are more likely related to a specific injury and demonstrate subchondral contusions on both articulating surfaces (kissing lesions). Although osteonecrosis associated with hemoglobinopathy, steroid, radiation, or chemotherapy can have a comparable clinical presentation, the specific etiology can usually be discerned through obtaining a focused history. Spontaneous osteonecrosis of the knee is likewise an idiopathic condition that may have a similar appearance on imaging but is more common in older patients (>50 years) and may be associated with subchondral insufficiency fractures or meniscal pathologies. Epiphyseal dysplasias are a group of inherited disorders that are often systemic, polyarticular, and accompanied by other unique clinical manifestations.[27,28]

History and Physical Examination

Patients may report a history of chronic overuse or mild injury to the knee but rarely an isolated significant traumatic event. The most common complaint on initial presentation is persistent, nonspecific knee pain with or without mechanical symptoms that is aggravated by vigorous activity and improved with rest. Variability in clinical presentation can be related to lesion location and stage. The presence of mechanical symptoms, such as crepitance, catching, locking, and a sense of giving way, along with knee effusion and restricted range of motion, is consistent with an unstable lesion or loose osteochondral fragment. Tenderness can be elicited with direct pressure applied to the lesion. This is demonstrated by a positive Wilson sign, when pain is reproduced with tibial internal rotation during knee extension from 90 to 30 degrees of flexion, which effectively impinges the tibial eminence against the lesion, and relieved with tibial external rotation.[29] However, this test has low diagnostic value and is only relevant to medial femoral condylar lesions.[30]

Imaging

Radiography is the first-line imaging modality for diagnostic workup and monitoring treatment response. An initial comprehensive knee series, including anteroposterior, lateral, intercondylar notch, and patellofemoral tangential views, is required to evaluate all predilection sites. Screening of the contralateral knee should be strongly considered because of the possibility for bilateral involvement. Standing full length lower extremity alignment films should be obtained to evaluate the mechanical axis as angular deformity may be a contributing factor. Early OCD lesions are characterized by an abnormal contour and radiolucency at the articular surface. More advanced OCD lesions are characterized by a well circumscribed and variably ossified "progeny" fragment separated from the underlying "parent" subchondral bone by a crescent-shaped radiolucent line. The progeny fragment can be unossified versus ossified, intact versus fragmented, and in situ versus displaced (**Fig. 2**). Distinction between the progeny fragment and parent subchondral bone will become less obvious with subsequent ossification and lesion healing.[11]

MRI is the standard-of-care imaging modality to confirm the diagnosis and characterize lesions (see **Fig. 2**). The combination of T1- and T2-weighted sequences provide clinically relevant information about articular cartilage integrity, marrow reaction in the parent subchondral bone, fluid or cystic changes at the parent-progeny interface, and composition of the progeny fragment. However, bright T2-signal around a lesion may

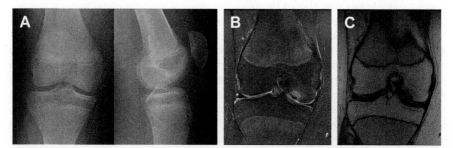

Fig. 2. A 16-year-old boy with OCD of the right knee at the medial femoral condyle. (*A*) Anteroposterior and lateral radiographs demonstrate a crescent shaped radiolucency outlining an ossified progeny fragment. (*B*) T2-weighted MRI reveals marrow reaction in the parent subchondral bone. (*C*), T1-weighted MRI allow more accurate lesion size measurement.

ambiguously represent either fluid that is concerning for lesion instability or vascular granulation tissue consistent with lesion healing.[31] In 2008, De Smet and colleagues published revised MRI criteria to better predict lesion instability: (1) bright T2-signal rim or cyst surrounding an adult OCD lesion are unequivocal signs of instability, (2) bright T2-signal rim surrounding a juvenile OCD lesion indicates instability only if it has the same signal intensity as adjacent joint fluid, is surrounded by a second outer rim with lower T2-signal, or is accompanied by multiple breaks in the subchondral bone, and (3) cysts surrounding a juvenile OCD lesion indicate instability only if they are multiple or large in size.[32] More recently, cartilage-specific MRI protocols, such as T2* mapping, have been implemented to improve the accuracy of characterizing lesions by providing additional information about soft tissue composition (**Fig. 3**).[11] They can also display a bone window that provides osseous detail comparable to

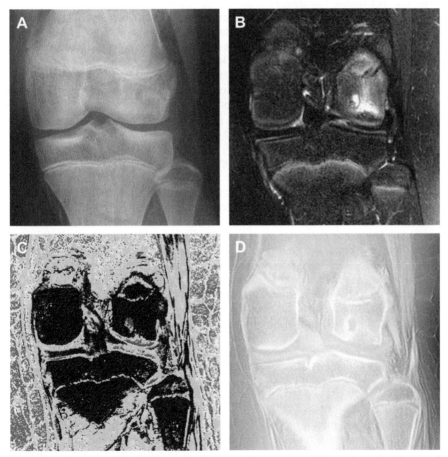

Fig. 3. Juvenile OCD of the left knee at the lateral femoral condyle evaluated with a cartilage specific 3T MRI protocol. (*A*) AP radiograph showing subchondral lucency and cysts. (*B*) T2-weighted MRI shows cystic changes and marrow edema. (*C*) T2* mapping with color coding intensities: blue to black is bone and mineralization, green to red is epiphyseal and articular cartilage, and red is fluid. (*D*) CT-like bone window image shows parent bone with cystic changes, sclerosis, and marginal mineralization surrounding an osteocartilaginous progeny fragment.

computed tomography (CT) without radiation exposure. This technology is currently not widely available and is primarily used at academic institutions for research purposes.[15]

Other imaging modalities include CT, ultrasound, and bone scan. CT is particularly useful for identifying osteochondral loose bodies and evaluating osseous healing after fragment fixation; however, it is limited by substantial radiation exposure and inability to adequately visualize soft tissue. Ultrasound has been described but is heavily operator dependent with a steep learning curve and is not used in most practices for managing knee OCD.[33] Bone scan is mainly of historic relevance since the advent of MRI because of its relatively poor specificity and need for intravenous administration of radioisotope.[34]

Classification Systems

There are numerous radiographic, MRI, and arthroscopic classification systems described for knee OCD. No single classification system has been unanimously accepted due in part to the difficulty of interpreting lesion stability with imaging. The Berndt–Harty radiography classification was originally described for talar osteochondral lesions in 1959 but has also been used for knee OCD: (I) small subchondral compression, (II) partially detached osteochondral fragment, (III) completely detached but nondisplaced fragment, and (IV) completely detached and displaced fragment.[35] The Hefti MRI classification devised in 1999 continues to be referenced: (I) small change of signal without clear margins of fragment, (II) osteochondral fragment with clear margins but without fluid between fragment and underlying bone, (III) fluid is visible partially between fragment and underlying bone, (IV) fluid surrounds the fragment but the fragment is still in situ, and (V) fragment is completely detached and displaced.[36] In 2017, Ellermann and colleagues outlined an MRI classification based on natural history of the disease using the T2* mapping protocol: (1) epiphyseal cartilage lesion with necrotic center, (II) epiphyseal cartilage lesion with complete or incomplete rim calcification, (III) partially or completely ossified lesion, (IV) healed osseous lesion with a linear osseous scar, and (V) unhealed detached osseous lesion.[15] Diagnostic arthroscopy with direct visualization and probing is the gold standard for determining lesion stability. The ROCK arthroscopy classification system published in 2013 is currently the most comprehensive, has been shown to be very reliable, can be used to guide surgical treatment, and helps facilitate multicenter research.[37] It is divided into six mutually exclusive categories divided into immobile (cue ball, shadow, wrinkle in the rug) and mobile (locked door, trap door, crater) lesions. It purposefully omits determination of lesion salvageability, which can be subjective and depends on lesion size, amount of fragmentation, subchondral necrosis, and cartilage degeneration as well as clinical judgment regarding skeletal maturity, prior treatments, and imaging findings.

TREATMENT

The primary goals of managing knee OCD are to relieve symptoms, restore function, heal the lesion, preserve the joint in the long-term, and improve quality of life for the patient. The most appropriate treatment of knee OCD is not completely clear and remains an area of active clinical investigation.

In 2010, the American Academy of Orthopedic Surgeons (AAOS) published a clinical practice guideline (CPG) for the diagnosis and treatment of knee OCD using the highest quality research available.[38] It included evaluation of nonsurgical or surgical treatment of 4 patient populations: skeletally immature with stable lesions, skeletally immature with unstable lesions, skeletally mature with stable lesions, and skeletally mature with unstable lesions. Due to the lack of high-level evidence and prospective randomized clinical studies, few conclusive recommendations could be made. Of the 16 recommendations, none were graded strong, most were graded inconclusive, 2 were graded weak, and 4 were consensus statements of the workgroup. The benefit of nonsurgical treatment for symptomatic or asymptomatic skeletally immature patients with OCD was inconclusive. The use of counseling patients on whether activity modification and weight control prevent onset and progression of OCD to osteoarthritis was inconclusive. For patients being treated nonoperatively the benefit of physical therapy was inconclusive. However, there was consensus that postoperative physical therapy be offered to patients who received surgery. The CPG was unable to recommend for or against arthroscopic drilling in symptomatic skeletally immature patients with stable lesions who have failed to heal with nonsurgical treatment over 3 months. It was not possible to recommend for or against a specific cartilage repair technique in symptomatic skeletally immature or mature patients with unsalvageable fragments. There was consensus without reliable evidence that symptomatic skeletally immature and mature patients with salvageable unstable or displaced OCD lesions be offered the option of surgery.

Currently, the optimal treatment of knee OCD is incompletely defined and there is a scarcity of high-level evidenced-based data, which underscores the importance of patient–physician communication, shared decision-making, and experienced clinical judgment. In general, conventional treatment protocols are largely based on skeletal maturity, lesion stability, and patient symptoms.

Nonoperative Treatment

Indications for nonoperative treatment include open physes, stable lesions, and minimal symptoms. The general assumptions are that younger patients have a better biological capacity to heal and lesion mobility is disruptive for the healing process. There is substantial variability in nonoperative protocols without high-level supporting evidence. Treatment duration is usually a minimum of 3 to 6 months and interventions include activity modification (immediate cessation of sports with restrictions on running and jumping) with or without weightbearing restrictions (partial vs nonweight-bearing) and joint immobilization (brace or cast). Skeletally immature patients with stable lesions and minimal symptoms generally respond well to nonoperative treatment. Favorable outcomes have been reported in more than one-half of nonoperatively treated cases depending on the referenced study.[4,36,39,40] The risk of needing surgery is higher with increasing age of the patient and most adults who are symptomatic are offered surgery because of a relatively elevated risk of progression to osteoarthritis with nonoperative treatment. Other risk factors for failing nonoperative treatment are body mass index (BMI) greater than 25 kg/m^2 and less common sites for OCD lesions (patella and trochlea).[41] Clinical decision-making nomograms have been developed to predict the likelihood of healing with nonoperative treatment and take into consideration patient age, mechanical symptoms, lesion size, lesion location, and cystlike lesions.[39,40]

Operative Treatment

Indications for operative treatment include closed physes, unstable lesions, mechanical symptoms, and failure of 3 to 6 months of nonoperative treatment as defined by increasing severity of the lesion on imaging and persistent or worsening symptoms. Lesion "salvageability" is designated by clinical judgment at the time of diagnostic arthroscopy. A lesion may be considered unsalvageable due to the small size of the fragment, substantial osteochondral fragmentation, subchondral necrosis, or articular cartilage degeneration. As such, lesions can be grouped into 3 broad categories to help guide treatment: stable, unstable salvageable, and unstable unsalvageable. Additionally, concomitant pathology, such as mechanical malalignment, joint instability, or anatomic anomalies, should be evaluated and properly addressed to optimize outcomes.

Stable lesions with an intact articular surface in skeletally immature patients can be treated with epiphyseal drilling to promote healing by increasing local blood flow and concentration of mesenchymal cells and growth factors (**Fig. 4**).[11,42] Positive patient-oriented and radiographic outcomes have been reported with transarticular (ie, retrograde), transepiphyseal (ie, antegrade or retroarticular), and notch drilling techniques.[43] Transarticular and notch drilling are performed arthroscopically with direct visualization, while transepiphyseal drilling avoids penetrating articular cartilage but requires fluoroscopic proficiency and radiation exposure. Successful return to activities and signs of radiographic healing have been reported to be as early as 4.5 months postoperatively regardless of the drilling method.[44]

Unstable salvageable lesions with locked door, trapped door, or detached crater fragments can be treated with reduction and fixation. These are usually performed with adjunctive procedures, such as debridement of fibrous tissue at the parent-progeny interface, subchondral drilling, and autologous bone grafting (**Fig. 5**). Suture bridge for fixation include metal and bioabsorbable headless compression screws (partially threaded or variable pitch), noncompressive bioabsorbable devices (pins or nails), and bone sticks or pegs. The specific fixation method depends on surgeon preference as well as tissue composition (fibrocartilaginous vs osseous) and quality of the fragment. Metallic devices provide firm purchase but may need to be removed before ambulation and generate artifact on MRI. Bioabsorbable devices offer the advantage of MRI compatibility but have been associated with higher rates of loosening and can be complicated by synovitis and sterile cyst formation. Regardless of the method of fixation, lesion healing has been shown to occur by 6 months.[45] Fragment fixation has also been shown to be successful for both skeletally immature and mature patients at midterm follow-up, with survival rates of 70.4% and 78.3%, respectively, shown in one study.[46]

Unstable unsalvageable lesions with substantial osteochondral fragmentation, subchondral bone necrosis, or articular cartilage degeneration can be treated with cartilage resurfacing using a variety of methods. Marrow stimulation with abrasion chondroplasty, drilling, or microfracture down to bleeding bone can stimulate fibrocartilage coverage of smaller and more shallow defects less than 10 mm.[47] Autologous chondrocyte implantation (ACI) or matrix induced ACI (MACI) are viable alternatives

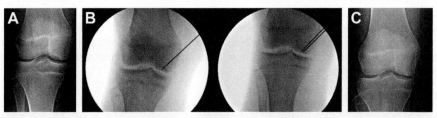

Fig. 4. Transepiphyseal (ie, antegrade or retroarticular) drilling of an OCD lesion at the medial femoral condyle of a skeletally immature patient. (*A*) Preoperative anteroposterior radiograph. (*B*) Fluoroscopy during transepiphyseal drilling using 0.062-in Kirschner wires to penetrate the lesion without penetrating the articular cartilage or violating the physis. (*C*) Radiography 3 months postoperatively showing interval healing. (Reproduced with permission, from: Heyworth BE, Kocher MS. Osteochondritis Dissecans of the Knee. JBJS Reviews. 2015 Jul;3[7]:e1.)

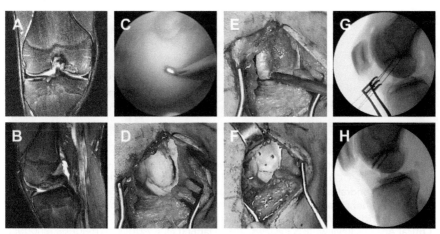

Fig. 5. An 18-year-old male with OCD of the right knee at the medial femoral condyle. (*A, B*) Coronal and sagittal T2-weighted MRI demonstrating an unstable lesion. (*C*) Diagnostic arthroscopy confirming a trap door lesion. (*D, E*) Clinical photograph showing an open medial parapatellar approach for fibrous tissue debridement and bone grafting at the parent–progeny interface. (*F*) Clinical photograph showing open reduction internal fixation of the progeny fragment. (*G, H*) Fluoroscopy during fixation of the progeny fragment using 3 cannulated, headless compression screws.

that can be used to cover larger defects with fibrocartilaginous tissue.[48] Good long-term survivorship of 82% at 20-year follow-up has been reported for ACI.[49] MACI coupled with bone grafting has also been shown to have satisfactory outcomes at 10-year follow-up.[50] Osteochondral transplantation using autograft or allograft is another feasible alternative (**Fig. 6**).[51] Autografts are obtained from less weight-bearing and articulating areas of the trochlear groove whereas allografts can be obtained from corresponding OCD sites thereby providing comparable articular surface contour. The main advantage of osteochondral transplantation over other cartilage resurfacing methods is the robust biomechanical properties of articular cartilage. However, donor site morbidity is a limitation, particularly for larger lesions, and potential complications include failure of graft integration and graft or adjacent articular cartilage degeneration. Osteochondral autograft transplantation was shown in a randomized clinical trial to be superior to microfracture at 4.2 years postoperatively.[52] Similarly, osteochondral allograft transplantation has been shown to have good to excellent outcomes after 7.7 years postoperatively.[53]

Lower extremity mechanical axis malalignment may generate undue stress in the affected compartment of the knee. In this scenario, an isolated cartilage procedure without correcting the biomechanical deformity will risk failure.[54] Realignment osteotomy can be performed either at the same time as the cartilage procedure or in a staged manner.[11] The decision of distal femur versus proximal tibia osteotomy depends on where the deformity is and knowing that the mechanical lateral distal femoral angle (mLDFA) and mechanical medial proximal tibial angle (mMPTA) with respect to the joint orientation line both approximate 87° in the average population. Furthermore, an opening wedge osteotomy will slightly lengthen the extremity whereas a closing wedge osteotomy will slightly shorten the extremity but may allow for earlier transition to full weightbearing. Guided growth or hemiepiphysiodesis (tension band plating or screw) can be considered for skeletally immature patients with at least 1 to 2 years of skeletal growth remaining as determined by hand or elbow radiographs (**Fig. 7**).

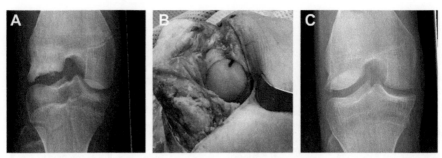

Fig. 6. Osteochondral allograft transplantation. (*A*) Preoperative tunnel radiograph demonstrating a juvenile OCD lesion of the lateral femoral condyle. (*B*) Clinical image of a fresh frozen osteochondral allograft restoring a large unstable unsalvageable OCD lesion. (*C*) Postoperative tunnel radiograph. (Reproduced with permission, from: Chan C, Richmond C, Shea KG, Frick SL. Management of Osteochondritis Dissecans of the Femoral Condyle: A Critical Analysis Review. JBJS Reviews. 2018 Mar;6[3]:e5.)

Gradual correction of angular limb deformity is less painful, requires shorter immobilization, and carries less surgical risk. Treatment of a concurrent discoid lateral meniscus may involve saucerization with repair as necessary for horizontal cleavage tears and to stabilize the peripheral rim, which theoretically normalizes the biomechanical stresses across the lateral compartment to allow healing of the OCD lesion. Conversely, subtotal and total resection of the discoid lateral meniscus has been

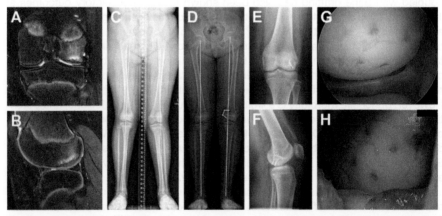

Fig. 7. A 13-year-old girl with OCD of the left knee at the lateral femoral condyle and concomitant genu valgum deformity. (*A*, *B*) Coronal and sagittal T2-weighted MRI demonstrating a lesion at the weightbearing surface. (*C*) Standing full length lower extremity alignment radiograph demonstrating left genu valgum with the mechanical axis traversing the lesion. (*D*), Guided growth with tension band plating 1 year postoperatively achieved correction of the mechanical axis to neutral. (*E*, *F*) After tension band plate removal, open reduction internal fixation of the lesion was performed using four headless compression screws with supplemental fibrous debridement and bone grafting at the parent–progeny interface. AP and lateral radiographs 6 months postoperatively demonstrated a healed lesion. (*G*), Diagnostic arthroscopy 6 months postoperatively during hardware removal demonstrated a smooth articular surface without step-off or screw prominence. (*H*), Clinical photograph at the time of open hardware removal.

reported to be a predisposing factor in the development of postoperative lateral femoral condyle OCD.[55,56]

Complications

Delayed diagnosis and inappropriate management of knee OCD are correlated with worse outcomes. Young athletes may have a high pain tolerance or attribute their symptoms with normal soreness from physical training and therefore initially present at a later disease stage. Nonadherence to treatment or rehabilitation can result in slowed or incomplete lesion healing. Failure of initial treatment may require multiple subsequent surgeries with each successive procedure being more salvage like. Non-healing of the lesion and progressive cartilage degeneration over time leading to premature osteoarthritis requiring arthroplasty is the most dreaded outcome for young athletes. One study showed that the rates of osteoarthritis and arthroplasty were 30% and 8% at 35 years, respectively, after nonoperative treatment.[41] Combining patients who were treated either nonoperatively or operatively another study estimated the rates to be 14% for persistent knee pain, 6% for symptomatic osteoarthritis, and 3% for conversion to total knee arthroplasty at 14 years follow-up.[57]

REHABILITATION

Physical therapy plays an important role in both nonoperative and postoperative management of knee OCD. The main goal is to maximize function by enhancing strength and flexibility while protecting the lesion against further degeneration. Comprehensive rehabilitation programs are designed on an individual basis by considering previous surgeries, lesion stage, skeletal maturity, symptoms, and concomitant injuries. Protocols are typically multiphasic and follow a stepwise progression of activity restriction, limited weightbearing, limited range of motion, strengthening, and return to activity. Criteria for progression from one stage to the next and a general overall timeline are provided by the physical therapist. Symptoms of OCD worsening that should prompt patients to communicate with their care team include increased pain, loss of range of motion, development of mechanical symptoms, and new onset or recalcitrant swelling.

A nonoperative therapy program can comprise three phases: initial (limited joint loading), intermediate (loading the joint), and advanced (progress functional activities).[58,59] In the initial phase, the lesion is protected with a period of immobilization and restricted weight bearing. Use of an unloader brace that selectively decreases compressive forces in the lateral or medial compartment has been described.[40] As the patient progresses through the initial phase, muscle strengthening interventions can be implemented with closed or open kinetic chain exercises. Balance and proprioception interventions can also be performed. Criteria to progress to the next phase include no pain or effusion, normal range of motion, muscle strength at least 4 out of 5, and painless weight bearing. In the intermediate phase, normal ambulation is resumed, gait training is implemented to reestablish normal kinematics, and further muscle strengthening of the extremity and core are performed. Criteria for phase progression include maintenance of prior criteria, muscle strength at least 4+ out of 5, normal gait, and stable mechanics such as during single limb stance. In the advanced phase, the patient progresses to their desired level of activity with continued strengthening, dynamic tasks to maximize neuromuscular control, and simulated sport-specific movements. Criteria before return to activity include maintenance of prior criteria, symmetric strength, normal mobility, and neuromuscular control without irregular movements while performing vigorous tasks and movements.

The ROCK physical therapy protocol for postoperative management of juvenile knee OCD is comprised of three phases: acute, neuromuscular strengthening, and return to activity.[60] The acute phase (postoperative weeks 0–6) recommends progression from nonweight-bearing to toe-touch weight bearing, full range of motion without restriction, and initiation of closed kinetic chain exercises. Criteria to progress after 6 weeks include range of motion within normal limits, straight leg raise without extensor lag, and no pain or effusion with exercise. In the neuromuscular strengthening phase (weeks 6–12), the patient progresses to full weightbearing as tolerated over a period of 1 to 2 weeks and closed kinetic chain interventions without weight-bearing restriction. Criteria to progress after 12 weeks include no symptoms with activity and quadriceps strength deficit less than 20% compared with the contralateral extremity. Advancing to the return-to-activity phase is permitted when complete lesion healing is achieved and involves continued strengthening, initiation of agility, jogging, and light impact activities, and progression to plyometric activities in line with future athletic goals. Criteria before return to activity are quadriceps strength within 10% of the contralateral limb, functional hop performance within 10% of the contralateral limb, and final clearance by the care team.

There is currently no widely accepted or validated rehabilitation protocol for the management of knee OCD. The overall timeline for nonoperative and postoperative rehabilitation varies and should be guided by best clinical judgment. For stable lesions, rehabilitation programs may last 6 weeks to 6 months regardless of treatment type. Cartilage fixation and restoration procedures for unstable lesions usually require longer rehabilitation programs from 6 to 12 months. The successful completion of an individualized program should indicate a safe return to activity. Optimized outcomes for young athletes with knee OCD depend on effective collaboration between the patient, family, coach, personal trainer, physical therapist, and physician.

SUMMARY

OCD of the knee is a relatively rare condition in young athletes that can lead to chronic pain and dysfunction. Compared with the general population young athletes are at an increased risk for developing knee OCD. Timely diagnosis and appropriate management are important for achieving successful outcomes. The primary goals of treatment include symptomatic relief, lesion healing, joint preservation, and return to activities. Although the optimal treatment strategy is currently unknown, most recommendations are based on skeletal maturity, lesion stability, and patient symptoms. Nonoperative and postoperative rehabilitation play critical roles for overall success. Although most patients recover and do well, it is essential for sports medicine specialists to appropriately guide management and avoid potential complications.

CLINICS CARE POINTS

- Osteochondritis dissecans of the knee in young athletes may result in premature osteoarthritis.
- Bilateral disease is not uncommon and should prompt contralateral evaluation despite symptoms.
- Radiography and MRI are the conventional modes of diagnostic and follow up imaging.
- Diagnostic arthroscopy with probing is the gold standard for determining lesion stability.

- Treatment decision making largely depends on skeletal maturity, lesion stability, and patient symptoms.
- Lesion salvageability is subjectively based on best clinical judgement.
- A proper rehabilitation and return to sport program is important for successful outcomes.

REFERENCES

1. Paget J. On the production of some of the loose bodies in joints. St Bartholomew's Hosp Rep 1870;6:1–4.
2. König F. The Classic: On Loose Bodies in the Joint. Clin Orthop Relat Res 2013; 471:1107–15.
3. Edmonds EW, Shea KG. Osteochondritis dissecans: editorial comment. Clin Orthop Relat Res 2013;471:1105–6.
4. Cahill BR. Osteochondritis Dissecans of the Knee: Treatment of Juvenile and Adult Forms. J Am Acad Orthop Surg 1995;3:237–47.
5. Lindén B. The incidence of osteochondritis dissecans in the condyles of the femur. Acta Orthop Scand 1976;47:664–7.
6. Kessler JI, Nikizad H, Shea KG, et al. The Demographics and Epidemiology of Osteochondritis Dissecans of the Knee in Children and Adolescents. Am J Sports Med 2014;42:320–6.
7. Pareek A, Sanders TL, Wu IT, et al. Incidence of symptomatic osteochondritis dissecans lesions of the knee: a population-based study in Olmsted County. Osteoarthr Cartil 2017;25:1663–71.
8. Price MJ, Tuca M, Nguyen J, et al. Juvenile Osteochondritis Dissecans of the Trochlea: A Cohort Study of 34 Trochlear Lesions Associated With Sporting Activities That Load the Patellofemoral Joint. J Pediatr Orthop 2020;40:103–9.
9. Wall EJ, Heyworth BE, Shea KG, et al. Trochlear Groove Osteochondritis Dissecans of the Knee Patellofemoral Joint. J Pediatr Orthop 2014;1. https://doi.org/10.1097/BPO.0000000000000212.
10. Kocher MS, Tucker R, Ganley TJ, et al. Management of Osteochondritis Dissecans of the Knee: Current Concepts Review. Am J Sports Med 2006;34:1181–91.
11. Chau MM, Klimstra MA, Wise KL, et al. Osteochondritis Dissecans: Current Understanding of Epidemiology, Etiology, Management, and Outcomes. J Bone Joint Surg 2021;103:1132–51.
12. Uozumi H, Sugita T, Aizawa T, et al. Histologic findings and possible causes of osteochondritis dissecans of the knee. Am J Sports Med 2009;37:2003–8.
13. Shea KG, Jacobs JC, Carey JL, et al. Osteochondritis dissecans knee histology studies have variable findings and theories of etiology. Clin Orthop Relat Res 2013;471:1127–36.
14. Yonetani Y, Nakamura N, Natsuume T, et al. Histological evaluation of juvenile osteochondritis dissecans of the knee: a case series. Knee Surg Sports Traumatol Arthrosc 2010;18:723–30.
15. Ellermann J, Johnson CP, Wang L, et al. Insights into the Epiphyseal Cartilage Origin and Subsequent Osseous Manifestation of Juvenile Osteochondritis Dissecans with a Modified Clinical MR Imaging Protocol: A Pilot Study. Radiology 2017; 282:798–806.
16. Tóth F, Tompkins MA, Shea KG, et al. Identification of Areas of Epiphyseal Cartilage Necrosis at Predilection Sites of Juvenile Osteochondritis Dissecans in Pediatric Cadavers. J Bone Joint Surg 2018;100:2132–9.

17. Tóth F, Johnson CP, Mills B, et al. Evaluation of the Suitability of Miniature Pigs as an Animal Model of Juvenile Osteochondritis Dissecans. J Orthop Res 2019;37: 2130–7.

18. Ellermann JM, Ludwig KD, Nissi MJ, et al. Three-Dimensional Quantitative Magnetic Resonance Imaging of Epiphyseal Cartilage Vascularity Using Vessel Image Features: New Insights into Juvenile Osteochondritis Dissecans. JB JS Open Access 2019;4. https://doi.org/10.2106/JBJS.OA.19.00031.

19. Jacobi M, Wahl P, Bouaicha S, et al. Association between mechanical axis of the leg and osteochondritis dissecans of the knee: radiographic study on 103 knees. Am J Sports Med 2010;38:1425–8.

20. Cooper T, Boyles A, Samora WP, et al. Prevalence of Bilateral JOCD of the Knee and Associated Risk Factors. J Pediatr Orthop 2015;35:507–10.

21. Backes JR, Durbin TC, Bentley JC, et al. Multifocal Juvenile Osteochondritis Dissecans of the Knee: A Case Series. J Pediatr Orthop 2014;34:6.

22. Wall E, Von Stein D. Juvenile osteochondritis dissecans. Orthop Clin North Am 2003;34:341–53.

23. Brown ML, McCauley JC, Gracitelli GC, et al. Osteochondritis Dissecans Lesion Location Is Highly Concordant With Mechanical Axis Deviation. Am J Sports Med 2020;48:871–5.

24. Kramer DE, Yen Y-M, Simoni MK, et al. Surgical Management of Osteochondritis Dissecans Lesions of the Patella and Trochlea in the Pediatric and Adolescent Population. Am J Sports Med 2015;43:654–62.

25. Deie M, Ochi M, Sumen Y, et al. Relationship between osteochondritis dissecans of the lateral femoral condyle and lateral menisci types. J Pediatr Orthop 2006;26: 79–82.

26. Takigami J, Hashimoto Y, Tomihara T, et al. Predictive factors for osteochondritis dissecans of the lateral femoral condyle concurrent with a discoid lateral meniscus. Knee Surg Sports Traumatol Arthrosc 2018;26:799–805.

27. Ribbing S. The hereditary multiple epiphyseal disturbance and its consequences for the aetiogenesis of local malacias–particularly the osteochondrosis dissecans. Acta Orthop Scand 1955;24:286–99.

28. Jackson GC, Marcus-Soekarman D, Stolte-Dijkstra I, et al. Type IX collagen gene mutations can result in multiple epiphyseal dysplasia that is associated with osteochondritis dissecans and a mild myopathy. Am J Med Genet A 2010;152A: 863–9.

29. Bronstein RD, Schaffer JC. Physical Examination of the Knee: Meniscus, Cartilage, and Patellofemoral Conditions. [Review]. J Am Acad Orthop Surg 2017; 25:365–74.

30. Conrad JM, Stanitski CL. Osteochondritis Dissecans: Wilson's Sign Revisited. Am J Sports Med 2003;31:777–8.

31. O'Connor MA, Palaniappan M, Khan N, et al. Osteochondritis dissecans of the knee in children. A comparison of MRI and arthroscopic findings. J Bone Joint Surg Br 2002;84:258–62.

32. Kijowski R, Blankenbaker DG, Shinki K, et al. Juvenile versus Adult Osteochondritis Dissecans of the Knee: Appropriate MR Imaging Criteria for Instability. Radiology 2008;248:571–8.

33. Jungesblut OD, Berger-Groch J, Meenen NM, et al. Validity of Ultrasound Compared with Magnetic Resonance Imaging in Evaluation of Osteochondritis Dissecans of the Distal Femur in Children. Cartilage 2021;12:169–74.

34. Cahill BR, Phillips MR, Navarro R. The results of conservative management of juvenile osteochondritis dissecans using joint scintigraphy. A prospective study. Am J Sports Med 1989;17:601–5 [discussion: 605–6].
35. Berndt AL, Harty M. Transchondral fractures (osteochondritis dissecans) of the talus. J Bone Joint Surg Am 1959;41-A:988–1020.
36. Hefti F, Beguiristain J, Krauspe R, et al. Osteochondritis dissecans: a multicenter study of the European Pediatric Orthopedic Society. J Pediatr Orthop B 1999;8: 231–45.
37. Carey JL, Wall EJ, Shea KG, et al. Reliability of the ROCK Osteochondritis Dissecans Knee Arthroscopy Classification System - Multi-center Validation Study. Orthop J Sports Med 2013;1. https://doi.org/10.1177/2325967113S00074.
38. Chambers HG, Shea KG, Anderson AF, et al. AAOS Clincial Practice Guideline - Diagnosis and Treatment of Osteochondritis Dissecans. J Am Acad Orthop Surg 2011;19:297–306.
39. Krause M, Hapfelmeier A, Möller M, et al. Healing Predictors of Stable Juvenile Osteochondritis Dissecans Knee Lesions After 6 and 12 Months of Nonoperative Treatment. Am J Sports Med 2013;41:2384–91.
40. Wall EJ, Vourazeris J, Myer GD, et al. The Healing Potential of Stable Juvenile Osteochondritis Dissecans Knee Lesions. J Bone Joint Surg Am 2008;90:2655–64.
41. Sanders TL, Pareek A, Johnson NR, et al. Nonoperative Management of Osteochondritis Dissecans of the Knee: Progression to Osteoarthritis and Arthroplasty at Mean 13-Year Follow-up. Orthop J Sports Med 2017;5. 232596711770464.
42. Heyworth BE, Kocher MS. Osteochondritis Dissecans of the Knee. JBJS Rev 2015;3:1.
43. Heyworth BE, Edmonds EW, Murnaghan ML, et al. Drilling Techniques for Osteochondritis Dissecans. Clin Sports Med 2014;33:305–12.
44. Gunton MJ, Carey JL, Shaw CR, et al. Drilling Juvenile Osteochondritis Dissecans: Retro- or Transarticular? Clin Orthop Relat Res 2013;471:1144–51.
45. Kocher MS, Czarnecki JJ, Andersen JS, et al. Internal Fixation of Juvenile Osteochondritis Dissecans Lesions of the Knee. Am J Sports Med 2007;35:712–8.
46. Wu IT, Custers RJH, Desai VS, et al. Internal Fixation of Unstable Osteochondritis Dissecans: Do Open Growth Plates Improve Healing Rate? Am J Sports Med 2018;46:2394–401.
47. Pascual-Garrido C, McNickle AG, Cole BJ. Surgical Treatment Options for Osteochondritis Dissecans of the Knee. Sports Health 2009;1:326–34.
48. Grimm N, Danilkowicz R, Shea K. OCD Lesions of the Knee: An Updated Review on a Poorly Understood Entity:, JPOSNA®. 1 (2019). Available at: https://www.jposna.org/ojs/index.php/jposna/article/view/35. Accessed November 25, 2021.
49. Carey JL, Shea KG, Lindahl A, et al. Autologous Chondrocyte Implantation as Treatment for Unsalvageable Osteochondritis Dissecans: 10- to 25-Year Follow-up. Am J Sports Med 2020;48:1134–40.
50. Roffi A, Andriolo L, Di Martino A, et al. Long-term Results of Matrix-assisted Autologous Chondrocyte Transplantation Combined With Autologous Bone Grafting for the Treatment of Juvenile Osteochondritis Dissecans. J Pediatr Orthop 2020;40. e115–e121.
51. Chan C, Richmond C, Shea KG, et al. Management of Osteochondritis Dissecans of the Femoral Condyle: A Critical Analysis Review. JBJS Rev 2018;6:e5.
52. Gudas R, Simonaitytė R, Čekanauskas E, et al. A Prospective, Randomized Clinical Study of Osteochondral Autologous Transplantation Versus Microfracture for the Treatment of Osteochondritis Dissecans in the Knee Joint in Children. J Pediatr Orthop 2009;29:741–8.

53. Lyon R, Nissen C, Liu XC, et al. Can fresh osteochondral allografts restore function in juveniles with osteochondritis dissecans of the knee? Clin Orthop Relat Res 2013;471:1166–73.

54. Perkins CA, Willimon SC. Management of the Failed OCD. Curr Rev Musculoskelet Med 2020;13:173–9.

55. Mizuta H, Nakamura E, Otsuka Y, et al. Osteochondritis dissecans of the lateral femoral condyle following total resection of the discoid lateral meniscus. Arthroscopy 2001;17:608–12.

56. Hashimoto Y, Nishino K, Reid JB, et al. Factors Related to Postoperative Osteochondritis Dissecans of the Lateral Femoral Condyle After Meniscal Surgery in Juvenile Patients With a Discoid Lateral Meniscus. J Pediatr Orthop 2020;40. e853–e859.

57. Hevesi M, Sanders TL, Pareek A, et al. Osteochondritis Dissecans in the Knee of Skeletally Immature Patients: Rates of Persistent Pain, Osteoarthritis, and Arthroplasty at Mean 14-Years' Follow-Up. Cartilage 2020;11:291–9.

58. Paterno MV, Prokop TR, Schmitt LC. Physical therapy management of patients with osteochondritis dissecans: a comprehensive review. Clin Sports Med 2014;33:353–74.

59. Wilk KE, Briem K, Reinold MM, et al. Rehabilitation of Articular Lesions in the Athlete's Knee. J Orthop Sports Phys Ther 2006;36:815–27.

60. Research in OsteoChondritis of the Knee, ROCK PT Protocol Following Operative Management for Juvenile Osteochondritis Dissecans of the Knee, (n.d.). Available at: https://kneeocd.org/rock-studies/rct/pt-protocol/. Accessed January 15, 2022.

Psychological Aspects of Adolescent Knee Injuries

Aneesh G. Patankar, BS[a], Melissa A. Christino, MD[b], Matthew D. Milewski, MD[b],*

KEYWORDS

- Psychological • Adolescent • Pediatric • Knee • Injury • Treatment • Recovery

KEY POINTS

- Knee injuries are prevalent and impactful to the adolescent population, leading to both physical and psychological disturbances.
- Following knee injury, adolescents are at risk for developing or exacerbating underlying psychological disorders.
- Maladaptive psychological beliefs, which can potentially be identified preoperatively, can negatively affect the efficacy and rate of recovery, return-to-sport, and reinjury.
- Locus of control, self-efficacy, and social support, among other factors, contribute to improved rates of recovery and full progression to preinjury levels of activity.
- Orthopedic surgeons should be cognizant of the overall psychological status of their patients preoperatively and intra-recovery so a psychological care team can potentially develop an adjunctive treatment plan for those who are struggling with recovery or at high risk of negative outcomes.

INTRODUCTION
Epidemiology of Knee Injuries in Adolescents

Knee injuries are one of the most prevalent musculoskeletal injuries affecting adolescents. In 2008, this young population made up approximately 40% of more than 6.6 million knee injuries seen in emergency departments (EDs).[1] The age groups composed of 5- to 14-year olds and 15- to 24-year olds consistently held the two highest annual rates of ED knee injuries from 1999 to 2008, with sports and recreational activities being reported as the most common injury mechanisms.[1] More recent estimates place the current prevalence of adolescent knee injuries at 10% to 25% and higher.[2–4] Knee pain, while commonly considered a problem of the older population, also significantly affects the youth, with greater than20% of adolescents aged 10 to 17 year old experiencing knee painwithin a week.[5]

This is especially true for anterior cruciate ligament (ACL) injuries. Annual rates of ACL injury per population have increased by approximately 150% from 2005 to 2015,[6] with

[a] Rutgers Robert Wood Johnson Medical School, New Brunswick, 125 Paterson St, New Brunswick, NJ, USA; [b] Division of Sports Medicine, Department of Orthopaedic Surgery, Boston Children's Hospital, 300 Longwood Ave., Boston, MA, USA
* Corresponding author.
E-mail address: matthew.milewski@childrens.harvard.edu

Clin Sports Med 41 (2022) 595–609
https://doi.org/10.1016/j.csm.2022.05.003
0278-5919/22/© 2022 Elsevier Inc. All rights reserved.
sportsmed.theclinics.com

girls' soccer and boys' football contributing the highest rates of ACL injury per amount of time playing the sport.[7] A variety of factors also contribute to differences in adolescent knee injury rates among the sexes, leading to adolescent girls experiencing a 1.4 times higher rate of ACL injury compared with their male counterparts.[7] Of the adolescents who injure their ACL, up to 32% can go on to suffer a second ACL injury within two years,[8] showing the recurrent impact this type of knee injury can have on this population. Other studies have reported significantly higher rates of lower extremity injurie-samong young athletes who specialize in a single sport, play their primary sport for more than eight months per year, or participate in high competition volume. Specifically, these athletes experience 1.5 times the risk of patellofemoral pain diagnoses and four times the risk of patellar tendinopathy and Osgood–Schlatter disease.[9–11]

Many of the athletes who injure their ACL undergo an operative ACL reconstruction (ACLR), with adolescents aged 13 to 17 making up approximately 23% of all ACLRs from 2002 to 2014 and annual ACLR rates increasing substantially in this age group over these years.[12] Unfortunately, insurance and socioeconomic status (SES) can affect ACLR timing; low SES and government-issued insurance were associated with longer times to orthopedic evaluation, imaging, surgery, and discharge.[13,14] Racially, approximately 50% of patients that undergo ACLR are White, followed in prevalence by Hispanic (27%), Asian (13%), and Black (7%) patients.[15,16]

With more than eight million students from a variety of racial, ethnic, and socioeconomic backgrounds participating in competitive athletics in high school alone[17] and many students participating in multiple sports in the same year, increased focus should be placed on addressing the effect of knee injury and recovery on this vulnerable population.

Although literature addressing the impact of knee injuries in adolescents is expansive, the analysis of the psychological aspects of injury and recovery in this population is limited. In the systematic review by Dietvorst and colleagues, they analyzed 26 studies regarding adolescent return-to-sport (RTS) following ACLR. However, the review only considers the strength tests, movement quality, and subjective outcome measures as factors of interest without mention of the significant psychological burden that pediatric patients experience following a knee injury.[18] Other reviews do not address these psychological aspects, specifically following a knee injury, or are not focused on the adolescent population.[19–24] This narrative review attempts to compile relevant studies addressing the psychological aspects of both the preoperative and postoperative recovery phases of adolescent knee injuries.

PSYCHOLOGICAL EFFECTS OF ADOLESCENT KNEE INJURY IN THE PREOPERATIVE PHASE

Adolescence is characterized by change, both physically—as adolescents' bodies grow and strengthen—and psychologically—as they encounter new situations in life and begin to mature emotionally and socially. As such, this population is especially vulnerable to substantial changes in their lives, such as a significant knee injury that impacts their day-to-day activities. The psychological effects of adolescent knee injuries can manifest themselves at various timepoints following the initial injury. Here, we first discuss the immediate effects of the knee injury on the young athlete, before any operative or therapeutic options are performed.

Post-Traumatic Stress Disorder

Studies have found that adolescents are at increased risk of developing symptoms of post-traumatic stress disorder (PTSD) following a traumatic injury, regardless of the athlete's current injury status.[25] Padaki and colleagues[26] specifically showed that at least three out of every four young athletes who have experienced an ACL rupture suffer from symptoms of avoidance (87.5%), intrusive thoughts (83.3%), or hyperarousal (75%). These traumatic experiences differentially affect the adolescent population; athletes aged 15 to 21 years old experienced more significant psychological trauma as compared with their younger counterparts, whereas female athletes were more severely affected than male athletes.[26]

The culpability and intentionality of an inflicted injury can also affect the intensity of PTSD symptoms experienced by the young athlete. Injuries resulting from an intent to do harm and those that are associated with rule violations or lack of punishment for the offending player have been associated with more significant psychological disturbance.[27,28] In a case report by McArdle, an 18-year-old athlete suffered a medial collateral ligament and ACL tear which he believed was caused intentionally and maliciously. Following the injury, he experienced significant symptoms consistent with PTSD, exacerbated by the blame and guilt he placed on the opposing player.[27] These studies suggest that the physical trauma associated with knee injuries can also bring psychological trauma to the young athlete.

Depression

Examining rates of major depressive disorder and its exacerbation by sport-related knee injury further illustrates the psychological sensitivity of the adolescent population. Studies from the late 1990s to 2000s show an average prevalence of depression of 2.2% in children aged 9 to 16 years old, increasing as the adolescent ages.[29–31] However, rates of depression have been increasing over the years,[32,33] with US Department of Health and Human Services reporting the prevalence of a depressive episode in adolescents in 2019 at 15.7%.[34] The new estimates, which are consistent with findings in older studies, report that 10.5% of 12- to 13-year-olds experience a depressive episode versus 20.1% of 16- to 17-year olds.[34] Female adolescents also experience depression at much higher rates than male adolescents at 23.0% versus 8.8%, respectively.[34] Costello and colleagues[29] further showed that those with depression are 28.9 times more likely to have comorbid anxiety as compared with those without depression. These studies describe the differential impact that depression has even within this young population, with older, female adolescents experiencing these symptoms at high rates.

Although some studies have shown that participation in athletics can be a protective factor against depression,[35,36] the possibility of sports-related knee injuries risks exacerbation of the already high level of depression in adolescents. In the study by Manuel and colleagues,[37] they report a postinjury prevalence of depression as high as 27% in its sample of young athletes; there was no significant decrease in these postinjury depressive symptoms until 6 to 12 weeks following the injury. Similarly, adult athletes have seven times higher depression scores following a knee injury versus a concussion[38] and exhibit greater rates of depression, higher levels of anxiety, and lower self-esteem up to two months following injury.[39]

These studies in the adolescent athlete, substantiated by similar findings in adults, show that depression—which is already on the rise in this young population—should be monitored closely following a knee injury in this population.

Athletic Identity

Athletic identity is the extent of self-identity derived from participation and success in sports. This begins developing in childhood and increases throughout adolescence into adulthood, with significant drops only being seen after an athlete ends their competitive career.[40] The level of athletic identity was also correlated with various postinjury psychological disturbances. Following a knee injury, adolescent athletes with increased levels of athletic identity experienced increased rates of depression,[37] greater risks of injury,[41] and trended toward experiencing more severe symptoms of PTSD.[26] Strong social support seemed to mitigate the severity of depressive symptoms in adolescents with elevated athletic identity,[37] whereas adult athletes experienced significant decreases in it over the two years following a knee injury, likely as a psychologically self-protective measure.[42] Further exploration should be done to investigate other psychologically mitigating factors in adolescent athletes with increased athletic identity.

Other Psychological Effects of Knee Injury

Knee injuries have specifically been shown to have overall detrimental effects on the mental health of the young athlete. Two studies by McGuine and colleagues showed decreases in the mental health component of the Health-Related Quality of Life survey in young female athletes following a variety of knee injuries, and particularly in ACL injuries, diseases causing anterior knee pain, patellar instability, and iliotibial band syndrome.[43,44] Boykin and colleagues also reported the negative impact of pediatric and adolescent knee injuries on the social and emotional health of this population, seeing significant impacts on expected categories such as physical function and pain but also on emotions, mental health, self-esteem, and the physical aspects of socializing. These findings were consistent between those treated nonoperatively, patients before surgery, and even postoperative patients.[45]

When analyzing adolescent versus adult athlete responses to an ACL injury, Udry and colleagues[46] found that the youth athletes reported higher levels of mood disturbance as compared with their older counterparts. However, the study also found that adolescents envisioned more benefits to surgical reconstruction and more frequently used processes of change in the preoperative period to help them cope with and adapt to their injury.[46] In this way, although adolescent athletes were more psychologically affected by their injury than adult athletes, they were also more cognitively flexible in order to adapt to their newly injured state.

Young athletes can have a variety of psychological responses to a knee injury that may negatively skew their postinjury experience. Following an injury, many athletes face high levels of fear avoidance (ie, engaging in behaviors to avoid pain- or fear-related emotions),[47] kinesiophobia (ie, the fear of movement due to worry of reinjury),[48] and pain catastrophizing (ie, magnification of thoughts about and the threat level of pain).[49] Selhorst and colleagues showed that in an adolescent population suffering from patellofemoral pain, those that scored higher in fear avoidance, kinesiophobia, and pain catastrophizing suffered from higher subjective pain and experienced lower function and strength from the injured knee.[50] These findings illustrate that regardless of the objective measures of knee injury severity, psychological factors can significantly impact the young athlete's experience of their injury. These responses to an injury can also feed back and affect the rate and efficacy of recovery in these adolescent athletes, as will be discussed in the following sections. In these ways, significant psychological disorders in adolescents may be further exacerbated by knee injuries that they experience.

PSYCHOLOGICAL ASPECTS ASSOCIATED WITH WORSE RECOVERY AFTER KNEE INJURY

The psychological impact of a knee injury in an adolescent can encompass nearly all aspects of an athlete's postinjury experience, from immediately following the injury to years into the postoperative recovery. In this section, we discuss how these psychological factors negatively affect the young athlete's postoperative recovery course and prevent a complete RTS.

Following a knee injury, kinesiophobia is one of the most common symptoms keeping adolescent athletes from full RTS. McCullough and colleagues[51] showed that approximately 50% of high school to collegiate athletes who underwent an ACLR and did not return to play their sport cited "fear of reinjury or further damage" as a contributing factor; this is further supported by similar rates of kinesiophobia (60%) in adult athletes following an ACL rupture.[26] Similarly, a 2021 study by Coronado and colleagues analyzed various aspects of recovery in athletes who were organized into subgroups based on preoperative fear of movement/reinjury, self-efficacy, and pain catastrophizing. Those who scored higher in kinesiophobia and pain catastrophizing and scored lower in self-efficacy had lower rates of RTS, sports participation, knee function, and quality of life at 6- or even 12-month postoperatively, depending on the measure.[52] Adolescents with higher levels of kinesiophobia also reported lower overall levels of activity as well as muscle and functional asymmetries at 1-year following ACLR.[53] Of significance, those who scored 19 or higher on the Tampa Scale of Kinesiophobia (TSK) were found to be 13 times more likely to reinjure the ipsilateral ACL within two years.[53]

A small cross-sectional study by DiSanti and colleagues[54] also identified psychological factors such as lack of motivation, uncertainty of recovery, and frustration with recovery speed as well as social aspects such as direct comparison to others and loss of athletic identity as other common barriers to RTS for adolescent athletes. During the recovery process, negative remarks by family, lack of attention by the care team, and the use of overly generalized—rather than individual- or sport-oriented—treatment approaches were reported to impede recovery.[54] These findings can help structure therapeutic regimens to focus on addressing these barriers to recovery.

In a retrospective study of adolescent athletes that had suffered a second ACL injury following an initial ACLR, the athletes reported increased fear of reinjury as well as frustration and hesitancy when playing sports due to concern for their knee.[55] In addition, over the 12 months following their operation, the reinjury group saw no change to their ACL Return to Sport After Injury (ACL-RSI) score, which measures psychological readiness to RTS in multiple domains.[55] This indicates that although the adolescent athletes may have been recovering physically after the reconstruction, they had psychologically plateaued, potentially increasing their risk for reinjury.

Sports-related coping strategies, measured by the Athletic Coping Skills Inventory-28 (ACSI-28), have also been correlated with response to recovery in adolescent athletes following ACLR. The ACSI-28 measures athlete's psychological skills in a variety of subscales, such as "peaking under pressure" and "coachability" among others; young athletes that had lower baseline scores correlated with slower rates of recovery.[56] Ellis and colleagues[56] found specific score-recovery associations, with those whose baseline ACSI-28 score was less than 58 experiencing recovery from ACLR that lasted two months longer than high ASCI-28 scorers. In particular, adolescents that scored lower in "coachability" and "coping with adversity" also experienced delayed levels and rates of recovery.[56] These findings reveal that athletes can be screened preoperatively to predict their response to treatment and can be targeted with more intensive therapy as needed.

Studies in adult athletes corroborate these results and offer guidance for future directions of exploration in the adolescent population. Following ACL injury and reconstruction, these older athletes showed similarly increased levels of kinesiophobia and functional deficits in both those who failed to RTS and those who reinjured their ACL.[57–60] Mood disturbances following ACLR also followed unique postoperative patterns, with negative mood peaks immediately following surgery and four to six months into recovery.[61] Frequent preoperative maladaptive beliefs (eg, pain catastrophizing, lower acceptance, neuroticism [ie, a predisposition to experiencing negative emotions and responding poorly to stress[62]]) were also associated with increased postoperative mood disturbances, high reported pain, and worse recovery.[63,64] Such patterns should be explored in adolescent athletes to proactively target the negative beliefs and mitigate the rates of these negative outcomes.

PSYCHOLOGICAL ASPECTS ASSOCIATED WITH IMPROVED RECOVERY AFTER KNEE INJURY

Equally important for therapeutic recommendations are the psychological factors associated with positive recovery outcomes following an adolescent knee injury. The study by DiSanti and colleagues identified some of these positive factors in young athletes: a good rapport and trusting relationship between patient and physician, an individualized therapeutic approach (eg, sport-specific exercises, considering patient motivators), and patient knowledge of the injury and recovery process.[54] Although these factors were not specifically analyzed for association with improved recovery time or knee function, they increased patient satisfaction and outlook during the recovery process that has been shown to correlate with full RTS, improved knee function, and improved knee-related quality of life in adult athletes.[65,66]

Following a significant knee injury, athletes can develop several coping strategies to help mitigate psychological disturbances and to improve their own outlook on recovery. Such strategies include self-distraction, venting, use of emotional or instrumental support, positive reframing, and acceptance.[67] Everhart and colleagues found that positive reframing—thinking about a negative situation or outcome with a more optimistic lens—was the only coping strategy associated with increased rates of RTS, decreased levels of kinesiophobia, and improved overall postoperative satisfaction in athletes under 20 year old who were recovering from a sports-related knee injury.[67] However, the study also found that this same age group used positive reframing least frequently compared with the other age groups.[67] These findings reveal a disconnect between the recovery strategies used by the young athlete and those that are most effective for them, which can be easily addressed by focusing therapeutic efforts on encouraging this strategy's use in this population.

Other psychological factors can also contribute to an improved recovery course. Adolescent athletes that scored higher in the "concentration" and "peaking under pressure" subscales of the ACSI-28 achieved faster recovery times than their counterparts with low scores in these categories.[56] In adult athletes, psychological factors such as high internal locus of control (ie, the belief that health and outcomes are patient-controlled rather than driven by uncontrollable external factors), high levels of self-efficacy (ie, the belief in one's ability to succeed), and greater preoperative confidence and readiness for eventual RTS were associated with greater knee function, higher rates of full RTS, decreased pain, and greater knee-related quality of life.[65,66,68–72] These findings can serve as directions for future investigation to address optimizing recovery through psychological factors in adolescent athletes. By focusing efforts on maximizing these measures and minimizing the previously-discussed negative influences on recovery, young athletes can help lessen the psychological distress associated with their injury.

TREATMENT RECOMMENDATIONS

Although most rehabilitation programs and treatments focus on the physical recovery of the knee, this review has shown that more focus should be placed on the psychological aspects of knee injury in the adolescent population.

Before the initiation of any treatment or therapeutic modality, injured young athletes can be screened with various preoperative measures that quantify their risk of psychological disturbance due to the injury, their predicted rate and response of recovery, and their likelihood to have a full RTS, among others. For example, athletes with an ACSI-28 score less than 58,[56] an ACL-RSI score less than 56,[71] a TSK score of 17 or higher,[53] or patients with high levels of fear avoidance,[52] kinesiophobia,[50,57,60] or pain catastrophizing[50,63] have been shown to have poorer recovery outcomes and thus can be targeted with more intensive therapeutic strategies. Similar strategies can be initiated for those with low health locus of control,[69,70,72] low levels of self-efficacy,[52] strong athletic identity,[42,63] or personality traits of neuroticism.[64] Intra-recovery measures can also indicate the future success of recovery, such as an unchanged ACL-RSI score at 12-month postoperatively[55] as well as the measurement of the aforementioned psychological variables at weeks or even months postoperatively.[70] In addition, adolescents who have injured their ACL that score 19 or higher on the TSK should be informed of their significantly higher risk of reinjury and can be enrolled in therapeutic regimens that focus on addressing feelings of kinesiophobia.[53]

Selhorst and colleagues showed that in adolescents suffering from patellofemoral pain, psychologically informed videos reduced their scores in fear avoidance, kinesiophobia, and pain catastrophizing.[73,74] As described previously, these measures of an adolescent patient's psychological state of mind regarding their injury can both predict likelihood of RTS and can even negatively impact the recovery itself. As such, these psychologically informed videos may have some efficacy in targeting maladaptive psychological beliefs and in improving recovery in this adolescent population. Similarly, in adult athletes, guided imagery sessions and therapy focused on relaxation techniques helped improve knee strength, decrease knee laxity, and reduce injury-related anxiety and pain.[75,76] Comparable therapeutic regimens should be explored in the adolescent population.

Gender-specific recovery themes also emerged in Lisee and colleagues' study of high school athletes following ACLR. During recovery, male athletes focused their motivations on the physical limitations of their injury, whereas the female athletes' motivational focus was on staying in shape.[77] Male adolescent athletes were also frustrated with the speed and length of recovery, used positive reinforcement, reported high internal locus of control, and feared sports-specific movements causing reinjury.[77] Conversely, young female athletes monitored their emotions more closely throughout recovery, used social support more frequently, maintained a balance of internal and external loci of control, and feared activities of daily living more than sports-specific fears.[77] With these responses to knee injury and gender-specific fears and motivations in mind, care teams can initially target these beliefs with specific cognitive-behavioral, motivational, and physical therapy techniques. However, care should be taken not to overgeneralize the beliefs of any athlete and to instead provide individualized therapy to achieve optimal recovery results.

Otsuki and colleagues further add to the gender-specific treatment recommendations, showing that by enrolling prepubertal females in injury prevention programs, movement patterns associated with ACL injury could be decreased.[78] This finding is especially important because of the disproportionate rates of knee injury in young female athletes[7] and the overall negative effects of knee injury on an adolescent's psychology which can be avoided. Otsuki and colleagues' findings suggest that young females who are found to be at increased risk of experiencing significant psychological disturbances from knee injury could also be targeted with injury prevention programs to prophylactically reduce the risk of developing a knee injury.

Olmedilla-Zafra and colleagues showed that adolescent athletes who participate in a psychologically based therapy program that focused on learning how to cope with and react to stressful situations showed significant decreases in sports injuries.[79] Similar to Otsuki and colleagues, this program can be targeted toward youths who are identified to be at higher risk of psychological distress following knee injury; this program can help to reduce injury rates and limit the psychological impact a knee injury can have on this at-risk population.

As discussed in this review, many surveys and questionnaires exist to help screen for adolescents prone to adverse psychological reactions following knee injury **(Table 1)**. With this in mind, orthopedic surgeons can be more cognizant of the mood and psychological status of their young patients, grossly gauging their affect, engagement with therapy, and overall satisfaction with recovery during follow-up appointments. If young athletes seem to be struggling with rehabilitation, they can potentially be referred to a trained psychological care team; here, the formal scales analyzing self-efficacy, kinesiophobia, and fear avoidance can be used to identify those whose recovery may benefit from individualized psychologically focused rehabilitation as an adjunct to the standard treatment options provided. These treatment recommendations are summarized in **Box 1**.

Table 1	
Surveys used to analyze psychological and functional measures following a knee injury	
Survey Name	**Measure of Interest**
Tampa Scale of Kinesiophobia	Kinesiophobia, fear of movement due to worry of reinjury[48]
Knee Injury and Osteoarthritis Outcome Score	Knee-related function[80]
Pain Catastrophizing Score	Pain catastrophizing, magnification of thoughts about and perceived threat level of pain[49]
Knee Self-Efficacy Scale	Subjective perception of ability to participate in physical activity at level before anterior cruciate ligament (ACL) injury[81]
Health-Related Quality of Life	Quality of life with regard to health[82]
ACL Return to Sport After Injury	Psychological readiness to return-to-sport after ACL injury and reconstruction[83]
International Knee Documentation Committee	Subjective knee function[84]
Profile of Mood States	Mood/emotional response with a variety of subscales (eg, tension, depression, anger, fatigue)[85]
Tegner Activity Scale	Level of activity (eg, to quantify patient baseline before knee injury)[86]
Medical Outcomes Study 36-Item Short-Form Health Survey	General health[87]
Athletic Coping Skills Inventory-28	Athletic psychological skills with subscales in a variety of domains (eg, coachability, concentration, and peaking under pressure)[88]

Box 1
Treatment recommendations

Treatment approaches can look to address the following:

- Screen for:
  - Athletic Coping Skills Inventory-28 score less than 58[56]
  - Anterior cruciate ligament Return to Sport After Injury (ACL-RSI) score less than 56[71]
  - Tampa Scale of Kinesiophobia score $\geq$ 17 (or $\geq$ 19 for risk of reinjury to ACL)[53]
  - High levels of fear avoidance,[52] kinesiophobia,[50,57,60] or pain catastrophizing[50,63]
  - Low health locus of control[69,70,72]
  - Low self-efficacy[52]
  - High athletic identity[42,63]
  - Personality traits of neuroticism[64]
  - Poor perception of rehabilitation[65,66]

- If screen positive:
  - More aggressive/frequent rehabilitation programs with focus on psychological aspects in these patients
    - Cognitive-behavioral-based physical therapy to enhance return-to-sport (RTS)[52]
  - Use psychologically informed videos in this population[73,74]
  - Continue to monitor and track maladaptive psychological scores (eg, unchanging ACL-RSI[53]) during recovery to predict outcomes

- Encourage self-efficacy and maintenance of athletic identity while beneficial

- Encourage positive recovery factors[54]
  - Thoroughly discuss the injury with patient
  - Develop trusting relationships and rapport
  - Individualize rehabilitation approach
    - Use sport-specific exercises
    - Incorporate patient-reported motivators

- Avoid negative recovery factors[54]
  - Instruct parents to avoid over-sympathy and encourage (rather than shy away from) utilization of injured knee and full RTS
  - Do not compare injured athletes to others
  - Avoid overly-generalized therapeutic approaches

- Assess for neurotic personality traits and gender-specific differences in fears and motivators to target-specific populations more aggressively

---

SUMMARY

Adolescents are a sensitive population who can experience significant psychological disturbances following a knee injury, and much of the current literature fails to adequately address the mental health aspects of this subset of the population. This narrative review aimed to summarize the psychological effects of a knee injury throughout its time course, from preinjury screening considerations to postoperative recovery recommendations. Recovery from a knee injury in any population, but especially in adolescents, is a multifaceted process that involves numerous objective and subjective measures to best optimize its rate and efficacy. Using findings from the current literature, therapeutic recommendations were made which aim to mitigate post-injury psychological disturbances, address potential causes of negative recovery outcomes, and bolster qualities that optimize recovery. We hope these findings and recommendations can guide the future study of knee injury in this population and help these young athletes recover from their injury so they can fearlessly return to playing the sports they love.

DISCLOSURE

M.D. Milewski—Elsevier, Inc. Editorial Royalties.

REFERENCES

1. Gage BE, McIlvain NM, Collins CL, et al. Epidemiology of 6.6 million knee injuries presenting to united states emergency departments from 1999 through 2008. Acad Emerg Med 2012;19(4):378–85.
2. Louw QA, Manilall J, Grimmer KA. Epidemiology of knee injuries among adolescents: A systematic review. Br J Sports Med 2008;42(1):2–10.
3. Jones D, Louw Q, Grimmer K. Recreational and sporting injury to the adolescent knee and ankle: Prevalence and causes. Aust J Physiother 2000;46(3):179–88.
4. Powell JW, Barber-Foss KD. Injury patterns in selected high school sports: A review of the 1995-1997 seasons. J Athl Train 1999;34(3):277–84.
5. Saes MO, Soares MCF. Knee pain in adolescents: Prevalence, risk factors, and functional impairment. Braz J Phys Ther 2017;21(1):7–14.
6. Shaw L, Finch CF. Trends in pediatric and adolescent anterior cruciate ligament injuries in Victoria, Australia 2005-2015. Int J Environ Res Public Health 2017; 14(6). https://doi.org/10.3390/ijerph14060599.
7. Bram JT, Magee LC, Mehta NN, et al. Anterior cruciate ligament injury incidence in adolescent athletes: A systematic review and meta-analysis. Am J Sports Med 2021;49(7):1962–72.
8. Dekker TJ, Godin JA, Dale KM, et al. Return to sport after pediatric anterior cruciate ligament reconstruction and its effect on subsequent anterior cruciate ligament injury. J Bone Joint Surg Am 2017;99(11):897–904.
9. Post EG, Trigsted SM, Riekena JW, et al. The association of sport specialization and training volume with injury history in youth athletes. Am J Sports Med 2017; 45(6):1405–12.
10. Post EG, Bell DR, Trigsted SM, et al. Association of competition volume, club sports, and sport specialization with sex and lower extremity injury history in high school athletes. Sports Health 2017;9(6):518–23.
11. Hall R, Barber Foss K, Hewett TE, et al. Sport specialization's association with an increased risk of developing anterior knee pain in adolescent female athletes. J Sport Rehabil 2015;24(1):31–5.
12. Herzog MM, Marshall SW, Lund JL, et al. Trends in incidence of ACL reconstruction and concomitant procedures among commercially insured individuals in the united states, 2002-2014. Sports Health 2018;10(6):523–31.
13. Patel AR, Sarkisova N, Smith R, et al. Socioeconomic status impacts outcomes following pediatric anterior cruciate ligament reconstruction. Medicine (Baltimore) 2019;98(17):e15361.
14. Leveille LA, Ladner TV, Sidhu P, et al. Delay in diagnosis and management of adolescent anterior cruciate ligament injuries in a publicly funded healthcare system. Orthop J Sports Med 2020;8(4). 2325967120S00229. Available at: https://www.ncbi.nlm.nih.gov/pmc/articles/PMC7225814/ https://www.ncbi.nlm.nih.gov/pmc/articles/PMC7225814/.
15. Navarro RA, Prentice HA, Inacio MCS, et al. The association between race/ethnicity and revision following ACL reconstruction in a universally insured cohort. J Bone Joint Surg Am 2019;101(17). Available at: https://journals.lww.com/jbjsjournal/subjects/sportsmedicine/Fulltext/2019/09040/The_Association_Between_Race_Ethnicity_and.4.aspx.

16. Navarro RA, Inacio MC, Maletis GB. Does racial variation influence preoperative characteristics and intraoperative findings in patients undergoing anterior cruciate ligament reconstruction? Am J Sports Med 2015;43(12):2959–65.

17. Niehoff KL. 2021-2022 NFHS Handbook. National Federation of State High School Associations; 2021. p. 56. https://www.nfhs.org/media/4119446/2021-22-nfhs-handbook-10_21.pdf.

18. Dietvorst M, Brzoskowski MH, van der Steen M, et al. Limited evidence for return to sport testing after ACL reconstruction in children and adolescents under 16 years: A scoping review. J Exp Orthop 2020;7(1):83–8.

19. Truong LK, Mosewich AD, Holt CJ, et al. Psychological, social and contextual factors across recovery stages following a sport-related knee injury: A scoping review. Br J Sports Med 2020;54(19):1149–56.

20. Ardern CL, Kvist J, Webster KE. Psychological aspects of anterior cruciate ligament injuries. Oper Tech Sports Med 2016;24(1):77–83. Available at: https://www.sciencedirect.com/science/article/pii/S1060187215001161.

21. Podlog L, Eklund RC. The psychosocial aspects of a return to sport following serious injury: A review of the literature from a self-determination perspective. Psychol Sport Exerc 2007;8(4):535–66. Available at: https://www.sciencedirect.com/science/article/pii/S1469029206000902.

22. Christino MA, Fantry AJ, Vopat BG. Psychological aspects of recovery following anterior cruciate ligament reconstruction. J Am Acad Orthop Surg 2015;23(8):501–9.

23. Daley MM, Griffith K, Milewski MD, et al. The mental side of the injured athlete. J Am Acad Orthop Surg 2021;29(12). Available at: https://journals.lww.com/jaaos/Fulltext/2021/06150/The_Mental_Side_of_the_Injured_Athlete.1.aspx.

24. Haraldsdottir K, Watson AM. Psychosocial impacts of sports-related injuries in adolescent athletes. Curr Sports Med Rep 2021;20(2):104–8.

25. Newcomer RR, Perna FM. Features of posttraumatic distress among adolescent athletes. J Athl Train 2003;38(2):163–6.

26. Padaki AS, Noticewala MS, Levine WN, et al. Prevalence of posttraumatic stress disorder symptoms among young athletes after anterior cruciate ligament rupture. Orthop J Sports Med 2018;6(7). 2325967118787159.

27. McArdle S. Psychological rehabilitation from anterior cruciate ligament-medial collateral ligament reconstructive surgery: A case study. Sports Health 2010; 2(1):73–7.

28. Heil J. The injured athlete. In: Hanin YL, editor. Emotions in sport. Champaign (IL): Human Kinetics; 2000. p. 245–67.

29. Costello EJ, Mustillo S, Erkanli A, et al. Prevalence and development of psychiatric disorders in childhood and adolescence. Arch Gen Psychiatry 2003;60(8): 837–44.

30. Merikangas KR, Nakamura EF, Kessler RC. Epidemiology of mental disorders in children and adolescents. Dialogues Clin Neurosci 2009;11(1):7–20.

31. Lewinsohn PM, Rohde P, Seeley JR. Major depressive disorder in older adolescents: Prevalence, risk factors, and clinical implications. Clin Psychol Rev 1998;18(7):765–94.

32. Bitsko RH, Holbrook JR, Ghandour RM, et al. Epidemiology and impact of health care provider-diagnosed anxiety and depression among US children. J Dev Behav Pediatr 2018;39(5):395–403.

33. Mojtabai R, Olfson M, Han B. National trends in the prevalence and treatment of depression in adolescents and young adults. Pediatrics 2016;138(6):e20161878.

34. Substance Abuse and Mental Health Services Administration. Key substance use and mental health indicators in the united states: Results from the 2019 national survey on drug use and health Center for Behavioral Health Statistics and Quality, Substance Abuse and Mental Health Services Administration. 2020.
35. Choi WS, Patten CA, Gillin JC, et al. Cigarette smoking predicts development of depressive symptoms among U.S. adolescents. Ann Behav Med 1997;19(1):42–50.
36. Snyder AR, Martinez JC, Bay RC, et al. Health-related quality of life differs between adolescent athletes and adolescent nonathletes. J Sport Rehab 2010;19(3):237–48. Available at: https://journals.humankinetics.com/view/journals/jsr/19/3/article-p237.xml.
37. Manuel JC, Shilt JS, Curl WW, et al. Coping with sports injuries: An examination of the adolescent athlete. J Adolesc Health 2002;31(5):391–3. Available at: https://www.sciencedirect.com/science/article/pii/S1054139X02004007.
38. Mainwaring LM, Hutchison M, Bisschop SM, et al. Emotional response to sport concussion compared to ACL injury. Brain Inj 2010;24(4):589–97.
39. Leddy MH, Lambert MJ, Ogles BM. Psychological consequences of athletic injury among high-level competitors. Res Q Exerc Sport 1994;65(4):347–54.
40. Houle JLW, Brewer BW, Kluck AS. Developmental trends in athletic identity: A two-part retrospective study. J Sport Behav 2010;33(2):146–59.
41. McKay C, Campbell T, Meeuwisse W, et al. The role of psychosocial risk factors for injury in elite youth ice hockey. Clin J Sport Med 2013;23(3):216–21. https://doi.org/10.1097/JSM.0b013e31826a86c9 [doi].
42. Brewer BW, Cornelius AE. Self-protective changes in athletic identity following anterior cruciate ligament reconstruction. Psychol Sport Exerc 2010;11(1):1–5. Available at: https://pubmed.ncbi.nlm.nih.gov/20161402 https://www.ncbi.nlm.nih.gov/pmc/articles/PMC2783627/.
43. McGuine TA, Winterstein AP, Carr K, et al. Changes in health-related quality of life and knee function after knee injury in young female athletes. Orthop J Sports Med 2014;2(4). 2325967114530988.
44. McGuine TA, Winterstein A, Carr K, et al. Changes in self-reported knee function and health-related quality of life after knee injury in female athletes. Clin J Sport Med 2012;22(4):334–40.
45. Boykin RE, McFeely ED, Shearer D, et al. Correlation between the child health questionnaire and the international knee documentation committee score in pediatric and adolescent patients with an anterior cruciate ligament tear. J Pediatr Orthop 2013;33(2):216–20.
46. Udry E, Donald Shelbourne K, Gray T. Psychological readiness for anterior cruciate ligament surgery: Describing and comparing the adolescent and adult experiences. J athletic Train 2003;38(2):167–71. Available at: https://pubmed.ncbi.nlm.nih.gov/12937530 https://www.ncbi.nlm.nih.gov/pmc/articles/PMC164908/.
47. Fischerauer SF, Talaei-Khoei M, Bexkens R, et al. What is the relationship of fear avoidance to physical function and pain intensity in injured athletes? Clin Orthop 2018;476(4):754–63. Available at: https://pubmed.ncbi.nlm.nih.gov/29480885 https://www.ncbi.nlm.nih.gov/pmc/articles/PMC6260093/.
48. Larsson C, Ekvall Hansson E, Sundquist K, et al. Kinesiophobia and its relation to pain characteristics and cognitive affective variables in older adults with chronic pain. BMC Geriatr 2016;16:128. https://pubmed.ncbi.nlm.nih.gov/27387557. https://www.ncbi.nlm.nih.gov/pmc/articles/PMC4936054/.
49. Quartana PJ, Campbell CM, Edwards RR. Pain catastrophizing: A critical review. Expert Rev Neurother 2009;9(5):745–58. Available at: https://pubmed.ncbi.nlm.

nih.gov/19402782 https://www.ncbi.nlm.nih.gov/pmc/articles/PMC2696024/. doi: 10.1586/ern.09.34.

50. Selhorst M, Fernandez-Fernandez A, Schmitt L, et al. Adolescent psychological beliefs, but not parent beliefs, associated with pain and function in adolescents with patellofemoral pain. Phys Ther Sport 2020;45:155–60.

51. McCullough KA, Phelps KD, Spindler KP, et al. Return to high school- and college-level football after anterior cruciate ligament reconstruction: A multicenter orthopaedic outcomes network (MOON) cohort study. Am J Sports Med 2012; 40(11):2523–9.

52. Coronado RA, Bley JA, Huston LJ, et al. Composite psychosocial risk based on the fear avoidance model in patients undergoing anterior cruciate ligament reconstruction: Cluster-based analysis. Phys Ther Sport 2021;50:217–25.

53. Paterno MV, Flynn K, Thomas S, et al. Self-reported fear predicts functional performance and second ACL injury after ACL reconstruction and return to sport: A pilot study. Sports Health 2018;10(3):228–33.

54. DiSanti J, Lisee C, Erickson K, et al. Perceptions of rehabilitation and return to sport among high school athletes with anterior cruciate ligament reconstruction: A qualitative research study. J Orthop Sports Phys Ther 2018;48(12):951–9.

55. McPherson AL, Feller JA, Hewett TE, et al. Smaller change in psychological readiness to return to sport is associated with second anterior cruciate ligament injury among younger patients. Am J Sports Med 2019;47(5):1209–15.

56. Ellis HB, Sabatino M, Nwelue E, et al. The use of psychological patient reported outcome measures to identify adolescent athletes at risk for prolonged recovery following an ACL reconstruction. J Pediatr Orthop 2020;40(9):e844–52.

57. Tagesson S, Kvist J. Greater fear of re-injury and increased tibial translation in patients who later sustain an ACL graft rupture or a contralateral ACL rupture: A pilot study. J Sports Sci 2016;34(2):125–32.

58. Flanigan DC, Everhart JS, Pedroza A, et al. Fear of reinjury (kinesiophobia) and persistent knee symptoms are common factors for lack of return to sport after anterior cruciate ligament reconstruction. Arthroscopy 2013;29(8):1322–9.

59. Kvist J, Ek A, Sporrstedt K, et al. Fear of re-injury: A hindrance for returning to sports after anterior cruciate ligament reconstruction. Knee Surg Sports Traumatol Arthrosc 2005;13(5):393–7.

60. Tajdini H, Letafatkar A, Brewer BW, et al. Association between kinesiophobia and gait asymmetry after ACL reconstruction: Implications for prevention of reinjury. Int J Environ Res Public Health 2021;18(6):3264.

61. Morrey MA, Stuart MJ, Smith AM, et al. A longitudinal examination of athletes' emotional and cognitive responses to anterior cruciate ligament injury. Clin J Sport Med 1999;9(2):63–9.

62. Widiger TA, Oltmanns JR. Neuroticism is a fundamental domain of personality with enormous public health implications. World Psychiatry 2017;16(2):144–5.

63. Baranoff J, Hanrahan SJ, Connor JP. The roles of acceptance and catastrophizing in rehabilitation following anterior cruciate ligament reconstruction. J Sci Med Sport 2015;18(3):250–4.

64. Shapiro JL, Brewer BW, Cornelius AE, et al. Patterns of emotional response to ACL reconstruction surgery. J Clin Sport Psychol 2017;11(3):169–80.

65. Thomeé P, Währborg P, Börjesson M, et al. Self-efficacy of knee function as a preoperative predictor of outcome 1 year after anterior cruciate ligament reconstruction. Knee Surg Sports Traumatol Arthrosc 2008;16(2):118–27.

66. Langford JL, Webster KE, Feller JA. A prospective longitudinal study to assess psychological changes following anterior cruciate ligament reconstruction surgery. Br J Sports Med 2009;43(5):377–81.

67. Everhart JS, DiBartola AC, Blough C, et al. Positive reframing: An important but underutilized coping strategy in youth athletes undergoing sports-related knee surgery. J Athl Train 2021. https://doi.org/10.4085/1062-6050-0618.20.

68. Chmielewski TL, Zeppieri G Jr, Lentz TA, et al. Longitudinal changes in psychosocial factors and their association with knee pain and function after anterior cruciate ligament reconstruction. Phys Ther 2011;91(9):1355–66.

69. Nyland J, Cottrell B, Harreld K, et al. Self-reported outcomes after anterior cruciate ligament reconstruction: An internal health locus of control score comparison. Arthroscopy 2006;22(11):1225–32.

70. Ardern CL, Taylor NF, Feller JA, et al. Psychological responses matter in returning to preinjury level of sport after anterior cruciate ligament reconstruction surgery. Am J Sports Med 2013;41(7):1549–58.

71. Ohji S, Aizawa J, Hirohata K, et al. The psychological readiness to return to sports of patients with anterior cruciate ligament reconstruction preoperatively and 6 months postoperatively. Phys Ther Sport 2021;50:114–20.

72. Christino MA, Fleming BC, Machan JT, et al. Psychological factors associated with anterior cruciate ligament reconstruction recovery. Orthop J Sports Med 2016;4(3). 2325967116638341.

73. Selhorst M, Hoehn J, Degenhart T, et al. Psychologically-informed video reduces maladaptive beliefs in adolescents with patellofemoral pain. Phys Ther Sport 2020;41:23–8.

74. Selhorst M, Fernandez-Fernandez A, Schmitt L, et al. Effect of a psychologically informed intervention to treat adolescents with patellofemoral pain: A randomized controlled trial. Arch Phys Med Rehabil 2021;102(7):1267–73.

75. Maddison R, Prapavessis H, Clatworthy M, et al. Guided imagery to improve functional outcomes post-anterior cruciate ligament repair: Randomized-controlled pilot trial. Scand J Med Sci Sports 2012;22(6):816–21.

76. Cupal DD, Brewer BW. Effects of relaxation and guided imagery on knee strength, reinjury anxiety, and pain following anterior cruciate ligament reconstruction. Rehabil Psychol 2001;46(1):28–43.

77. Lisee CM, DiSanti JS, Chan M, et al. Gender differences in psychological responses to recovery after anterior cruciate ligament reconstruction before return to sport. J Athl Train 2020;55(10):1098–105.

78. Otsuki R, Benoit D, Hirose N, et al. Effects of an injury prevention program on anterior cruciate ligament injury risk factors in adolescent females at different stages of maturation. J Sports Sci Med 2021;20(2):365–72.

79. Olmedilla-Zafra A, Rubio VJ, Ortega E, et al. Effectiveness of a stress management pilot program aimed at reducing the incidence of sports injuries in young football (soccer) players. Phys Ther Sport 2017;24:53–9.

80. Roos EM, Lohmander LS. The knee injury and osteoarthritis outcome score (KOOS): From joint injury to osteoarthritis. Health Qual Life Outcomes 2003;1:64.

81. Thomeé P, Währborg P, Börjesson M, et al. A new instrument for measuring self-efficacy in patients with an anterior cruciate ligament injury. Scand J Med Sci Sports 2006;16(3):181–7.

82. Filbay SR, Ackerman IN, Russell TG, et al. Health-related quality of life after anterior cruciate ligament reconstruction: A systematic review. Am J Sports Med 2014;42(5):1247–55.

83. Webster KE, Feller JA, Lambros C. Development and preliminary validation of a scale to measure the psychological impact of returning to sport following anterior cruciate ligament reconstruction surgery. Phys Ther Sport 2008;9(1):9–15. Available at: https://www.sciencedirect.com/science/article/pii/S1466853X07000971.
84. Greco NJ, Anderson AF, Mann BJ, et al. Responsiveness of the international knee documentation committee subjective knee form in comparison to the western ontario and McMaster universities osteoarthritis index, modified cincinnati knee rating system, and short form 36 in patients with focal articular cartilage defects. Am J Sports Med 2010;38(5):891–902.
85. Grove JR, Prapavessis H. Preliminary evidence for the reliability and validity of an abbreviated profile of mood states. Int J Sport Psychol 1992;23(2):93–109.
86. Briggs KK, Lysholm J, Tegner Y, et al. The reliability, validity, and responsiveness of the lysholm score and tegner activity scale for anterior cruciate ligament injuries of the knee: 25 years later. Am J Sports Med 2009;37(5):890–7.
87. Stewart AL, Hays RD, Ware JE Jr. The MOS short-form general health survey. reliability and validity in a patient population. Med Care 1988;26(7):724–35.
88. Smith RE, Schutz RW, Smoll FL, et al. Development and validation of a multidimensional measure of sport-specific psychological skills: The athletic coping skills inventory-28. J Sport Exerc Psychol 1995;17(4):379–98. Available at: https://journals.humankinetics.com/view/journals/jsep/17/4/article-p379.xml.

Multiligament Knee Injuries in Young Athletes

Crystal A. Perkins, MD*, Samuel Clifton Willimon, MD

KEYWORDS

- Multiligament knee injury • Dislocation • Adolescent • Reconstruction • Arthroscopy
- ACL • PCL • FCL

KEY POINTS

- Evaluation and management of multiligament knee injuries (MLKI) require a comprehensive understanding of anatomy and biomechanics.
- In addition to a thorough history and physical examination, stress radiographs provide a reliable method to assess knee stability.
- Single-stage anatomic reconstruction techniques should be performed, as they restore native knee kinematics and enable early knee range of motion and superior outcomes.

Knee dislocations and multiligament knee injuries (MLKI) are potentially devastating injuries that occur most commonly as a result of sports or high energy trauma. As compared with isolated anterior cruciate ligament (ACL) injuries, MLKI account for a smaller proportion of acute knee injuries. Knee dislocations may spontaneously reduce before evaluation and present only with a large effusion and multidirectional instability. Recognition and management of these injuries are important, as failure to recognize and treat concomitant injuries at the time of ACL reconstruction has been demonstrated to increase the risk of subsequent revision surgery.[1,2]

ANATOMY

The medial and lateral knee is composed of numerous static and dynamic stabilizers (**Figs. 1** and **2**) and a thorough understanding of the anatomy, function, and relationship of these structures is critical for the assessment and management of MLKI. The fibular collateral ligament (FCL) is the primary static stabilizer to varus stress of the knee, most important from 0° to 30° of knee flexion, and a secondary restraint against tibial internal and external rotation.[3] The FCL originates 1.4 mm proximal and 3.1 mm posterior to the lateral epicondyle, extends a length of 70 mm, and inserts on the

Children's Orthopedics and Sports Medicine, Children's Healthcare of Atlanta, 5445 Meridian Mark Road, Suite 250, Atlanta, GA 30342, USA
* Corresponding author.
E-mail address: crystalperkins11@gmail.com
Twitter: @crystal_perkins (C.A.P.); @cliffwillimonMD (S.C.W.)

Clin Sports Med 41 (2022) 611–625
https://doi.org/10.1016/j.csm.2022.05.004
0278-5919/22/© 2022 Elsevier Inc. All rights reserved.

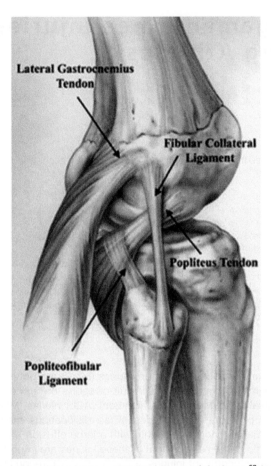

Fig. 1. The primary posterolateral corner static stabilizers of the knee.[69] (*From* LaPrade RF, Ly TV, Wentorf FA, Engebretsen L. The posterolateral attachments of the knee: a qualitative and quantitative morphologic analysis of the fibular collateral ligament, popliteus tendon, popliteofibular ligament, and lateral gastrocnemius tendon. Am J Sports Med 2003;31:854-60.)

lateral aspect of the fibular head. The popliteus is the primary lateral knee restraint against tibial external rotation and provides additional resistance against internal rotation, varus angulation, and anterior translation.[4] It attaches to the anterior fifth of the popliteus sulcus of the femur (18.5 mm from the FCL femoral origin) and extends distally to the musculotendinous junction.[4,5] The popliteofibular ligament courses lateral and distal from the musculotendinous junction to attach on the posteromedial aspect of the fibular styloid, serving as a secondary restraint to external rotation at 30° and 60° and varus at 30°.[6] The mid-third lateral capsular ligament, or anterolateral ligament, is a thickening of the lateral capsule of the knee. It includes meniscofemoral and mensicotibial components and is an important secondary stabilizer to varus stress.[4] The biceps femoris consists of a long and short head. The long head attaches to the fibula via a direct and anterior arm and the FCL-biceps bursa is formed between these 2 arms and is the interval through which the distal FCL attachment is identified at the time of FCL reconstruction.[7] The numerous attachments of the biceps femoris contribute to the dynamic stability of the posterolateral knee. The iliotibial band is a

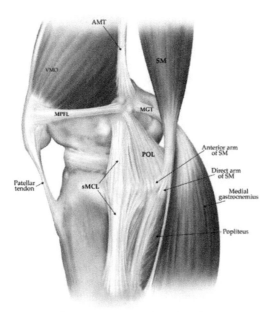

Fig. 2. Medial knee structures.[9] AMT, adductor magnus tendon; MGT, medial gastrocnemius tendon; MPFL, medial patellofemoral ligament; POL, posterior oblique ligament; SM, semimembranosus muscle; sMCL, superficial medial collateral ligament; VMO, vastus medialis obliquus. (*From* LaPrade RF, Engebretsen AH, Ly TV, Johansen S, Wentorf FA, Engebretsen L. The anatomy of the medial part of the knee. J Bone Joint Surg Am 2007;89:2000-10.)

broad fascial band extending from the pelvis to the anterolateral tibia at Gerdy's tubercle. The deep (Kaplan) fibers of the iliotibial band have strong osseous attachments to the distal femur and contribute to rotational knee stability.[8]

Three bony prominences serve as key anatomic landmarks on the medial femur: the medial epicondyle, adductor tubercle (proximal and posterior to the medial epicondyle), and the gastrocnemius tubercle (distal and posterior to the adductor tubercle).[9] The superficial medial collateral ligament (sMCL), the primary restraint to valgus stress and external rotation at 30° and internal rotation at all flexion angles, originates in a depression on the distal femur 3.2 mm proximal and 4.8 mm posterior to the medial epicondyle. Distally it has 2 distinct tibial attachments, the first located 1.2 cm distal to the joint line and the second 6.1 cm distal to the joint line and just anterior to the posteromedial crest of the tibia. The proximal tibial insertion primarily resists valgus stress, while the distal tibial attachment limits the external rotation of the knee at 30° of flexion. Because of their distinct functions, both insertions should be reproduced at the time of sMCL reconstruction. The deep medial collateral ligament is a thickening of the middle-third medial capsular ligament and consists of meniscofemoral and meniscotibial components, both acting to resist valgus gapping. The posterior oblique ligament consists of 3 fascial attachments extending from the semimembranosus tendon. The central arm is the largest and most functionally important of these and inserts 1.4 mm distal and 2.9 mm anterior to the medial gastrocnemius tubercle.

The posterior cruciate ligament (PCL) extends from the superolateral aspect of the medial femoral condyle adjacent to the articular cartilage margin to the depression on the posterior aspect of the proximal tibia. It is composed of 2 bundles—the larger anterolateral and smaller posteromedial—named based on their femoral attachment. The anterolateral bundle is the primary restraint to posterior translation with greatest tension at 90° of flexion. The posteromedial bundle provides maximal stability in full extension and is a secondary restraint to knee rotation. The unique functions of each bundle explain the biomechanical superiority of double-bundle PCL reconstruction as compared with the single-bundle technique.[10,11]

INJURY PATTERNS

The direction of force and position of the limb at the time of knee injury determines the ligaments injured. The classification of knee dislocations is based on the position of the tibia relative to the femur at the time of dislocation. The classification and the respective multiligamentous injuries were developed by Schenck and modified by Wascher (**Table 1**).[12]

ASSOCIATED INJURIES

The popliteal artery is tethered within the adductor hiatus proximal to the knee and in the arch of the soleus distally and is at risk for injury with knee dislocations. The reported incidence of popliteal artery injury in association with these injuries is 2% to 30%,[13–15] with the highest incidence among posterior dislocations and posterolateral corner (PLC) injuries. All patients with a knee dislocation and MLKI should have an examination of the peripheral pulses, and for those presenting acutely with a dislocation, the ankle-brachial index (ABI) was calculated. Strong collateral circulation around the knee can result in normal pulses despite a significant popliteal artery injury, thus palpable pulses do not absolutely exclude the presence of a popliteal artery injury. Studies demonstrate that an ABI less than 0.9 has a sensitivity and specificity of 100% in predicting a significant arterial injury, while no patient with an ABI greater than 0.9 had a vascular injury on follow-up ultrasound and angiography.[16,17] An abnormal ABI postreduction should prompt emergent duplex ultrasound or computed tomography angiography (CTA). Both CTA and magnetic resonance arteriography (MRA) have been shown to be highly accurate for popliteal artery injury.[18,19] In the setting of an acute vascular injury, CTA is preferred as it is the fastest advanced imaging modality. In contrast, vascular imaging to evaluate for intimal injury in the setting of a normal ABI and peripheral pulses can be performed as an MRA in conjunction with an MRI to evaluate the ligamentous injuries.

A careful neurologic assessment, including motor function and sensation, is important in all suspected multiligament knee injuries. The peroneal nerve is injured in 14%

Table 1	
Classification of knee dislocations based on the pattern of ligament injury[12]	
Class	**Ligament Injuries**
KD I	ACL or PCL with PMC and/or PLC
KD II	ACL and PCL
KD III	ACL and PCL with PMC or PLC
KD IV	ACL, PCL, PMC, and PLC
KD V	MLKI with periarticular fracture

From Wascher DC. High-velocity knee dislocation with vascular injury. Treatment principles. Clin Sports Med 2000;19:457-77.

to 40% of MLKI.[20] The odds of having a common peroneal nerve injury is 42 times higher among those patients with a PLC injury as compared with those without.[15] The presence of a peroneal nerve injury correlates with a higher incidence of vascular injury.[17]

Postreduction radiographs should be assessed for associated fractures, which can include those of the tibial spine, anterolateral proximal tibia (segond fracture), fibular head, lateral epicondyle, and medial epicondyle. In skeletally immature patients, the MCL and FCL originate on the distal femoral epiphysis, and unique physeal fractures can occur as energy is transmitted through the ligaments to the relatively weaker physis.[21]

CLINICAL ASSESSMENT

Acute management of a knee dislocation in the emergency department should include prompt reduction with appropriate sedation. Pre and postreduction neurovascular status should be documented. Skin puckering, most common in dislocations with a rotational component, can indicate femoral condyle entrapment in the soft tissues and may necessitate open reduction if irreducible. A grossly stable reduction without signs of vascular injury can be immobilized in a knee immobilizer or hinged knee brace locked in extension. If emergent vascular intervention is necessary, then a knee-spanning external fixator can be applied if necessary for the grossly unstable knee. In the absence of vascular injury, the authors recommend 12 to 24 hours of inpatient hospital observation postreduction with serial examinations to ensure no changes in the neurovascular status.

The physical examination of the knee is critical in the diagnosis and management of MLKI. In these young patients, examination of the uninjured knee is essential to allow the assessment of physiologic laxity, often present in this age group. Additionally, an examination of the well-leg allows the patient to experience the examination maneuvers performed on the uninjured limb often relaxing the patient and decreasing their anxiety and guarding that can otherwise limit the examination of an acutely painful knee injury. Dynamic examinations, such as the Lachman, anterior and posterior drawer testing, pivot shift, varus/valgus stress, and dial testing should be compared with the uninjured knee. In the setting of an acute injury whereby pain and apprehension limit the examination, focal areas of tenderness can heighten concern for areas of injury. As pain and guarding improve, a more thorough ligamentous examination is tolerated, thus serial examinations are important.

Among patients with an acute knee injury and hemarthrosis, isolated PCL injuries and PLC injuries are rare, accounting for 5% and 2% of injuries, respectively.[22] For this reason, these injuries should be presumed to represent a MLKI. Posterolateral corner injuries most frequently occur in association with ACL injuries, with studies identifying an incidence of 5% to 39% among adult ACL injuries[22,23] and 13 to 52%[24] of pediatric patients with ACL injuries.

Initial imaging should include AP, lateral, notch, and sunrise views of the injured knee to assess for physeal status, symmetry of joint spaces, fractures, and other underlying conditions. In skeletally immature patients, standing long-leg alignment radiographs are important preoperatively to assess for limb length inequalities or angular deformities. A posteroanterior left-hand radiograph is also necessary for skeletally immature patients to determine skeletal age and the shorthand bone age assessment[25] is the authors' favored method for calculating skeletal age and growth remaining. MRI is the gold-standard imaging modality for the diagnosis of ligament, meniscus, and chondral injuries of the knee and is obtained for surgical planning.

Stress radiographs should be performed to quantify laxity and guide the treatment of collateral and posterior cruciate ligament injuries. Varus, valgus, and PCL stress radiographs are highly reliable and valid.[26,27] The indication for FCL reconstruction is a side-to-side difference of 2.0 mm or greater on varus stress radiographs at 20° of knee flexion, while a difference of >/ = 4 mm represents a complete PLC injury.[27] Valgus stress radiographs at 20° of flexion with a side-to-side difference of 3.2 to 9.8 mm indicates a complete superficial MCL tear, while a difference greater than 9.8 mm indicates a complete tear of all medial knee structures.[26] **Figs. 3** and **4** provide examples of varus and valgus stress radiographs. A complete PCL tear produces 8 to 11 mm of increased posterior translation on stress radiographs, while PCL injuries combined with a PLC or medial knee injury result in 12 mm or more of posterior translation.[28]

Some PCL and medial knee injuries are amenable to nonoperative treatment with 4 to 6 weeks of brace immobilization. Knee range of motion and quad activation should be encouraged during this phase through the use of formal physical therapy and home exercises to achieve terminal knee extension as well as flexion. Modifications are made to avoid valgus stress in MCL injuries and to include the use of prone knee flexion in patients with PCL injuries to avoid posterior tibial sag. In these patients, valgus and PCL stress radiographs should be repeated after a period of bracing and before surgery, once the range of motion has been regained, to assess for residual laxity and potential need for reconstruction.

In those patients with peroneal nerve palsy, serial examinations should be performed to monitor for changes in motor and sensory function. The most distal extent of a Tinel's sign over the peroneal nerve can be monitored in reference to the distance from the fibular head to gauge nerve recovery. Patients should be encouraged to perform stretching of the gastrocsoleus complex to prevent an equinus contracture, and the use of a carbon-fiber ankle-foot orthosis aids in ambulation.

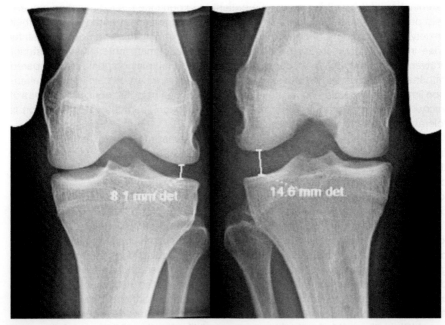

Fig. 3. Varus stress radiographs with 6.5 mm side to side difference in a 16-year-old male with a knee dislocation and complete posterolateral corner injury.

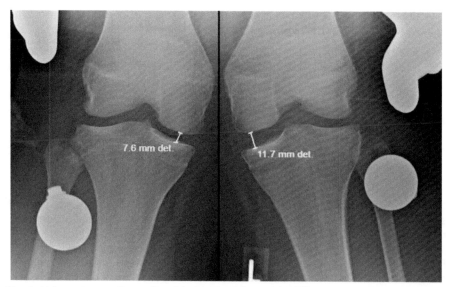

Fig. 4. Valgus stress radiographs with 4.1 mm side-to-side difference in a 16-year-old male patient with an ACL and sMCL tear.

SURGERY

The complexity of lateral and medial knee anatomy and injury patterns has resulted in a multitude of reconstruction techniques. Primary repair is a treatment option that should be reserved for very select injuries, most notably acute avulsion injuries within the first 3 weeks following injury.[29] In the pediatric population, repair may be considered for acute bony avulsions without midsubstance tearing or attenuation. Otherwise, numerous studies have illustrated inferior repair outcomes as compared with the reconstruction of the posterolateral corner does, as it does not restore native knee stability and results in high rates of failure.[29–33]

Numerous anatomic and nonanatomic techniques have been described for each ligament reconstruction. In general, anatomic reconstruction techniques are preferred secondary to their ability to restore native knee biomechanics, allowing early postoperative knee motion with improved outcomes and stability.[31,32,34,35] Failure to reconstruct some ligaments during a staged procedure can result in nonphysiologic loading of reconstruction grafts. Biomechanical studies have reported significantly increased force on the cruciates when the PLC is insufficient.[36,37] Therefore, single-stage reconstructive procedures are favored when possible to minimize the risk of graft failure and to allow for early knee range of motion.[38]

Timing of surgery can be broadly categorized as early versus late. The definition of early surgery has been somewhat arbitrary, but generally less than 3 weeks after injury. In contrast, late surgery occurs more than 3 weeks after injury and also includes chronic instability. Historically, early surgical treatment has been shown to result in higher outcome scores and sports activity scores as compared with delayed treatment.[38,39] Multiple factors, however, can impact surgical timing, including concomitant neurovascular injuries, avulsion injuries amenable to early repair, and MCL and PCL injuries treated with an initial phase of bracing. In reality, performing a single-stage anatomic reconstruction with early knee range of motion is likely more critical to optimal outcomes than reconstruction within a specific time frame.

Graft options for adolescent multiligament knee reconstructions are numerous. The authors' preference for grafts is as follows:

- ACL reconstruction with quadriceps tendon autograft, which is notable for lower rates of graft failure as compared with other autografts[40,41] and allografts[42–44] in this population
- Double-bundle PCL reconstruction with Achilles allograft with calcaneus bone block for the anterolateral bundle and tibialis posterior allograft for the postero-medial bundle
- Isolated FCL reconstruction with semitendinosus autograft
- Full PLC reconstruction with a split Achilles allograft with bone blocks for both the FCL and popliteus
- MCL reconstruction with semitendinosus autograft or allograft

For skeletally immature patients with significant growth remaining, physeal sparing,[45–50] partial transphyseal,[51] and transphyseal[52,53] ACL reconstruction techniques have been described and are also detailed in this edition.

The anatomic posterolateral corner reconstruction has been described in detail by Robert LaPrade.[54] The key surgical steps include posterolateral dissection, peroneal nerve neurolysis, identification of the FCL remnant and attachment on the fibula, drilling of the fibular tunnel, identification and drilling of the tibial tunnel, identification and drilling of the femoral insertions of the FCL and popliteus, proximal fixation and distal passage of the grafts, and distal fixation of the grafts. Peroneal nerve neurolysis is a critical initial step in posterolateral reconstruction. The neurolysis is conducted to allow for safe drilling of an anatomic FCL tunnel in the fibula and to minimize the risk of peroneal nerve neuropraxia postoperatively. The neurolysis extends from post-eromedial to the long head of biceps proximally to the peroneal fascia distally. Several millimeters of peroneal fascia must be incised to avoid compression of the nerve at this level. In patients with a preoperative peroneal nerve palsy and significant postero-lateral corner injury, the peroneal nerve is typically in continuity, but can be signifi-cantly enlarged and encased in adhesions. In these patients, meticulous peroneal nerve neurolysis and decompression can be followed by the use of a nerve wrap to prevent further adhesions and compression. In cases of known nerve disruption, oper-ative planning should be performed in conjunction with a microvascular surgeon.

For acute medial knee injuries that fail to improve with bracing and have valgus instability in flexion, augmented repair can be performed using a semitendinosus auto-graft with suture anchor or socket fixation at the tibial and femoral attachments.[32] For those medial injuries with instability in both flexion and full extension, anatomic MCL and posterior oblique ligament reconstruction is performed.[55] This technique uses 2 grafts, 4 separate closed-socket tunnels, and suture anchors to restore the proximal attachment of the sMCL.

Posterior cruciate reconstruction techniques have also evolved due to recent ad-vances in the understanding of the contributions of each PCL bundle, anterolateral (AL) and posteromedial (PM), to knee stability. Historically, PCL reconstruction used single bundle techniques to reconstruct more of the AL bundle and postoperatively mild to moderate knee laxity persisted.[56] More recently, double-bundle technique has resulted in improved restoration of knee kinematics and ultimately improved pa-tient outcomes.[57] This technique, as published by LaPrade and colleagues, uses a sin-gle transtibial tunnel and 2 sockets in the center of the AL and PM bundle footprints.[58]

In multiligament reconstruction, the risk of tunnel convergence increases secondary to the limited total area within the distal femur. The highest risk of tunnel convergence is with combined ACL and FCL reconstruction and sMCL/POL and PCL reconstruction. To minimize these risks, the FCL tunnel should be aimed approximately 35° anteriorly to avoid convergence with the ACL tunnel.[59] To avoid convergence between the sMCL, POL, and PCL tunnels, the sMCL is aimed at 40° proximally and anteriorly and the POL 20° proximally and anteriorly.

POSTOPERATIVE CARE

Postoperative management of patients following complex knee reconstruction requires careful attention, equal to that of the technical skill and focus required for surgery. Weight bearing is guided by the concomitant meniscal and chondral procedures performed in addition to multiligament knee reconstruction, but typically includes touch-down weight bearing for 6 weeks in a hinged knee brace locked in extension, 50% weight-bearing for week 7, 1-crutch for week 8, and then weight bearing as tolerated. Early knee range of motion is encouraged, typically 0° to 90° for 4 weeks, then progression as tolerated. If PCL reconstruction is performed, then prone range motion or supine range of motion in a dynamic PCL brace is performed to avoid posterior tibial sag which may stretch the PCL grafts in the early postoperative period. A structured rehabilitation program with experienced physical therapists is important to ensure optimal outcomes following multiligament knee reconstruction. Standard rehabilitation protocols include a range of motion, progressive strengthening, proprioception, and endurance. A running progression is typically initiated around month 4, with side to side motions limited until 6 months. A functional test guides the initiation of a return to play progression, with full return to play no sooner than 9 to 12 months postoperatively depending on the extent of the MLKI. Establishing clear patient and family expectations regarding restrictions and estimated return to play is critical to successful outcomes and maximizing compliance and should be a routine part of the preoperative discussion.

Pain management following complex knee surgery should use a multimodal approach that is both patient and procedure specific. Multiple strategies can be used to minimize postoperative pain, including nerve blocks, peri-articular injections, oral pain medications, and cryotherapy. First-line therapies to treat postoperative pain are pharmacologic, including anesthetics, opioids, nonsteroidal antiinflammatory medications, and acetaminophen.

Complex knee surgeries are highly variable in terms of open and arthroscopic techniques, surgical and tourniquet times, weight-bearing precautions, and concomitant fractures, vascular injuries, and neurologic injuries. As such, there is minimal data to definitively recommend for or against deep vein thrombosis (DVT) prophylaxis following these surgeries. Although rates of symptomatic venothromboembolic (VTE) have been reported to be less than 1% following knee arthroscopy and ACL reconstruction,[60] asymptomatic VTE is alarmingly high (8.5%) in some studies.[61] Two largely adult studies have assessed the risk of thromboembolism after multiligament knee reconstruction, reporting rates of symptomatic DVT of 2.2%[62] and 3.5%.[63] A risk assessment for each individual patient, including comorbidities, family history, surgical details, and postoperative restrictions should be performed routinely. Although there are no guidelines for VTE prophylaxis specific to multiligament knee reconstruction in adolescents, procedures associated with lengthy surgical times, large soft tissue dissections, or prolonged postoperative weight-bearing restrictions in postpubescent patients should strongly be considered for combined mechanical (early mobilization, foot pumps, graduated compression stockings) and chemical prophylaxis.

Complications, although rare, should not be underestimated. Fever, infection, and frostbite are the most frequently cited early complications, and recognition and prompt treatment are essential to minimizing their impact on long-term patient outcomes. If patients have a concern about infection or any postoperative wound complication, they should be encouraged to contact their surgeon rather than their primary care physician or urgent care/emergency department to ensure proper management. Arthrofibrosis, in the setting of complex knee reconstruction surgery, can be a potentially devastating complication with significant impacts on patient function and outcomes. Multiple risk factors for arthrofibrosis have been described, including age less than 18 years, concomitant meniscal and/or chondral procedures, female sex, surgery within 28 days of injury, and quadriceps tendon and patellar tendon grafts.[64] Historically, ligament repair, unnecessarily staged procedures, nonanatomic reconstructions, and improper rehabilitation protocols required prolonged immobilization, delayed range of motion, and weight-bearing restrictions which likely contributed to the development of arthrofibrosis and graft failure. Anatomic reconstruction techniques of the medial and lateral knee ligaments allow for early motion and thus minimize the risk for arthrofibrosis.[30,65,66] For this reason, the authors recommend anatomic single-stage reconstructions with early range of motion as allowed based on the patient's specific surgical procedure.

Outcomes

Many studies on the outcomes of multiligament knee reconstruction are limited by heterogeneous populations, injury patterns, and reconstruction techniques. Notably, sports-related MLKI can be vastly different than high-energy knee dislocations. Concomitant neurovascular injuries, including popliteal artery injuries requiring repair and complete peroneal nerve palsies have the potential to dramatically impact both short- and long-term outcomes. Additionally, undiagnosed injuries, unnecessarily staged procedures, and nonanatomic techniques compromise outcomes.

Outcomes following anatomic multiligament knee reconstruction in adolescent patients are scarce as compared with adults.[67,68] Among a cohort of 20 patients less than 19 years of age (mean age 1.7 years) undergoing anatomic multiligament reconstruction with a minimum 2-year follow-up, Lysholm, Tegner, SF-12, and WOMAC scores all improved significantly.[68] Median patient satisfaction was 10. Two patients (10%) had a secondary ligament surgery—one for a PCL graft tear and the other for an ACL graft tear. 95% of patients returned to the same level of the sport. None of the patients had arthrofibrosis, infection, or deep vein thrombosis and no differences in outcomes were noted for medial versus lateral reconstructions. Similar outcomes have been described for 194 adult sports-related MLKI treated with anatomic reconstruction, with significant improvements in all outcome scores and low rates of graft failure (4.6%).[65]

SUMMARY

Evaluation and management of MLKI require a comprehensive understanding of anatomy and biomechanics. In addition to a thorough history and physical examination, stress radiographs provide a reliable method to assess knee stability. Single-stage anatomic reconstruction techniques should be performed, as they restore native knee kinematics and enable early knee range of motion and superior outcomes.[69]

CLINICS CARE POINTS

- Stress radiographs provide a reliable method to assess multiligament knee stability.

- Single-stage anatomic reconstruction techniques restore native knee kinematics and enable early knee range of motion and superior outcomes.

DISCLOSURE

The authors have nothing to disclose.

REFERENCES

1. Ho B, Edmonds EW, Chambers HG, et al. Risk Factors for Early ACL Reconstruction Failure in Pediatric and Adolescent Patients: A Review of 561 Cases. J Pediatr Orthop 2018;38:388–92.
2. Svantesson E, Hamrin Senorski E, Alentorn-Geli E, et al. Increased risk of ACL revision with non-surgical treatment of a concomitant medial collateral ligament injury: a study on 19,457 patients from the Swedish National Knee Ligament Registry. Knee Surg Sports Traumatol Arthrosc 2019;27:2450–9.
3. LaPrade RF, Wentorf F. Diagnosis and treatment of posterolateral knee injuries. Clin Orthop Relat Res 2002;(402):110–21.
4. Terry GC, LaPrade RF. The posterolateral aspect of the knee. Anatomy and surgical approach. Am J Sports Med 1996;24:732–9.
5. Staubli HU, Birrer S. The popliteus tendon and its fascicles at the popliteal hiatus: gross anatomy and functional arthroscopic evaluation with and without anterior cruciate ligament deficiency. Arthroscopy 1990;6:209–20.
6. LaPrade RF, Tso A, Wentorf FA. Force measurements on the fibular collateral ligament, popliteofibular ligament, and popliteus tendon to applied loads. Am J Sports Med 2004;32:1695–701.
7. Terry GC, LaPrade RF. The biceps femoris muscle complex at the knee. Its anatomy and injury patterns associated with acute anterolateral-anteromedial rotatory instability. Am J Sports Med 1996;24:2–8.
8. Godin JA, Chahla J, Moatshe G, et al. A comprehensive reanalysis of the distal iliotibial band: quantitative anatomy, radiographic markers, and biomechanical properties. Am J Sports Med 2017;45:2595–603.
9. LaPrade RF, Engebretsen AH, Ly TV, et al. The anatomy of the medial part of the knee. J Bone Joint Surg Am 2007;89:2000–10.
10. Race A, Amis AA. PCL reconstruction. In vitro biomechanical comparison of 'isometric' versus single and double-bundled 'anatomic' grafts. J Bone Joint Surg Br 1998;80:173–9.
11. Wijdicks CA, Kennedy NI, Goldsmith MT, et al. Kinematic analysis of the posterior cruciate ligament, part 2: a comparison of anatomic single- versus double-bundle reconstruction. Am J Sports Med 2013;41:2839–48.
12. Wascher DC. High-velocity knee dislocation with vascular injury. Treatment principles. Clin Sports Med 2000;19:457–77.
13. Sillanpaa PJ, Kannus P, Niemi ST, et al. Incidence of knee dislocation and concomitant vascular injury requiring surgery: a nationwide study. J Trauma Acute Care Surg 2014;76:715–9.
14. Stannard JP, Sheils TM, Lopez-Ben RR, et al. Vascular injuries in knee dislocations: the role of physical examination in determining the need for arteriography. J Bone Joint Surg Am 2004;86:910–5.

15. Moatshe G, Dornan GJ, Loken S, et al. Demographics and Injuries Associated With Knee Dislocation: A Prospective Review of 303 Patients. Orthop J Sports Med 2017;5. 2325967117706521.
16. Klineberg EO, Crites BM, Flinn WR, et al. The role of arteriography in assessing popliteal artery injury in knee dislocations. J Trauma 2004;56:786–90.
17. Mills WJ, Barei DP, McNair P. The value of the ankle-brachial index for diagnosing arterial injury after knee dislocation: a prospective study. J Trauma 2004;56: 1261–5.
18. Potter HG, Weinstein M, Allen AA, et al. Magnetic resonance imaging of the multiple-ligament injured knee. J Orthop Trauma 2002;16:330–9.
19. Seamon MJ, Smoger D, Torres DM, et al. A prospective validation of a current practice: the detection of extremity vascular injury with CT angiography. J Trauma 2009;67:238–43 [discussion: 43–4].
20. Johnson ME, Foster L, DeLee JC. Neurologic and vascular injuries associated with knee ligament injuries. Am J Sports Med 2008;36:2448–62.
21. Mayer S, Albright JC, Stoneback JW. Pediatric knee dislocations and physeal fractures about the knee. J Am Acad Orthop Surg 2015;23:571–80.
22. LaPrade RF, Wentorf FA, Fritts H, et al. A prospective magnetic resonance imaging study of the incidence of posterolateral and multiple ligament injuries in acute knee injuries presenting with a hemarthrosis. Arthroscopy 2007;23:1341–7.
23. Temponi EF, de Carvalho Junior LH, Saithna A, et al. Incidence and MRI characterization of the spectrum of posterolateral corner injuries occurring in association with ACL rupture. Skeletal Radiol 2017;46:1063–70.
24. Kinsella SD, Rider SM, Fury MS, et al. Concomitant posterolateral corner injuries in skeletally immature patients with acute anterior cruciate ligament injuries. J Pediatr Orthop 2020;40:271–6.
25. Heyworth BE, Osei DA, Fabricant PD, et al. The shorthand bone age assessment: a simpler alternative to current methods. J Pediatr Orthop 2013;33:569–74.
26. Laprade RF, Bernhardson AS, Griffith CJ, et al. Correlation of valgus stress radiographs with medial knee ligament injuries: an in vitro biomechanical study. Am J Sports Med 2010;38:330–8.
27. LaPrade RF, Heikes C, Bakker AJ, et al. The reproducibility and repeatability of varus stress radiographs in the assessment of isolated fibular collateral ligament and grade-III posterolateral knee injuries. An in vitro biomechanical study. J Bone Joint Surg Am 2008;90:2069–76.
28. Jackman T, LaPrade RF, Pontinen T, et al. Intraobserver and interobserver reliability of the kneeling technique of stress radiography for the evaluation of posterior knee laxity. Am J Sports Med 2008;36:1571–6.
29. Geeslin AG, LaPrade RF. Outcomes of treatment of acute grade-III isolated and combined posterolateral knee injuries: a prospective case series and surgical technique. J Bone Joint Surg Am 2011;93:1672–83.
30. Levy BA, Dajani KA, Morgan JA, et al. Repair versus reconstruction of the fibular collateral ligament and posterolateral corner in the multiligament-injured knee. Am J Sports Med 2010;38:804–9.
31. LaPrade RF, Johansen S, Agel J, et al. Outcomes of an anatomic posterolateral knee reconstruction. J Bone Joint Surg Am 2010;92:16–22.
32. Wijdicks CA, Michalski MP, Rasmussen MT, et al. Superficial medial collateral ligament anatomic augmented repair versus anatomic reconstruction: an in vitro biomechanical analysis. Am J Sports Med 2013;41:2858–66.
33. Black BS, Stannard JP. Repair versus reconstruction in acute posterolateral instability of the knee. Sports Med Arthrosc Rev 2015;23:22–6.

34. Laprade RF, Wijdicks CA. Surgical technique: development of an anatomic medial knee reconstruction. Clin Orthop Relat Res 2012;470:806–14.

35. LaPrade RF, Spiridonov SI, Coobs BR, et al. Fibular collateral ligament anatomical reconstructions: a prospective outcomes study. Am J Sports Med 2010;38: 2005–11.

36. LaPrade RF, Muench C, Wentorf F, et al. The effect of injury to the posterolateral structures of the knee on force in a posterior cruciate ligament graft: a biomechanical study. Am J Sports Med 2002;30:233–8.

37. LaPrade RF, Resig S, Wentorf F, et al. The effects of grade III posterolateral knee complex injuries on anterior cruciate ligament graft force. A biomechanical analysis. Am J Sports Med 1999;27:469–75.

38. Levy BA, Dajani KA, Whelan DB, et al. Decision making in the multiligament-injured knee: an evidence-based systematic review. Arthroscopy 2009;25:430–8.

39. Shelbourne KD, Haro MS, Gray T. Knee dislocation with lateral side injury: results of an en masse surgical repair technique of the lateral side. Am J Sports Med 2007;35:1105–16.

40. Gagliardi AG, Carry PM, Parikh HB, et al. Outcomes of Quadriceps Tendon With Patellar Bone Block Anterior Cruciate Ligament Reconstruction in Adolescent Patients With a Minimum 2-Year Follow-up. Am J Sports Med 2020;48:93–8.

41. Pennock AT, Johnson KP, Turk RD, et al. Transphyseal Anterior Cruciate Ligament Reconstruction in the Skeletally Immature: Quadriceps Tendon Autograft Versus Hamstring Tendon Autograft. Orthop J Sports Med 2019;7. 2325967119872450.

42. DeFrancesco CJ, Striano BM, Bram JT, et al. An In-Depth Analysis of Graft Rupture and Contralateral Anterior Cruciate Ligament Rupture Rates After Pediatric Anterior Cruciate Ligament Reconstruction. Am J Sports Med 2020;48: 2395–400.

43. Engelman GH, Carry PM, Hitt KG, et al. Comparison of allograft versus autograft anterior cruciate ligament reconstruction graft survival in an active adolescent cohort. Am J Sports Med 2014;42:2311–8.

44. Kaeding CC, Aros B, Pedroza A, et al. Allograft Versus Autograft Anterior Cruciate Ligament Reconstruction: Predictors of Failure From a MOON Prospective Longitudinal Cohort. Sports Health 2011;3:73–81.

45. Anderson AF. Transepiphyseal replacement of the anterior cruciate ligament in skeletally immature patients. A preliminary report. J Bone Joint Surg Am 2003; 85:1255–63.

46. Cruz AI Jr, Fabricant PD, McGraw M, et al. All-Epiphyseal ACL Reconstruction in Children: Review of Safety and Early Complications. J Pediatr Orthop 2017;37: 204–9.

47. Fabricant PD, McCarthy MM, Cordasco FA, et al. All-Inside, All-Epiphyseal Autograft Reconstruction of the Anterior Cruciate Ligament in the Skeletally Immature Athlete. JBJS Essent Surg Tech 2014;3:e9.

48. Lawrence JT, Bowers AL, Belding J, et al. All-epiphyseal anterior cruciate ligament reconstruction in skeletally immature patients. Clin Orthop Relat Res 2010;468:1971–7.

49. McCarthy MM, Graziano J, Green DW, et al. All-epiphyseal, all-inside anterior cruciate ligament reconstruction technique for skeletally immature patients. Arthrosc Tech 2012;1:e231–9.

50. Kennedy MI, Akamefula R, DePhillipo NN, et al. Fibular Collateral Ligament Reconstruction in Adolescent Patients. Arthrosc Tech 2019;8:e141–5.

51. Demange MK, Camanho GL. Nonanatomic anterior cruciate ligament reconstruction with double-stranded semitendinosus grafts in children with open physes: minimum 15-year follow-up. Am J Sports Med 2014;42:2926–32.

52. Cohen M, Ferretti M, Quarteiro M, et al. Transphyseal anterior cruciate ligament reconstruction in patients with open physes. Arthroscopy 2009;25:831–8.

53. Kocher MS, Smith JT, Zoric BJ, et al. Transphyseal anterior cruciate ligament reconstruction in skeletally immature pubescent adolescents. J Bone Joint Surg Am 2007;89:2632–9.

54. Serra Cruz R, Mitchell JJ, Dean CS, et al. Anatomic Posterolateral Corner Reconstruction. Arthrosc Tech 2016;5:e563–72.

55. Coobs BR, Wijdicks CA, Armitage BM, et al. An in vitro analysis of an anatomical medial knee reconstruction. Am J Sports Med 2010;38:339–47.

56. Lee DY, Kim DH, Kim HJ, et al. Biomechanical Comparison of Single-Bundle and Double-Bundle Posterior Cruciate Ligament Reconstruction: A Systematic Review and Meta-Analysis. JBJS Rev 2017;5:e6.

57. Chahla J, Moatshe G, Cinque ME, et al. Single-Bundle and Double-Bundle Posterior Cruciate Ligament Reconstructions: A Systematic Review and Meta-analysis of 441 Patients at a Minimum 2 Years' Follow-up. Arthroscopy 2017;33: 2066–80.

58. Chahla J, Nitri M, Civitarese D, et al. Anatomic Double-Bundle Posterior Cruciate Ligament Reconstruction. Arthrosc Tech 2016;5:e149–56.

59. Moatshe G, Brady AW, Slette EL, et al. Multiple Ligament Reconstruction Femoral Tunnels: Intertunnel Relationships and Guidelines to Avoid Convergence. Am J Sports Med 2017;45:563–9.

60. Gaskill T, Pullen M, Bryant B, et al. The Prevalence of Symptomatic Deep Venous Thrombosis and Pulmonary Embolism After Anterior Cruciate Ligament Reconstruction. Am J Sports Med 2015;43:2714–9.

61. Erickson BJ, Saltzman BM, Campbell KA, et al. Rates of Deep Venous Thrombosis and Pulmonary Embolus After Anterior Cruciate Ligament Reconstruction: A Systematic Review. Sports Health 2015;7:261–6.

62. Born TR, Engasser WM, King AH, et al. Low frequency of symptomatic venous thromboembolism after multiligamentous knee reconstruction with thromboprophylaxis. Clin Orthop Relat Res 2014;472:2705–11.

63. Engebretsen L, Risberg MA, Robertson B, et al. Outcome after knee dislocations: a 2-9 years follow-up of 85 consecutive patients. Knee Surg Sports Traumatol Arthrosc 2009;17:1013–26.

64. Huleatt J, Gottschalk M, Fraser K, et al. Risk Factors for Manipulation Under Anesthesia and/or Lysis of Adhesions After Anterior Cruciate Ligament Reconstruction. Orthop J Sports Med 2018;6. 2325967118794490.

65. LaPrade RF, Chahla J, DePhillipo NN, et al. Single-Stage Multiple-Ligament Knee Reconstructions for Sports-Related Injuries: Outcomes in 194 Patients. Am J Sports Med 2019;47:2563–71.

66. Mook WR, Miller MD, Diduch DR, et al. Multiple-ligament knee injuries: a systematic review of the timing of operative intervention and postoperative rehabilitation. J Bone Joint Surg Am 2009;91:2946–57.

67. Fanelli GC, Fanelli DG. Knee Dislocations and PCL-Based Multiligament Knee Injuries in Patients Aged 18 Years and Younger: Surgical Technique and Outcomes. J Knee Surg 2016;29:269–77.

68. Godin JA, Cinque ME, Pogorzelski J, et al. Multiligament Knee Injuries in Older Adolescents: A 2-Year Minimum Follow-up Study. Orthop J Sports Med 2017;5. 2325967117727717.
69. LaPrade RF, Ly TV, Wentorf FA, et al. The posterolateral attachments of the knee: a qualitative and quantitative morphologic analysis of the fibular collateral ligament, popliteus tendon, popliteofibular ligament, and lateral gastrocnemius tendon. Am J Sports Med 2003;31:854–60.

Patellar Instability in Young Athletes

Shital N. Parikh, MD[a],*, Matthew Veerkamp, BA[a], Lauren H. Redler, MD[b],
John Schlechter, DO[c], Brendan A. Williams, MD[d], Moshe Yaniv, MD[e],
Nicole Friel, MD[f], Sofia Hidalgo Perea, BS[g], Sara Rose Shannon[g],
Daniel W. Green, MD, MS[g]

KEYWORDS

- Pediatric • Patellar instability • Patellar dislocation • Children • Physis • MPFL
- Quadricepsplasty • Skeletally immature

KEY POINTS

- Besides patellofemoral anatomic risk factors, the rotational and coronal plane alignment of entire lower extremity should be evaluated.
- Prediction models should be used to estimate the rate of recurrent dislocation in young patients.
- Medial patellofemoral ligament reconstruction in skeletally immature patients is safe and effective for recurrent episodic patellar dislocation.
- Quadricepsplasty is necessary to address fixed or obligatory patellar dislocation.

INCIDENCE AND EPIDEMIOLOGY

Lateral patellar dislocation (LPD) is common during adolescence and represents one of the most frequent knee injuries in this age group.[1] The annual incidence of primary (first-time) LPD is estimated to range from 2.3 to 77.4 per 100,000 person-years, peaking during adolescence and young adulthood (**Fig. 1**). Longitudinal studies over several years have suggested that the incidence of injury is either stable or slowly rising in the adolescent age group (**Fig. 2**).[2–13] A recent report from 3 national administrative databases suggests increased rates of admission and surgical intervention for patellar instability.[13–15] These findings may be attributable either to trends toward earlier surgical

[a] Cincinnati Children's Hospital Medical Center, 3333 Burnet Avenue, Cincinnati, OH 45229, USA; [b] Columbia University, New York, NY, USA; [c] Children's Hospital of Orange County, Orange, CA, USA; [d] Children's Hospital of Philadelphia, Philadelphia, PA, USA; [e] Dana-Dwek Children's Hospital - Tel Aviv Sourasky Medical Center, Tel Aviv, Israel; [f] Shriners Hospital for Children Northern California, Sacramento, CA, USA; [g] Hospital for Special Surgery, New York, NY, USA
* Corresponding author.
E-mail address: Shital.Parikh@cchmc.org

Clin Sports Med 41 (2022) 627–651
https://doi.org/10.1016/j.csm.2022.05.005

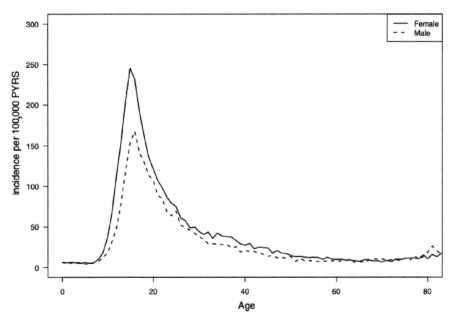

Fig. 1. Incidence of primary patellar dislocation. The figure shows the average, age-related incidence of suffering a primary patellar dislocation for the period 1994 to 2013. A primary patellar dislocation was defined as a patient with no earlier incidents in the same knee; hence, the calculation included the *International Classification of Diseases*, 10 the edition, code DS 83.0, and each individual could only be included in the analysis once with each knee. Incidence rates are reported per 100,000 person-year risk. (*From* Gravesen KS, Kallemose T, Blønd L, Troelsen A, Barfod KW. High incidence of acute and recurrent patellar dislocations: a retrospective nationwide epidemiological study involving 24.154 primary dislocations. Knee Surg Sports Traumatol Arthrosc. 2018;26(4):1204–1209. doi:10.1007/s00167-017-4594-7.)

management for this condition or perhaps a true increasing incidence of injury in response to increased youth sports participation or early sports specialization.[16]

More than one-half (55%–61%) of primary LPD events occur during sport participation in adolescents.[2,5,17,18] Much of our current understanding of the epidemiology of LPD injuries occurring during sport participation is derived from Mitchell and colleagues' study of high school athletes in the United States using the Reporting Information Online Athletic Trainers Injury Surveillance system. These researchers identified an overall LPD injury rate of 1.95 per 100,000 athletic exposures (AEs) over a 6-year period.[19] The majority (75.1%) were primary LPD events, whereas recurrent injuries from the same or prior academic year occurred in 5.7% and 17.8% of athletes, respectively. The highest rate of injury occurred during gymnastics in females (6.19/100,000 AEs) and during football (4.10/100,000 AEs) and wrestling (3.45/100,000 AEs) in males. The most common injury occurring concomitantly with LPD episodes were medial collateral ligament injuries (3.3%).

Although the overall rates of LPD seem to be similar between the sexes across numerous studies, females in the late adolescent period seem to be at greatest risk for first-time LPD with an estimated incidence as high as 100 to 150 per 100,000 in some cohorts.[2,3,8,11] Female predisposition to LPD is believed to be most attributable to sex-based anatomic differences including greater ligamentous laxity and increased

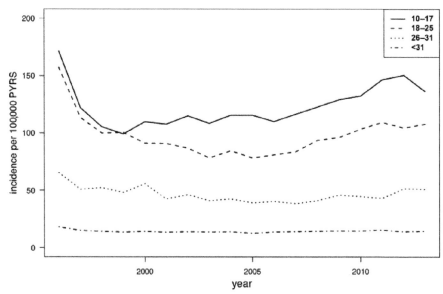

Fig. 2. Incidence rate in primary patellar dislocation from 1996 to 2013. The figure shows changes in the incidence of suffering a primary patellar dislocation from 1996 to 2013. A primary patellar dislocation was defined as a patient with no earlier incidents in the same knee; hence, the calculation included the *International Classification of Diseases*, 10 the edition, code DS 83.0, and each individual could only be included in the analysis once with each knee. Incidence rates are reported per 100,000 person-year (PYRS) risk. (*From* Gravesen KS, Kallemose T, Blønd L, Troelsen A, Barfod KW. High incidence of acute and recurrent patellar dislocations: a retrospective nationwide epidemiological study involving 24.154 primary dislocations. Knee Surg Sports Traumatol Arthrosc. 2018;26(4):1204–1209. doi:10.1007/s00167-017-4594-7.)

Q-angle owing to pelvic width and limb alignment. In their epidemiologic review of high school patellofemoral injuries, Mitchell and colleagues[19] found that the overall injury occurrence rate was lower for girls than boys (1.66 vs 2.15 per 100,000 AEs), but rates were higher for females in sex-comparable sports. Contact injuries occurred nearly twice as frequently as noncontact injuries, with contact injuries more common in male athletes and noncontact injuries more common in females. Together, these data indicate that the higher percentage of male participation in contact sports may explain gender differences in incidence of primary LPD, and that the female sport-related LPD events may be more related to their anatomic differences.

TYPES OF INSTABILITY AND CLASSIFICATION

Several classification systems for LPD have been proposed. Chotel and colleagues[20] focused on classifying patellar dislocation by extensively reviewing the anatomic, biomechanical, pathophysiological, and clinical patterns seen most commonly in children. It differentiated habitual dislocation during knee flexion from habitual dislocation during knee extension.

Parikh and Lykissas[21] published a comprehensive classification system of 4 types of patellar dislocation in addition to voluntary patellar instability and syndromic patellar instability. The 4 types were type 1 or first time patellar dislocation; type 2, or recurrent patellar instability; type 3, dislocatable; and type 4, dislocated. The classification system proposed by Green and his colleagues [1] is useful for surgical indications and

Table 1	
Classification of patellofemoral instability	
Type	**Features**
Syndromic	Connective tissue disorders predisposing to instability
Obligatory	Dislocates with every flexion
Fixed	Irreducible
Traumatic	First time vs recurrent

planning (**Table 1**). This classification system notes syndromic, obligatory (either in flexion or extension), fixed lateral, and traumatic types. Traumatic LPD represent the typical episodic dislocations seen in the majority of adolescent athletes.

Traumatic LPD by definition have an inciting event which disrupts the medial patellofemoral ligament (MPFL). Traumatic dislocations can be further subdivided into first-time (primary) or recurrent dislocations. Repeated traumatic LPD typically involve less energy with subsequent episodes owing to weakened medial supporting structures. Obligatory (habitual) patellar dislocations means that the patella dislocates with every episode of knee flexion and reduce when the knee is extended. This phenomenon is typically associated with a malpositioned and shortened quadriceps mechanism and tight lateral retinacular structures.[22,23] There is a rare subset of patients with obligatory patellar instability in extension that decreases in flexion; this finding is similar to an exaggerated J-sign. This subtype presents one of the more challenging cases to treat surgically. Fixed lateral dislocations remain laterally dislocated throughout the entire range of motion and are irreducible. This type is the rarest and is often associated with other congenital limb deficiency, but can be seen in patients with normal anatomy (**Fig. 3**). Treatment for both obligatory and fixed dislocations often requires a more extensive open reconstruction with a wide lateral release or lateral lengthening to address the tight lateral retinacular structures that are tethering the patella.[22] V–Y or other forms of quadriceps lengthening is often required for these cases as well.[23]

Syndromic dislocators have a genetic syndrome that predisposes the patient to recurrent instability, such as Marfan syndrome, Ehlers–Danlos syndrome, Down syndrome, nail–patella syndrome, or skeletal dysplasias.[1] Syndromic dislocators are predisposed to frequent or fixed patellar dislocations owing to connective tissue laxity, incompetent collagen supporting structures, trochlear dysplasia, and lower extremity deformity.[24] These patients will often present with falls during gait. Historic literature referring to cases of congenital dislocations have included cases of syndromic, obligatory, and fixed dislocations.

PATHOANATOMY

There are several pathoanatomic risk factors for patellar instability, including trochlear dysplasia, lateralization of the tibial tubercle or medialization of the trochlear groove represented by an increased tibial tubercle to trochlear groove (TT–TG) distance, patella alta, lower limb malalignment, excessive femoral anteversion and tibial torsion, hyperlaxity, and syndromic associations.

Trochlear Dysplasia

Trochlear dysplasia is an abnormal shape and depth of the trochlear groove. Dejour and colleagues[25] classified trochlear dysplasia into 1 of 4 different categories based upon a lateral radiograph and axial imaging on a computed tomography scan or MRI. Type A denotes a shallow trochlea with a sulcus angle greater than 145°, type

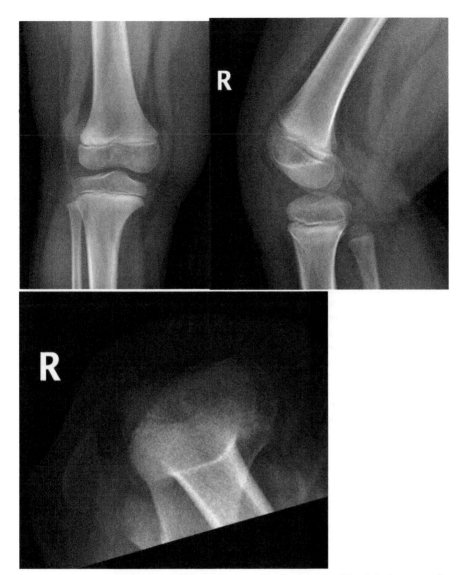

Fig. 3. Anteroposterior, lateral, and sunrise view of a fixed irreducible right knee patellar dislocation.

B has a flat trochlea, type C has a convex trochlea, and type D has a cliff pattern with a convex lateral trochlea and significantly hypoplastic medial femoral condyle. There are now more than 30 unique measurements to assess trochlear dysplasia, including lateral trochlea inclination, trochlear depth, and the ventral trochlea prominence (bump).[26] Trochlear dysplasia is most often cited as the greatest anatomic risk factor for recurrent patellar dislocation.[18,27,28]

Elevated Tibial Tubercle to Trochlear Groove Distance

An increased TT–TG distance predisposes one to patellar instability. A TT–TG of 20 mm measured on MRI has frequently been used as a cutoff value to direct surgical treatment towards a tibial tubercle osteotomy in adults, although this decision is multi-factorial. In the pediatric and adolescent populations, the normative values of TT–TG distance increases with chronologic age. Thus, a growth chart type of representation may be an appropriate way to describe normal TT–TG distance, and correspondingly an abnormal TT–TG distance, for a given age.[29] Some of the drawbacks of TT–TG, including changing values with knee flexion, difficulty in identifying the trochlear groove in patients with trochlear dysplasia, and difficulty in identifying the site of anatomic abnormality, can be addressed by an alternative measurement described as the tibial tubercule-to-posterior cruciate ligament (TT–PCL) distance.[30] The TT–PCL measurement has been validated in children and its value increases with patient age.[31]

Correction of an increased TT–TG in an adult can be accomplished by an osteotomy of the tibial tubercle and medial, anterior, and/or distal transposition of the tubercle. Management in the skeletally immature patient is more challenging owing to the risk of injury to the physis, but soft tissue realignment procedures such as the Roux–Goldthwait procedure or complete patellar tendon transposition have been utilized to avoid growth plate disruption.

Patella Alta

An increased patellar height is associated with patellar instability. With the knee in full extension, the patella remains proximal to the trochlear groove, and thus the patella alta keeps the patella away from the groove through a larger arc of knee range of motion. Multiple measurements are used to measure patella height; the Caton–Deschamps index is a simple and reliable index measure on lateral radiographs of the knee for evaluating patellar height in adults and also has been validated in children (**Fig. 4**).[32] A Caton–Deschamps index of greater than 1.2 predisposes to patellar instability in children.

Lower Limb Malalignment

Genu valgum is a risk factor for patellar instability, because it produces an increased Q angle and an increased lateral force on the patella. At 3 to 4 years of age, children can have up to 20° of genu valgum, but this should normalize and be no greater than 8° by

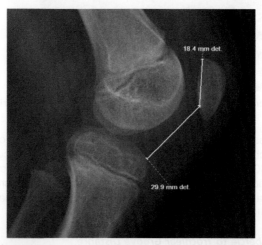

18.4 mm det.

29.9 mm det.

Fig. 4. Caton–Deschamps Index of 1.6 (29.9/18.4) in a 7-year-old girl with habitual patellar dislocation. As patella ossifies from proximal to distal, normative values of the Caton–Deschamps Index decrease with age.

age 12. Genu valgum in skeletally immature patients can be corrected by guided growth using a number of different methods, including a percutaneous transphyseal screw or by use of a physeal tethering device such as an 8-plate. However, the threshold value or what constitutes pathologic valgus is not known. In a recent study, guided growth of distal femur for correction of genu valgum in presence of patellar instability was performed when the lateral distal femoral angle was 84° or less, and the mechanical axis was in the lateral compartment.[33] In skeletally mature adolescents, an osteotomy, most often a lateral opening wedge distal femoral osteotomy, can achieve correction of the malalignment.

Lower Limb Torsion

The combination of excessive femoral anteversion and tibial torsion, often coupled with genu valgum, describes miserable malalignment. Excessive femoral anteversion increases strain in the MPFL, as well as increases contact pressure on the lateral aspect of the patellofemoral joint. There is no consensus regarding the acceptable tolerance of anteversion, but a derotational osteotomy can be considered in children with symptomatic patellofemoral instability and an increased femoral anteversion, based on both examination and imaging measurements.

Hyperlaxity

Hyperlaxity refers to increased joint mobility related to tissue elasticity, in which primarily type III collagen is increased. The Beighton score is a tool used to identify hyperlaxity. Traditionally, a score of 5 out of 9 or higher identifies joint hypermobility; however, it has been suggested that for children, a score of 7 out of 9 or higher should identify hypermobility. The most common diagnosis associated with hyperlaxity in this patient population is Ehlers–Danlos syndrome.

Syndromic Associations

Multiple syndromes have associated patellar instability, including Down's syndrome, Kabuki syndrome, and nail–patella syndrome.[1] The treatment approach is individualized for each syndrome, given that children with each of these syndromes may have different functional levels.

NATURAL HISTORY OF PATELLAR INSTABILITY IN YOUNG PATIENTS

The natural history following first-time episodes of LPD in children and adolescents runs the gamut. The instability event may occur in isolation or as a 1-time phenomenon. More often, however, there tends to be a recurrence of instability that ranges from lateral maltracking of the patella with apprehension during activities to recurrent subluxations and frank dislocations. Frank dislocations may reduce spontaneously or may require formal manipulation or reduction in an emergency department setting. Ipsilateral recurrence rates after a first-time LPD range from 15% to 71%.[12,27,34–39] Contralateral dislocations may occur in 5% to 8% of patients.[12,38]

Palmu and colleagues[35] reported on 62 patients (64 knees) less than 16 years of age with primary LPD who were randomized to nonoperative treatment (28 knees) or operative treatment (36 knees). Operative treatment consisted of direct repair of the damaged medial structures if the patella was dislocatable with the patient under anesthesia (29 knees) or lateral release alone if the patella was not dislocatable with the patient under anesthesia (7 knees). The rehabilitation protocol was the same for both groups. The patients were seen at 2 years, and a telephone interview was conducted at a mean of 6 years and again at a mean of 14 years. There were 58 patients (64 knees; 94%) who were reviewed at the time of the most recent follow-up. The rates of recurrent dislocation were 71% (20/28) for the nonoperative group and 67% (24/36) for the operative group. The first redislocation occurred within 2 years after the primary injury in 23 of the 44 knees (52%) with recurrent dislocation. Instability of the contralateral patella was noted in 30 of the 62 patients (48%).

In addition to recurrent dislocation, functional limitations after an acute LPD in children and adolescents may include persistent pain, mechanical symptoms, and an inability to return to sport. The occurrence of these limitations is variable and depends on many factors, such as the nature and force of the initial inciting event, underlying pathoanatomy, ligamentous laxity, and activity level.

Depending on underlying anatomic factors, acute LPD and relocation may produce major forces at the articular surfaces.[40,41] Articular injury is best assessed with MRI and arthroscopy. Acute LPDs result in predominantly lateral femoral condylar and medial patella facet lesions.[40,42] The incidence is high and ranges from 70% to 96%.[41] Stanitski and Paletta[40] assessed 48 patients, 24 boys and 24 girls (mean age, 14 years), with acute, initial, noncontact LPD. Eleven of the 48 patients (23%) had radiologic diagnoses of articular injuries. Thirty-four of the 48 patients (71%) had arthroscopic evidence of articular damage.[40] Nomura and Inoue[42] examined 70 knees in 57 patients with recurrent patellar instability and found that 67 knees (96%) had articular cartilage lesions of the patella. In a population-based cohort study of 232 skeletally immature patients who experienced a first-time LPD with a mean follow-up of 12.1 years, Sanders and colleagues[12] reported that 20% of patients developed arthritis by 20 years after the initial dislocation.

Numerous studies have compared outcomes after nonoperative versus operative treatment after primary LPD in adolescents.[36,39,43–47] In a randomized controlled trial, Askenberger and colleagues[39] examined whether arthroscopic-assisted repair of the MPFL in patients with an acute first-time traumatic LPD would decrease the recurrence rate and offer better objective and subjective knee function compared with a knee brace without repair. They found that the redislocation rate was significantly lower in the MPFL repair group than in the knee brace group at final follow-up, but surgery did not improve subjective or objective knee function compared with a knee brace without repair. The majority of the patients in both groups were satisfied with their knee function.

The fundamentals of a nonoperative treatment algorithm after an LPD include a period of rest, cryotherapy, nonsteroidal anti-inflammatory drugs, bracing, and physical therapy. The addition of a specific patellofemoral brace may improve joint mechanics and decrease the likelihood of future instability when worn.[48] The author's preferred method of nonoperative treatment after an acute LPD in children and adolescents without chondral or osteochondral fracture is a brief period (<21 days) of immobilization in a knee immobilizer for comfort and weight bearing as tolerated with the assistance of crutches. Often, after an acute patella dislocation, there will be a large knee effusion. In patients with a large effusion, therapeutic arthrocentesis is considered to relieve pressure and pain. The initiation of a formal physical therapy regimen commences in the first 3 weeks after the injury with a focus on restoration of range of motion, normalization of gait, proprioception, and strength. Functional progression to sport-specific rehabilitation follows with an anticipated return to sport 9 to 12 weeks after the injury. A patella-stabilizing brace is used for sport and activity for the first 12 months after the initial dislocation and at the patient's discretion thereafter. It is important to recognize that poor results after nonoperative treatment of LPD may involve nonrecognition of articular injuries.[40]

PREDICTION MODELS FOR PATELLAR INSTABILITY

Several demographic and anatomic risk factors for LPD and recurrence have been identified, of which the age (chronologic age and open physes) and anatomic factors (trochlear dysplasia and patella alta) are most consistently identified.[17,18,27,34] In patients with multiple risk factors, the risk of recurrent instability increases considerably, with rates as high as 88%.[18,27] Lewallen and colleagues[18] found open/closing physes and the presence of trochlear dysplasia to be the greater risk factors for recurrence in one of the largest cohorts of adolescent patellar instability. The authors identified a recurrence rate of 68.8% in patients having both of these risk factors indicating a 3-fold increase in risk compared with skeletally mature primary dislocators without dysplasia. Individuals without these risk factors had an estimated recurrence-free survival of 85%, 73%, and 73% at 1, 3, and 5 years, respectively.

Family history is also a significant factor to consider in the epidemiology of LPD. Even in the absence of inheritable conditions of ligamentous laxity such as Ehlers–Danlos syndrome, a positive family history of LPD alone is considered to be a risk factor for dislocation events. Palmu and colleagues[35] identified that a positive family history of LPD was a risk factor for both recurrent and contralateral instability. Fithian and colleagues[2] similarly identified that patients with a family history of instability carry an increased odds of contralateral dislocation after a primary instability episode.

Depending on the duration of follow-up and the population studied, recurrent ipsilateral LPD has been reported to occur in 15% to 54% of patients after primary dislocation in adolescent and young cohorts, with a pooled rate of 41.8% in a systematic review performed by Zhang and colleagues.[2,8,12,18,27,49–51] Episodes of recurrence appear to peak during adolescence with the vast majority occurring within the first 5 years of the primary event.[12,18] Contralateral dislocation can occur in as many as 10% to 11% of pediatric and adolescent patients.[2,8,12]

Several prediction models have been developed to evaluate the risk of recurrent instability after a first-time patellar dislocation.[52] The usefulness of such models is based on the hypothesis that, if recurrent instability can be predicted after a first-time dislocation, then surgical stabilization of the patella can be considered after a first-time dislocation in selected patients. This approach would be different from the standard recommendation of conservative treatment for all first-time patellar dislocation. To date, none of the models have been validated in a prospective study.

Balcarek and colleagues[53] developed the patellar instability severity score based on age, contralateral dislocation, trochlear dysplasia, a TT–TG distance of greater than 16 mm, a patellar tilt of greater than 20°, and patellar height (**Table 2**). If the score was 4 or higher, then the odds of recurrent dislocation were 5 times higher than if the scores were less than 4.

Jaquith and Parikh[27] identified 4 risk factors based on history and lateral knee radiographs: young age, contralateral dislocation, patella alta (Caton–Deschamps index of >1.45), and trochlear dysplasia. Based on the presence of the number of risk factors, the likelihood of patellar dislocation could be estimated (**Table 3**).

Arendt and colleagues[54] reported on 3 risk factors on MRI: sulcus angle of 154°or more, an Insall–Salvati rate of 1.3 or greater, and skeletal immaturity. The probability of recurrent dislocation was 5.8% in absence of any risk factor and 78.5% if all 3 factors were present.

Recently, Ling and colleagues[55] synthesized 4 prediction models and reported on 7 variables in their multivariate model: younger age, skeletal immaturity, contralateral dislocation, trochlear dysplasia, increased TT–TG distance, increased patellar tilt, and an increased Insall–Salvati ratio. Huntington and colleagues[56] performed a

Table 2
Patellar Instability Severity Score. Odds for recurrence are 5 times higher when total score of 4 or more points

Risk Factors (Odds Ratio)		Points
Age (11.2)	>16 y	0
	≤16 y	1
Bilateral instability (3.2)	No	0
	Yes	1
Trochlear dysplasia (4.2)	None	0
	Mild	1
	Severe	2
Patellar height (1.4)	≤1.2	0
	>1.2	1
TT–TG (1.5)	<16 mm	0
	≥16 mm	1
Patellar tilt (1.9)	≤20°	0
	>20	1
	Total score range	0–7

systematic review and meta-analysis of prognostic risk factors for LPD, based on 17 studies. The overall rate of recurrent dislocations after first-time LPD was 33.6%. Recurrent rates were 7.7% to 13.8% when no risk factors were present but increased to more than 70% when 3 risk factors were present.

MEDIAL PATELLOFEMORAL LIGAMENT RECONSTRUCTION

The MPFL plays an important role as a passive restraint against lateral displacement of the patella. Owing to its important role in the patellofemoral biomechanics and the high frequency of MPFL injuries after a traumatic LPD, its reconstruction has become a mainstay for treatment of patellofemoral instability. In LPD cases where the underlying pathoanatomy is not severe enough to justify anatomic corrections, isolated MPFL reconstruction can provide satisfactory outcomes.

The femoral insertion of the MPFL has been well-described in the adult population, with most investigators agreeing that it is located anterior to a midpoint between the

Table 3
Prediction model for recurrence after first-time patellar dislocation based on number of risk factors

Risk Factors	Average Predicted Risk of Recurrence (%)	Treatment Recommendation
0	13.8	Conservative treatment
1	30.1	
2	53.6	Surgery optional
3	74.8	Surgical treatment
4	88.4	

The 4 risk factors include trochlear dysplasia, history of contralateral dislocation, skeletal immaturity, and a Caton–Deschamps index of >1.45.

medial epicondyle and the adductor tubercle.[57–59] The MPFL femoral footprint anatomic relation to the distal femoral physis is critical for its reconstruction in the skeletally immature population, owing to the risk of femoral physis injury. In a radiological study of 27 children (mean age, 14.3 years; range, 12–16 years) the center of MPFL femoral insertion was a mean of 6 mm (range, 2.9–8.5 mm) distal to the physis.[60] In a cadaveric study of 6 knees (1 month to 11 years), Shea and colleagues[61] found significant variability of the femoral foot print of the MPFL in the skeletal immature specimens. With respect to the distal femoral physis, the MPFL origin was more anterior and proximal (0.8 mm) to the physis in specimens over the age of 7 years, and posterior and distal (4.7 mm) to the physis in specimens under the age of 7 years.[61]

Different techniques have been developed for reconstruction of the MPFL in skeletally immature patients with variations in terms of graft types and fixation methods. A free or distally attached hamstring graft, quadriceps tendon pedicle graft, adductor magnus pedicled graft, allograft, and synthetic graft have all been described as options for MPFL reconstruction, with no evidence of superiority of one over the other. The need to avoid distal femoral physeal injury during MPFL femoral attachment has generated 2 main concepts. Extraosseous soft tissue fixation may use the adductor tendon insertion or medial collateral ligament origin as an anchor or a pulley. Avikainen and colleagues[62] described MPFL reconstruction with extraosseous fixation on the femoral side, using the distal adductor magnus tendon as a graft and leaving the adductor insertion in place as the femoral fixation. A hamstring graft, left attached at its tibial insertion and looped around the adductor origin and then secured to the patella, has been described.[20,63] In contrast with extraosseous fixation, intraosseous femoral fixation involves drilling a tunnel through the medial femoral condyle epiphysis. The tunnel is created distal to the distal femoral physis and under image intensifier guidance.[64] An anatomic 3-dimensional study showed a technique for safe drilling paths across the distal femoral epiphysis, such that the distal femoral physis, intercondylar notch, and trochlear articular cartilage can be avoided.[64] The location of the femoral MPFL attachment distal to the femoral physis was demonstrated to result in a more isometric graft, compared with techniques using the attachment point proximal to the physis like adductor sling technique.[65]

In a cadaveric study of MPFL patellar attachment in skeletally immature subjects, the center of the MPFL insertion was found below the midpoint of the patella in some younger specimens. In older skeletally immature specimens, MPFL insertion was found in the proximal two-thirds of the patella, similar to the location in adult anatomic studies.[66] The options for patellar graft fixation include patellar bony socket, tunnel (single or double), or longitudinal slot with anchors. Free ends or the midportion of the graft can be docked to the patella. There is a small risk of patellar fracture after tunnel or anchor placement in the patella. The use of a pedicled quadriceps tendon graft for MPFL reconstruction can help to decrease the risk of patella fracture by avoiding such patellar drill holes.[67] The MPFL graft could be looped through the periosteum and sutured to itself on the anterior aspect of the patella.[68] The graft could be looped around the quadriceps tendon and the adductor tubercle (medial quadriceps tendon–femoral ligament) to avoid any drill holes in the patella or femur.[69]

True complication rates after MPFL reconstruction surgery in the skeletal immature patient are difficult to ascertain because most of the reports focus on the adult population with multiple procedures. Recurrent patellar instability, stiffness, limited flexion, patellar fractures, pain, and arthrosis were reported in 38 of 179 knees (16.2%) of adolescents and young patients (mean age 14.5 years; range, 6–21 years) who had undergone MPFL reconstruction. One-half of the complications were attributed to erroneous surgical techniques like patellar drill placement.[70]

The cause of MPFL reconstruction failure was evaluated in 19 young patients (aged 16–27 years). The most frequent complication was redislocation associated with trochlear dysplasia or graft failure. Medial pain was associated with overtensioning of the graft or femoral tunnel malposition. Patellofemoral pain was associated with chondral damage and limb malrotation.[71]

QUADRICEPSPLASTY

Fixed and obligatory (or habitual) lateral dislocators present with pathologic morphologic anatomic risk factors, tight lateral structures, and often with a shortened extensor mechanism that contributes to patellar instability.[72] Fixed dislocation refers to an irreducible lateral dislocation throughout the knee range of motion. Obligatory dislocation in flexion refers to patients whose patella dislocates laterally every time their knee flexes. If left untreated, both types of patellar instability may lead to degenerative arthritis.[73]

Different techniques have been published to guide treatment. However, owing to the uncommon nature of both fixed and obligatory instability, there is no standard treatment algorithm in the literature. Surgical treatment must account for the variety of underlying etiologies of these conditions and the presence of open physes. Typically, MPFL reconstruction is not enough to remove the deforming forces on the patella, resulting in the need for concomitant procedures. Our approach is typically to begin with an extensive lateral retinacular release (with a lateral lengthening of the retinacular tissues when possible), which often extends into the vastus lateralis tendon, and a lengthening of the vastus lateralis tendon. If, after lateral retinacular lengthening and vastus lateralis tendon lengthening the patella continues to dislocate laterally when the knee is flexed, then a formal quadriceps Z-lengthening can be performed to address the shortened extensor mechanisms and maintain the patella in the trochlear groove during knee flexion.

Various open quadriceps lengthening techniques have been described, often for congenital knee dislocations (not patella dislocations). Among these, the most frequently cited technique has been the V–Y quadricepsplasty described by Curtis and Fisher in 1969.[74] Quadriceps lengthening techniques for pediatric patellar instability are few (**Table 4**).[72,75–85] In 1976, Stanisavljevic and colleagues described a novel technique that included a proximal extensive subperiosteal realignment of the quadriceps mechanism, medial plication using the large overstretched medial capsule as a cover to the realigned patella, and an additional distal Roux–Goldthwait patellar tendon realignment procedure. At the 2-year follow-up they observed satisfactory results in 6 knees. However, there have been few, small cohort studies that have been able to replicate this technique with good outcomes, and the largest cohort to date reported an 80% recurrence of instability.[86–90]

In a study including 12 patients (15 knees), Sever and colleagues[75] performed a modified Stanisavljevic technique that included a Roux–Goldthwait distal realignment, subperiosteal quadriceps realignment, and soft tissue medial plication. One patient (8%) presented with recurrent patellar instability that occurred after a fall in the early postoperative stage. At 46.2 months of follow-up, postoperative knee extension and quality of life (measured by the Pediatric Outcome Data Collection Instrument) had significantly improved. Using a separate novel technique, Danino and colleagues[72] performed a "4-in-1" procedure on 34 patients (46 knees) that included a combination of the Roux–Goldthwait procedure, vastus medialis obliquus advancement, lateral release, and the Galeazzi procedure. Six patients presented with recurrent instability (18%). Sixteen patients (22 knees) responded to a phone interview and follow-up

Table 4
Quadriceps lengthening techniques for pediatric patellar instability

Author	No. of knees	Mean age (years)	Mean Follow-up (years)	Summarized Treatment
Williams,[77] 1968: Quadriceps contracture Obligatory dislocators Technique	NA	NA	NA	The tight lateral bands are released from the patella and the incision continued proximally, lateral to the rectus femoris tendon, thus fully releasing vastus lateralis. Vastus intermedius is inspected and divided if tight. When necessary, the rectus femoris is lengthened by extending the medial release proximally, medial to the rectus femoris tendon and dividing the rectus femoris at its musculotendinous junction. The knee is then flexed, lengthening the rectus femoris. The vastus lateralis and vastus medialis are sewn to each other and to the rectus femoris tendon in its lengthened position. If lateral dislocation is still not controlled, a medial advancement of the vastus medialis, medial plication, patellar tendon transfer, or sartorius to patella transfer is added.
Jones et al,[78] 1976: Congenital dislocation of the patella Fixed dislocators Case report	8	NA	NA	Lateral release of patella, medial transposition of patellar tendon, and plication of medial capsule or advancement of vastus medialis.
Stanisavljevic et al,[79] 1976: Congenital, irreducible, permanent lateral dislocation of the patella Fixed dislocators Therapeutic	6	NA	2	Proximal extensive subperiosteal realignment of the quadriceps mechanism, medial plication using the large overstretched medial capsule as a cover to the realigned patella, and an additional distal Roux-Goldthwait patellar tendon realignment procedure.
Gao et al,[80] 1990:	35	5	5	Extensive lateral release, medial plication, and transfer of the lateral one-

(continued on next page)

Table 4
(continued)

Author	No. of knees	Mean age (years)	Mean Follow-up (years)	Summarized Treatment
Surgical management of congenital and habitual dislocation of the patella Fixed and obligatory Therapeutic				half of the patella tendon. The vastus intermedius was released when required, and in extreme cases the rectus femoris was lengthened.
Gordon and Schoenecker,[81] 1999: Surgical treatment of congenital dislocation of the patella Fixed dislocators Therapeutic	17	7.8	5.1	Extensive procedure including lateral release and advancement of the vastus medialis obliquus. Skeletally immature children underwent medial transfer of the entire patellar tendon. Skeletally mature patients underwent medial transfer of the tibial tubercle.
Eilert,[82] 2001: Congenital Dislocation of the Patella Fixed dislocators Case report	3	NA	NA	Lateral retinaculum release, medialization of the patellar ligament followed by a Z or Z–Y quadricepsplasty and a medial plication of the quadriceps mechanism. The lengthening is done proximal to the patella through the tendinous fibers of the muscle as they insert into the patella. In older patients a Galeazzi procedure was also performed.
Martin et al,[83] 2013: Treatment of femoral lengthening-related knee stiffness with a novel quadricepsplasty Obligatory dislocators Therapeutic	6	18.7	6.2	Distal medial to proximal lateral oblique transection of the main quadriceps tendon and the transposition to the medial side of the proximal aspect of the tendon.
Inan et al,[84] 2015: A combined procedure for irreducible dislocation of patella in children with ligamentous laxity: a preliminary report Fixed dislocators Therapeutic	14	6.9	3.1	The tensor fascia was divided into 2 strips, and these strips were passed via the joint and sutured to themselves. The combined procedure additionally includes lateral capsular release, vastus lateralis resection, medial capsular plication, and Z-plasty of the rectus femoris tendon.

(continued on next page)

Table 4
(*continued*)

Author	No. of knees	Mean age (years)	Mean Follow-up (years)	Summarized Treatment
Niedzielski et al,[85] 2015: The results of an extensive soft tissue procedure in the treatment of obligatory patellar dislocation in children with ligamentous laxity: a postoperative isokinetic study Obligatory dislocators Therapeutic	11	NA	8.1	Extensive soft tissue procedure: vastus medialis advancement, lateral release, partial patellar ligament transposition and Galeazzi semitendinosus tenodesis.
Sever et al,[75] 2019: Surgical treatment of congenital and obligatory dislocation of the patella in children Fixed and obligatory dislocators Therapeutic	15	Fixed: 7.6 Obligatory: 7.3	3.9	Modified Stanisavljevic technique; fascia lata was split rather than excised and in patients in whom the insertion of the split lateral portion of the patellar tendon over (rather than under) the medial portion eliminated patellar tilt. Moreover, did not close the lateral fascial window created by the medial mobilization of the quadriceps muscle.
Danino et al,[72] 2020: Four-in-one extensor realignment for the treatment of obligatory or fixed, lateral patellar instability in skeletally immature knee Fixed and obligatory dislocators Therapeutic	46	10.3	4.3	The 4-in-1 extensor realignment procedure uses an extensive lateral release, Roux–Goldthwait procedure, Galeazzi procedure, and vastus medialis obliquus advancement.
Ellsworth et al,[76] 2021: Stepwise lengthening of the quadriceps extensor mechanism for severe obligatory and fixed patella dislocators Fixed and obligatory dislocators Technique	24	NA	NA	Stepwise lengthening of the extensor mechanism composed of a lateral retinaculum lengthening, followed by a vastus lateralis tendon lengthening and if the patella continues to dislocate in flexion a Z-lengthening quadricepsplasty. These 3 procedures are followed by an MPFL reconstruction.

questionnaire, of which 91% returned to sports at an average of 23.1 weeks of follow-up. After using the 4-in-1 technique in 6 knees, Joo and colleagues[91] observed no recurrence of instability at 54.5 months of follow-up. Both Sever and colleagues and Danino and colleagues reported a low incidence of patellar instability recurrence and neither reported extensor lag after surgery, demonstrating that there may be multiple techniques to treat these complex cases.[72,75]

These authors' preferred technique is the stepwise lengthening of the extensor mechanism previously described by Ellsworth and colleagues[76] and characterized by an extensive lateral release or lengthening, vastus lateralis lengthening, and a separate Z-lengthening of the rectus and intermedius tendon (if needed); this procedure permits the surgeon to preferentially lengthen the lateral aspect of the quadriceps tendon more than the medial aspect.

MANAGEMENT OF ANATOMIC RISK FACTORS

Several anatomic risk factors increase the likelihood of recurrent episodes of patellar instability, including but not limited to patella alta, trochlear dysplasia, elevated TT–TG, genu valgum, femoral anteroversion, and patellar tilt.[92]

Patella Alta

Patella alta is defined as the displacement of the patella within the trochlear groove of the femur, usually in an orientation that is considered high.[93,94] This instability is most commonly the result of an injury owing to overextension, quick and unnatural changes in movements, and frequently a predisposed developmental condition.[95] Patients can develop patella alta at any age, with many displacements occurring in active teenagers and adults. This instability contributes to overall anterior knee pain, demonstrated when patients simply walk.[96] Previous studies found that subjects with patella alta compared with the control group, when walking, had incrementally smaller amounts of patellofemoral contact area at the point of maximal stress.[97]

To improve patella alta, common options are used. The transfer of the tibial tuberosity is an option for skeletally mature patients.[98] However, children who have severe displacement will most likely achieve surgical stabilization through MPFL reconstruction.[99] Partial or complete distal transposition of patellar tendon, patellar tendon imbrication and patellar tendon shortening methods have been described to address patella alta in skeletally immature patients.

An MPFL reconstruction alone has been shown to decrease preoperative patella alta in patient presenting with patella instability.[24,100] In a study performed by Fabricant and colleagues[24] that included 27 pediatric patients, the Insall–Salvati Ratio, Modified Insall–Salvati Ratio, and Caton–Deschamps measures (patella alta indices) improved significantly ($P < .001$) after undergoing MPFL reconstruction without a distal realignment procedure. Lykissas and colleagues[100] observed similar outcomes when comparing preoperative and post-MPFL reconstruction Insall–Salvati ratio, Blackburne–Peel index, Caton–Deschamps index, and plateau–patella angle in 38 pediatric patients.

Trochlear Dysplasia

Trochlear dysplasia is one of the leading causes of patella instability in which a patient possesses a slightly flat or prominent trochlea, resulting in pain within the anterior femoral cortex.[28] Trochlear dysplasia is most commonly the result of genetic risk factors with morphologic trochlea changes leading to greater instability and further injury.[101] There are several different types of trochlear dysplasia, with type A demonstrating a shallow trochlea, type B displaying a flat trochlea, type C presenting a convex trochlea, and type D showing asymmetry of trochlear facets and a vertical cliff pattern.[102]

Many surgical treatments have been explored for the various types of trochlear dysplasia, with many being performed in association with other procedures. Trochleoplasty is suggested as the most common procedure for high-grade trochlear dysplasia.[103] Deepening trochleoplasty has been found to be a safe procedure that reduces patella instability.[104] In addition to this technique, recession-wedge trochleoplasty has shown improvement in patients by reducing the bump on the trochlea.[105] This trochleoplasty procedure has essentially only been reported in adults or adolescents near the end of growth; therefore, there is little literature to support this surgical approach in skeletally immature patients.

Tibial Tubercle to Trochlear Groove Distance

The TT–TG distance is defined as the lateral distance or deviation between the tibial tubercle relative to the center of the trochlea in the axial plane.[106] An abnormal TT–TG distance, defined as greater than or equal to 20 mm in adults, has a greater than 90% association with patellar instability.[28] However, Dickens and colleagues[29] demonstrated that, similar to other pediatric orthopedic assessments, the TT–TG depends on chronologic age. In their study, skeletally immature patients with patellar instability had an average TT–TG of 12.1 mm. Thus, clinicians must use an age-based approach when measuring this distance and defer from using the adult parameters.[29]

Although the TT–TG distance is a well-established indicator for patellar instability, there are multiple limitations to this measurement; it is confounded by age, gives no information about the anatomic malformation location, and varies with the degree of knee flexion on cross-sectional imaging.[29,30,107] To overcome these shortcomings, the TT–PCL has been proposed as an alternate measurement; it quantifies the position of the tibial tubercule in respect to the tibia alone and independent of the trochlea, better describing the lateralization of the tibial tubercle.[30] However, in a study of 566 pediatric patients, Clifton and colleagues[31] showed that, similar to the TT–TG, the TT–PCL was cofounded by age and did not correlate to recurrent patellar instability. Moreover, in 2018, Brady and colleagues[107] demonstrated that the TT–TG distance was superior at differentiating patellar instability compared with the TT–PCL. However, several studies have suggested that the TT–PCL may be a useful measurement to determine surgical treatment when used in conjunction with TT–TG.[107,108]

Genu Valgum

Genu valgum, also known as knocked knees, is a prevalent orthopedic deformity in the coronal plane of the lower extremity. This condition has been associated with patellofemoral instability, because it alters the forces on the lateral aspect of the patellofemoral joint.[109,110] If left uncorrected when performing an MPFL reconstruction, genu valgum and its subsequent increased tensile forces can lead to graft failure and poor clinical outcomes.[33] Typically corrected using a distal femoral osteotomy in adults, correction in skeletally immature patients can be achieved by growth modulation, such as implant-mediated guided growth.[22,111–113] In a recent study, Parikh and colleagues[33] demonstrated that performing an MPFL and implant-mediated guided growth simultaneously could correct the angular deformity without interfering with graft placement.

Femoral anteversion

The role of rotational malalignment such as femoral anteversion in relation to patellar instability has been recognized as an important anatomic risk factor.[28,114,115] A study conducted by Diederichs and colleagues[116] that compared rotational alignment on MRI of nontraumatic patellofemoral instability with healthy controls suggested that higher femoral anteversion and knee rotation can be associated to patellofemoral instability. Moreover, in a study including 70 knees with a mean of 28 months of follow-up, Zhang and colleagues[117] showed that patients with increased femoral anteversion had inferior clinical outcomes and worse patient-reported outcomes after MPFL reconstruction and combined tibial tubercle osteotomy. Given the adverse effect of elevated femoral anteversion, clinicians should consider performing a concomitant derotational distal femoral osteotomy.[117–120]

Patellar Tilt

Patellar tilt is a static radiographic measure of patellar tracking.[121] Once believed to have been the leading cause of patellar instability, recent studies have shown it to be a consequence of other pathologic anatomic risk factors, such as elevated TT–TG, patella alta, and trochlear dysplasia, rather than an independent factor.[122–124] A continuation of these studies performed by Kaiser and colleagues[125] demonstrated that patellar tilt is mainly influenced by knee torsion, TT–TG, and trochlear dysplasia, but not by femoral or tibial torsion. An abnormal patellar tilt, defined as more than 20° on axial computed tomography images, can be corrected surgically by performing a lateral retinacular release (or lengthening), in addition to an MPFL reconstruction, and distal realignment (if needed).[126]

Other Markers

The aforementioned risk factors are well-documented in the literature. Recent studies have shifted to novel measurements that will provide clinicians with a better understanding of the degree of patellofemoral instability and guide surgical treatment alongside the standard risk factors already used. In a study including 215 pediatric patients' MRIs, Mistovich and colleagues[127] proposed using the patellar tendon lateral to the lateral trochlear ridge distance. Their study demonstrated this measurement to be similarly sensitive to TT–TG but with higher specificity for patellofemoral dislocations.[127]

Moreover, Chassaing and colleagues[128] demonstrated that TT torsion correlated with the TT–TG and patellar tilt. In a 2021 study comparing fixed and obligatory dislocators, standard patellofemoral instability patients, and controls, Lin and colleagues[129] showed that the degree of tibiofemoral rotation correlated to the severity of patellofemoral instability. Both studies introduced these 2 novel parameters as reliable patellar instability risk factors.

SUMMARY

The management of patellar instability in young patients continues to evolve. Owing to its multifactorial nature, several demographic and anatomic risk factors need to be considered during medical decision making process. The role of MPFL is increasingly recognized and physeal-respecting MPFL reconstruction can be safely performed in skeletally immature patients. On the other hand, quadricepsplasty for fixed and habitual patellar dislocation is challenging. No single procedure is appropriate for all cases and treatment should be tailored to each patient.

DISCLOSURE

The authors have nothing to disclose.

REFERENCES

1. Weeks KD 3rd, Fabricant PD, Ladenhauf HN, et al. Surgical options for patellar stabilization in the skeletally immature patient. Sports Med Arthrosc Rev 2012; 20(3):194–202. Available at: https://www.ncbi.nlm.nih.gov/pubmed/23882722.
2. Fithian DC, Paxton EW, Stone ML, et al. Epidemiology and natural history of acute patellar dislocation. Am J Sports Med 2004;32(5):1114–21.
3. Sanders TL, Pareek A, Hewett TE, et al. Incidence of first-time lateral patellar dislocation: a 21-year population-based study. Sports Health 2018;10(2): 146–51.
4. Sillanpää P, Mattila VM, Iivonen T, et al. Incidence and risk factors of acute traumatic primary patellar dislocation. Med Sci Sports Exerc 2008;40(4):606–11.
5. Nietosvaara Y, Aalto K, Kallio PE. Acute patellar dislocation in children: incidence and associated osteochondral fractures. J Pediatr Orthop 1994;14(4): 513–5. Available at: https://www.ncbi.nlm.nih.gov/pubmed/8077438.
6. Buchner M, Baudendistel B, Sabo D, et al. Acute traumatic primary patellar dislocation: long-term results comparing conservative and surgical treatment. Clin J Sport Med 2005;15(2):62–6.
7. Kiviluoto O, Pasila M, Santavirta S, et al. Recurrences after conservative treatment of acute dislocation of the patella. Ital J Sport Traumatol 1986;3:159–62.
8. Gravesen KS, Kallemose T, Blønd L, et al. High incidence of acute and recurrent patellar dislocations: a retrospective nationwide epidemiological study involving 24.154 primary dislocations. Knee Surg Sports Traumatol Arthrosc 2018;26(4): 1204–9.
9. Atkin DM, Fithian DC, Marangi KS, et al. Characteristics of patients with primary acute lateral patellar dislocation and their recovery within the first 6 months of injury. Am J Sports Med 2000;28(4):472–9.
10. Hsiao M, Owens BD, Burks R, et al. Incidence of acute traumatic patellar dislocation among active-duty United States military service members. Am J Sports Med 2010;38(10):1997–2004.
11. Waterman BR, Belmont PJ Jr, Owens BD. Patellar dislocation in the United States: role of sex, age, race, and athletic participation. J Knee Surg 2012; 25(1):51–7.
12. Sanders TL, Pareek A, Hewett TE, et al. High rate of recurrent patellar dislocation in skeletally immature patients: a long-term population-based study. Knee Surg Sports Traumatol Arthrosc 2018;26(4):1037–43.
13. McFarlane KH, Coene RP, Feldman L, et al. Increased incidence of acute patellar dislocations and patellar instability surgical procedures across the United States in paediatric and adolescent patients. J Child Orthop 2021; 15(2):149–56.
14. Poorman MJ, Talwar D, Sanjuan J, et al. Increasing hospital admissions for patellar instability: a national database study from 2004 to 2017. Phys Sportsmed 2020;48(2):215–21.
15. Arshi A, Cohen JR, Wang JC, et al. Operative management of patellar instability in the United States: an evaluation of national practice patterns, surgical trends, and complications. Orthop J Sports Med 2016;4(8). 2325967116662873.

16. Anderson FL, Knudsen ML, Ahmad CS, et al. Current trends and impact of early sports specialization in the throwing athlete. Orthop Clin North Am 2020;51(4): 517–25.
17. Lewallen L, McIntosh A, Dahm D. First-time patellofemoral dislocation: risk factors for recurrent instability. J Knee Surg 2015;28(4):303–9.
18. Lewallen LW, McIntosh AL, Dahm DL. Predictors of recurrent instability after acute patellofemoral dislocation in pediatric and adolescent patients. Am J Sports Med 2013;41(3):575–81.
19. Mitchell J, Magnussen RA, Collins CL, et al. Epidemiology of patellofemoral instability injuries among high school athletes in the United States. Am J Sports Med 2015;43(7):1676–82.
20. Chotel F, Bérard J, Raux S. Patellar instability in children and adolescents. Orthop Traumatol Surg Res 2014;100(1 Suppl):S125–37.
21. Parikh SN, Lykissas MG. Classification of lateral patellar instability in children and adolescents. Orthop Clin North Am 2016;47(1):145–52.
22. Redler LH, Wright ML. Surgical management of patellofemoral instability in the skeletally immature patient. J Am Acad Orthop Surg 2018;26(19):e405–15.
23. Schlichte LM, Sidharthan S, Green DW, et al. Pediatric management of recurrent patellar instability. Sports Med Arthrosc Rev 2019;27(4):171–80.
24. Fabricant PD, Ladenhauf HN, Salvati EA, et al. Medial patellofemoral ligament (MPFL) reconstruction improves radiographic measures of patella alta in children. Knee 2014;21(6):1180–4.
25. Dejour H, Walch G, Neyret P, et al. [Dysplasia of the femoral trochlea]. Rev Chir Orthop Reparatrice Appar Mot 1990;76(1):45–54.
26. Paiva M, Blønd L, Hölmich P, et al. Quality assessment of radiological measurements of trochlear dysplasia; a literature review. Knee Surg Sports Traumatol Arthrosc 2018;26(3):746–55.
27. Jaquith BP, Parikh SN. Predictors of recurrent patellar instability in children and adolescents after first-time dislocation. J Pediatr Orthop 2017;37(7):484–90.
28. Dejour H, Walch G, Nove-Josserand L, et al. Factors of patellar instability: an anatomic radiographic study. Knee Surgery, Sport Traumatol Arthrosc 1994; 2(1):19–26.
29. Dickens AJ, Morrell NT, Doering A, et al. Tibial tubercle-trochlear groove distance: defining normal in a pediatric population. J Bone Jt Surg 2014;96(4): 318–24.
30. Seitlinger G, Scheurecker G, Högler R, et al. Tibial tubercle-posterior cruciate ligament distance: a new measurement to define the position of the tibial tubercle in patients with patellar dislocation. Am J Sports Med 2012;40(5):1119–25.
31. Clifton B, Richter DL, Tandberg D, et al. Evaluation of the tibial tubercle to posterior cruciate ligament distance in a pediatric patient population. J Pediatr Orthop 2017;37(6):e388–93.
32. Thévenin-Lemoine C, Ferrand M, Courvoisier A, et al. Is the Caton-Deschamps index a valuable ratio to investigate patellar height in children? J Bone Jt Surg 2011;93(8):e35.
33. Parikh SN, Redman C, Gopinathan NR. Simultaneous treatment for patellar instability and genu valgum in skeletally immature patients: a preliminary study. J Pediatr Orthop B 2019;28(2):132–8.
34. Christensen TC, Sanders TL, Pareek A, et al. Risk factors and time to recurrent ipsilateral and contralateral patellar dislocations. Am J Sports Med 2017;45(9): 2105–10.

35. Palmu S, Kallio PE, Donell ST, et al. Acute patellar dislocation in children and adolescents: a randomized clinical trial. J Bone Joint Surg Am 2008;90(3):463–70.
36. Dixit S, Deu RS. Nonoperative treatment of patellar instability. Sports Med Arthrosc Rev 2017;25(2):72–7.
37. Martinez-Cano JP, Chica J, Rincón-Escobar E, et al. Patellofemoral dislocation recurrence after a first episode: a case-control study. Orthop J Sports Med 2021;9(1). 2325967120981636.
38. Hevesi M, Heidenreich MJ, Camp CL, et al. The recurrent instability of the patella score: a statistically based model for prediction of long-term recurrence risk after first-time dislocation. Arthroscopy 2019;35(2):537–43.
39. Askenberger M, Bengtsson Moström M, Ekström W, et al. Operative repair of medial patellofemoral ligament injury versus knee brace in children with an acute first-time traumatic patellar dislocation: a randomized controlled trial. Am J Sports Med 2018;46(10):2328–40.
40. Stanitski CL, Paletta GA. Articular cartilage injury with acute patellar dislocation in adolescents. Arthroscopic and radiographic correlation. Am J Sports Med 1998;26(1):52–5.
41. Farr J, Covell DJ, Lattermann C. Cartilage lesions in patellofemoral dislocations: incidents/locations/when to treat. Sports Med Arthrosc Rev 2012;20(3):181–6.
42. Nomura E, Inoue M. Cartilage lesions of the patella in recurrent patellar dislocation. Am J Sports Med 2004;32(2):498–502.
43. Schlechter JA, Nguyen SV, Fletcher KL. Utility of bioabsorbable fixation of osteochondral lesions in the adolescent knee: outcomes analysis with minimum 2-year follow-up. Orthop J Sports Med 2019;7(10). 2325967119876896.
44. Sherman B, Vardiabasis N, Schlechter JA. Suture tape augmentation repair of the medial patellofemoral ligament. Arthrosc Tech 2019;8(10):e1159–62.
45. Beasley LS, Vidal AF. Traumatic patellar dislocation in children and adolescents: treatment update and literature review. Curr Opin Pediatr 2004;16(1):29–36.
46. Fuller JA, Hammil HL, Pronschinske KJ, et al. Operative versus nonoperative treatment after acute patellar dislocation: which is more effective at reducing recurrence in adolescents? J Sport Rehabil 2018;27(6):601–4.
47. Pagliazzi G, Napoli F, Previtali D, et al. A meta-analysis of surgical versus nonsurgical treatment of primary patella dislocation. Arthroscopy 2019;35(8): 2469–81.
48. Becher C, Schumacher T, Fleischer B, et al. The effects of a dynamic patellar realignment brace on disease determinants for patellofemoral instability in the upright weight-bearing condition. J Orthop Surg Res 2015;10:126.
49. Stefancin JJ, Parker RD. First-time traumatic patellar dislocation: a systematic review. Clin Orthop Relat Res 2007;455:93–101.
50. Mäenpää H, Lehto MU. Patellar dislocation. The long-term results of nonoperative management in 100 patients. Am J Sports Med 1997;25(2):213–7.
51. Zhang K, Jiang H, Li J, et al. Comparison between surgical and nonsurgical treatment for primary patellar dislocations in adolescents: a systematic review and meta-analysis of comparative studies. Orthop J Sports Med 2020;8(9). 2325967120946446.
52. Parikh SN, Lykissas MG, Gkiatas I. Predicting risk of recurrent patellar dislocation. Curr Rev Musculoskelet Med 2018;11(2):253–60.
53. Balcarek P, Oberthür S, Hopfensitz S, et al. Which patellae are likely to redislocate? Knee Surg Sports Traumatol Arthrosc 2014;22(10):2308–14.

54. Arendt EA, Askenberger M, Agel J, et al. Risk of redislocation after primary patellar dislocation: a clinical prediction model based on magnetic resonance imaging variables. Am J Sports Med 2018;46(14):3385–90.
55. Ling DI, Brady JM, Arendt E, et al. Development of a multivariable model based on individual risk factors for recurrent lateral patellar dislocation. J Bone Joint Surg Am 2021;103(7):586–92.
56. Huntington LS, Webster KE, Devitt BM, et al. Factors associated with an increased risk of recurrence after a first-time patellar dislocation: a systematic review and meta-analysis. Am J Sports Med 2020;48(10):2552–62.
57. Tuxøe JI, Teir M, Winge S, et al. The medial patellofemoral ligament: a dissection study. Knee Surg Sports Traumatol Arthrosc 2002;10(3):138–40.
58. Kang HJ, Wang F, Chen BC, et al. Functional bundles of the medial patellofemoral ligament. Knee Surg Sports Traumatol Arthrosc 2010;18(11):1511–6.
59. Nomura E, Inoue M, Osada N. Anatomical analysis of the medial patellofemoral ligament of the knee, especially the femoral attachment. Knee Surg Sports Traumatol Arthrosc 2005;13(7):510–5.
60. Nelitz M, Dornacher D, Dreyhaupt J, et al. The relation of the distal femoral physis and the medial patellofemoral ligament. Knee Surg Sports Traumatol Arthrosc 2011;19(12):2067–71.
61. Shea KG, Martinson WD, Cannamela PC, et al. Variation in the medial patellofemoral ligament origin in the skeletally immature knee: an anatomic study. Am J Sports Med 2018;46(2):363–9.
62. Avikainen VJ, Nikku RK, Seppänen-Lehmonen TK. Adductor magnus tenodesis for patellar dislocation. Technique and preliminary results. Clin Orthop Relat Res 1993;(297):12–6.
63. Deie M, Ochi M, Sumen Y, et al. Reconstruction of the medial patellofemoral ligament for the treatment of habitual or recurrent dislocation of the patella in children. J Bone Joint Surg Br 2003;85(6):887–90.
64. Nguyen CV, Farrow LD, Liu RW, et al. Safe drilling paths in the distal femoral epiphysis for pediatric medial patellofemoral ligament reconstruction. Am J Sports Med 2017;45(5):1085–9.
65. Black SR, Meyers KN, Nguyen JT, et al. Comparison of ligament isometry and patellofemoral contact pressures for medial patellofemoral ligament reconstruction techniques in skeletally immature patients. Am J Sports Med 2020;48(14):3557–65.
66. Shea KG, Polousky JD, Jacobs JC Jr, et al. The patellar insertion of the medial patellofemoral ligament in children: a cadaveric study. J Pediatr Orthop 2015;35(4):e31–5.
67. Nelitz M, Williams SR. Anatomic reconstruction of the medial patellofemoral ligament in children and adolescents using a pedicled quadriceps tendon graft. Arthrosc Tech 2014;3(2):e303–8.
68. Parikh SN. Medial Patellofemoral ligament reconstruction in skeletally immature patients. Tech Knee Surg 2011;10(3):171–7.
69. Spang RC, Tepolt FA, Paschos NK, et al. Combined reconstruction of the medial patellofemoral ligament (MPFL) and medial quadriceps tendon-femoral ligament (MQTFL) for patellar instability in children and adolescents: surgical technique and outcomes. J. Pediatr Orthop 2019;39(1):e54–61.
70. Parikh SN, Nathan ST, Wall EJ, et al. Complications of medial patellofemoral ligament reconstruction in young patients. Am J Sports Med 2013;41(5):1030–8.

71. Nelitz M, Williams RS, Lippacher S, et al. Analysis of failure and clinical outcome after unsuccessful medial patellofemoral ligament reconstruction in young patients. Int Orthop 2014;38(11):2265–72.

72. Danino B, Deliberato D, Abousamra O, et al. Four-in-one extensor realignment for the treatment of obligatory or fixed, lateral patellar instability in skeletally immature knee. J Pediatr Orthop 2020;40(9). https://doi.org/10.1097/BPO. 0000000000001610.

73. Crosby EB, Insall J. Recurrent dislocation of the patella. Relation of treatment to osteoarthritis. J Bone Jt Surg - Ser A 1976;58(1):9–13.

74. Curtis BH, Fisher RL. Congenital hyperextension with anterior subluxation of the knee. Surgical treatment and long-term observations. J Bone Joint Surg Am 1969;51(2):255–69.

75. Sever R, Fishkin M, Hemo Y, et al. Surgical treatment of congenital and obligatory dislocation of the patella in children. J Pediatr Orthop 2019;39(8):436–40.

76. Ellsworth B, Hidalgo Perea S, Green DW. Stepwise lengthening of the quadriceps extensor mechanism for severe obligatory and fixed patella dislocators. Arthrosc Tech 2021;10(5):e1327–31.

77. Williams PF. Quadriceps contracture. J Bone Joint Surg Br 1968;50(2):278–84.

78. Jones RWS, Fisher RL, Curtis BH. Congenital dislocation of the patella. Clin Orthop Relat Res 1976;119(119):177–83.

79. Stanisavljevic S, Zemenick G, Miller D. Congenital, irreducible, permanent lateral dislocation of the patella. Clin Orthop Relat Res 1976;116:190–9.

80. Gao G, Lee E, Bose K. Surgical management of congenital and habitual dislocation of the patella. J Pediatr Orthop 1990;10(2):255–60.

81. Gordon JE, Schoenecker PL. Surgical treatment of congenital dislocation of the patella. J Pediatr Orthop 1999;19(2):260–4.

82. Eilert RE. Congenital dislocation of the patella. In: Atik OS, editor. Clinical orthopaedics and related research. Philadelphia, PA: Lippincott Williams and Wilkins; 2001. p. 22–9.

83. Martin BD, Cherkashin AM, Tulchin K, et al. Treatment of femoral lengthening-related knee stiffness with a novel quadricepsplasty. J Pediatr Orthop 2013; 33(4):446–52.

84. Inan M, Sarikaya IA, Şeker A, et al. A combined procedure for irreducible dislocation of patella in children with ligamentous laxity: a preliminary report. Acta Orthop Traumatol Turc 2015;49(5):530–8.

85. Niedzielski KR, Malecki K, Flont P, et al. The results of an extensive soft-tissue procedure in the treatment of obligatory patellar dislocation in children with ligamentous laxity: a post-operative isokinetic study. Bone Joint J 2015;97-B(1): 129–33.

86. Marumo K, Fujii K, Tanaka T, et al. Surgical management of congenital permanent dislocation of the patella in nail patella syndrome by Stanisavljevic procedure. J Orthop Sci 1999;4(6):446–9.

87. Ceynowa M, Mazurek T. Congenital patella dislocation in a child with Rubinstein–Taybi syndrome. J Pediatr Orthop B 2009;18(1):47–50.

88. Ghanem I, Wattincourt L, Seringe R. Congenital dislocation of the patella. Part II: orthopaedic management. J Pediatr Orthop 2000;20(6):817–22.

89. Wada A, Fujii T, Takamura K, et al. Congenital dislocation of the patella. J Child Orthop 2008;2(2):119–23.

90. Camathias C, Rutz E, Götze M, et al. Poor outcome at 7.5 years after Stanisavljevic quadriceps transposition for patello-femoral instability. Arch Orthop Trauma Surg 2014;134(4):473–8.

91. Joo SY, Park KB, Kim BR, et al. The "four-in-one" procedure for habitual dislocation of the patella in children: Early results in patients with severe generalised
ligamentous laxity and aplasis of the trochlear groove. J Bone Jt Surg - Ser B
2007;89(12):1645–9.
92. Wolfe S, Varacallo M, Thomas J, et al. Patellar instability. StatPearls Publishing;
2020.
93. Brattström H. Patella alta in non-dislocating knee joints. Acta Orthop 1970;41(5):
578–88.
94. Holtzman GW, Harris-Hayes M. Treatment of patella alta with taping, exercise,
mobilization, and functional activity modification: a case report. Physiother
Theor Pract 2012;28(1):71–83.
95. Jacobsen K, Bertheussen K. the vertical location of the patella: fundamental
views on the concept patella alta, using a normal sample. Acta Orthop 1974;
45(1–4):436–45.
96. Ward SR, Terk MR, Powers CM. Influence of patella alta on knee extensor mechanics. J Biomech 2005;38(12):2415–22.
97. Ward SR, Powers CM. The influence of patella alta on patellofemoral joint stress
during normal and fast walking. Clin Biomech 2004;19(10):1040–7.
98. Otsuki S, Nakajima M, Fujiwara K, et al. Influence of age on clinical outcomes of
three-dimensional transfer of the tibial tuberosity for patellar instability with patella alta. Knee Surgery, Sport Traumatol Arthrosc 2017;25(8):2392–6.
99. Antinolfi P, Bartoli M, Placella G, et al. Acute patellofemoral instability in children
and adolescents. Joints 2016;4(1):47–51.
100. Lykissas MG, Li T, Eismann EA, et al. Does medial patellofemoral ligament
reconstruction decrease patellar height? A preliminary report. J Pediatr Orthop
2014;34(1):78–85.
101. Bollier M, Fulkerson JP. The role of trochlear dysplasia in patellofemoral instability. J Am Acad Orthop Surg 2011;19(1):8–16.
102. Batailler C, Neyret P. Trochlear dysplasia: imaging and treatment options.
EFORT Open Rev 2018;3(5):240–7.
103. Fucentese SF, Zingg PO, Schmitt J, et al. Classification of trochlear dysplasia as
predictor of clinical outcome after trochleoplasty. Knee Surgery, Sport Traumatol
Arthrosc 2011;19(10):1655–61.
104. Balcarek P, Zimmermann F. Deepening trochleoplasty and medial patellofemoral
ligament reconstruction normalize patellotrochlear congruence in severe trochlear dysplasia. Bone Joint J 2019;101-B(3):325–30.
105. Thaunat M, Bessiere C, Pujol N, et al. Recession wedge trochleoplasty as an
additional procedure in the surgical treatment of patellar instability with major
trochlear dysplasia: early results. Orthop Traumatol Surg Res 2011;97(8):
833–45.
106. Green DW. Surgical treatment of pediatric patella instability. In: Die therapie der
instabilen patella. AGA-Komitee-Knie-Patellofemoral; 2016. p. 80–90.
107. Brady JM, Rosencrans AS, Shubin Stein BE. Use of TT-PCL versus TT-TG. Curr
Rev Musculoskelet Med 2018;11(2):261–5.
108. Heidenreich MJ, Camp CL, Dahm DL, et al. The contribution of the tibial tubercle
to patellar instability: analysis of tibial tubercle–trochlear groove (TT-TG) and
tibial tubercle–posterior cruciate ligament (TT-PCL) distances. Knee Surgery,
Sport Traumatol Arthrosc 2017;25(8):2347–51.
109. Maquet P. Biomechanics of the knee: with application to the pathogenesis and
the surgical treatment of osteoarthritis. 2nd edition. Springer-Verlag; 1984.
110. Paley D. Principles of deformity correction. 1st edition. Springer; 2002.

111. Brauwer V De, Moens P. Temporary hemiepiphysiodesis for idiopathic genua valga in adolescents: percutaneous transphyseal screws (PETS) versus stapling. J Pediatr Orthop 2008;28(5):549–54.
112. Castañeda P, Urquhart B, Sullivan E, et al. Hemiepiphysiodesis for the correction of angular deformity about the knee. J Pediatr Orthop 2008;28(2):188–91.
113. Lin KM, Thacher RR, Apostolakos JM, et al. Implant-mediated guided growth for coronal plane angular deformity in the pediatric patient with patellofemoral instability. Arthrosc Tech 2021;10(3):e913–24.
114. Lee T, Anzel S, Bennett K, et al. The influence of fixed rotational deformities of the femur on the patellofemoral contact pressures in human cadaver knees. Clin Orthop Relat Res 1994;302:69–74.
115. Dejour D, Le Coultre B. Osteotomies in patello-femoral instabilities. Sports Med Arthrosc 2007;15(1):39–46.
116. Diederichs G, Köhlitz T, Kornaropoulos E, et al. Magnetic resonance imaging analysis of rotational alignment in patients with patellar dislocations. Am J Sports Med 2013;41(1):51–7.
117. Zhang ZJ, Zhang H, Song GY, et al. Increased femoral anteversion is associated with inferior clinical outcomes after MPFL reconstruction and combined tibial tubercle osteotomy for the treatment of recurrent patellar instability. Knee Surg Sport Traumatol Arthrosc 2020;28(7):2261–9.
118. Dickschas J, Harrer J, Pfefferkorn R, et al. Operative treatment of patellofemoral maltracking with torsional osteotomy. Arch Orthop Trauma Surg 2012;132(3): 289–98.
119. Ateschrang A, Freude T, Grünwald L, et al. Patellaluxation: Diagnostik- und Behandlungsalgorithmus unter Berücksichtigung der Torsion. Z Orthop Unfall 2014;152(1):59–67.
120. Hinterwimmer S, Rosenstiel N, Lenich A, et al. Femorale Osteotomien bei patellofemoraler Instabilität. Unfallchirurg 2012;115(5):410–6.
121. Fulkerson JP, Shea KP. Disorders of patellofemoral alignment. J Bone Jt Surg - Ser A 1990;72(9):1424–9.
122. Saggin PRF, Saggin JI, Dejour D. Imaging in patellofemoral instability: An abnormality-based approach. Sports Med Arthrosc 2012;20(3):145–51.
123. Waldt S, Rummeny EJ. Bildgebung der patellofemoralen Instabilität. Radiologe 2012;52(11):1003–11.
124. Fucentese SF. Patellainstabilität. Orthopade 2018;47(1):77–86.
125. Kaiser P, Loth F, Attal R, et al. Static patella tilt and axial engagement in knee extension are mainly influenced by knee torsion, the tibial tubercle-trochlear groove distance (TTTG), and trochlear dysplasia but not by femoral or tibial torsion. Knee Surg Sports Traumatol Arthrosc 2020;28(3):952–9.
126. Fithian DC, Neyret P, Servien E. Patellar instability: the Lyon experience. Tech Knee Surg 2007;6(2):112–23.
127. Mistovich RJ, Urwin JW, Fabricant PD, et al. Patellar tendon–lateral trochlear ridge distance: a novel measurement of patellofemoral instability. Am J Sports Med 2018;46(14):3400–6.
128. Chassaing V, Zeitoun JM, Camara M, et al. Tibial tubercle torsion, a new factor of patellar instability. Orthop Traumatol Surg Res 2017;103(8):1173–8.
129. Lin KM, James EW, Aitchison AH, et al. Increased tibiofemoral rotation on MRI with increasing clinical severity of patellar instability. Knee Surgery, Sport Traumatol Arthrosc 2021. https://doi.org/10.1007/s00167-020-06382-x.

Tibial Spine Fractures in Young Athletes

Aristides I. Cruz Jr, MD, MBA[a],*, Rushyuan Jay Lee, MD[b], Indranil Kushare, MD[c], Soroush Baghdadi, MD[d], Daniel W. Green, MD, MS[e], Theodore J. Ganley, MD[f], Henry B. Ellis Jr, MD[g], PRiSM[i], Tibial Spine Research Interest Group[j] Ronald Justin Mistovich, MD, MBA[h]

KEYWORDS

- Eminence • Sports • Injury • Knee • ACL

KEY POINTS

- Tibial spine fractures are a relatively uncommon injury accounting for 2% to 5% of traumatic knee arthroses in adolescents and most commonly occur at an average age of 11 to 12 years.
- Definitive management depends on the amount of fracture displacement and the presence of associated injuries.
- Arthroscopic treatment offers the advantage of addressing concomitant intraarticular injury.
- Arthrofibrosis is the most common complication after operative treatment, but others include hardware related complications and subsequent anterior cruciate ligament tear.
- Further research is needed with regards to the role of diagnostic magnetic resonance imaging, amount of acceptable fracture displacement, and optimal fixation options.

[a] Department of Orthopedics, Warren Alpert Medical School of Brown University, Hasbro Children's Hospital, Providence, RI, USA; [b] Department of Orthopedic Surgery, The Johns Hopkins Hospital/Johns Hopkins Bloomberg Children's Center, Baltimore, MD, USA; [c] Department of Orthopedic Surgery, Texas Children's Hospital, Houston, TX, USA; [d] Children's Hospital of Philadelphia, Philadelphia, PA, USA; [e] Weill Cornell Medical College, Hospital for Special Surgery, New York, NY, USA; [f] Perelman School of Medicine at the University of Pennsylvania, Children's Hospital of Philadelphia, Philadelphia, PA, USA; [g] Department of Orthopaedic Surgery, UT Southwestern Medical Center, Texas Scottish Rite Hospital for Children, Dallas, TX, USA; [h] Case Western Reserve University School of Medicine, Rainbow Babies & Children's Hospital, Cleveland, OH, USA; [i] Pediatric Research in Sports Medicine; [j] Julien Aoyama, BA, Peter D. Fabricant, MD, MPH, Daniel W. Green, MD, Benjamin Johnson, PA-C, Scott D. McKay, MD, Todd A. Millbrandt, MD, Neeraj M. Patel, MD, MPH, MBS, Jason T. Rhodes, MD, Brant C. Sachleben, MD, Gregory A. Schmale, MD, Jessica L. Traver, MD, Yi-Meng Yen, MD, PhD
* Corresponding author. 1 Kettle Point Avenue, East Providence, RI 02914.
E-mail address: aristides.cruz@gmail.com

Clin Sports Med 41 (2022) 653–670
https://doi.org/10.1016/j.csm.2022.05.006
0278-5919/22/© 2022 Elsevier Inc. All rights reserved.

INTRODUCTION

Tibial spine fractures (TSFs) represent an avulsion injury of the anterior cruciate liga-ment (ACL) from its insertion on the proximal tibia that typically occurs in early adoles-cence. These injuries are relatively rare and historically were considered as analogous to a pediatric ACL injury, which were thought to be even less common. However, with more recent studies examining both pediatric ACL injuries and TSFs, these two in-juries are now understood to be distinct entities. Although there may be some overlap between these two diagnoses, the clinical presentation, diagnostic evaluation, and treatment principles often differ.

ANATOMY

The tibial spines (or tibial intercondylar eminences) of the knee consist of two promi-nences (medial and lateral) located in the intercondylar region of the tibial plateau (**Fig. 1**). Although a TSF represents an avulsion of the ACL from the tibia, the ACL does not actually insert directly onto either the medial or lateral tibial spine.[1–3] Both the posterolateral (PL) and anteromedial (AM) bundles of the ACL insert anterior and between the medial and lateral tibial spines in the intercondylar region. The lateral tibial eminence is posterior and lateral to the ACL center (11.0 ± 0.3 mm), AM bundle center (14.1 ± 0.5 mm), and PL bundle center (8.9 ± 0.4 mm).[1] The lateral tibial spine is commonly anterior to the medial tibial spine and because of this, the lateral tibial spine is commonly used as an anatomic landmark during arthroscopy. The medial tibial spine is directly anterior to the posterior medial meniscal root (**Fig. 2**).

The intercondylar region is the non-articulating area between the medial and lateral tibial spine. Although a TSF typically occurs in the intercondylar region, fracture prop-agation can extend onto the weight bearing tibial plateau, with the medial tibial plateau most frequently involved.[4,5] The ossification pattern of the immature skeleton may pre-dispose young patients to this injury. In skeletally immature patients, the intercondylar region is incompletely ossified and thus weaker than the ACL complex. The location of a TSF is commonly deep to the subchondral plate in the cancellous, epiphyseal, non-ossified bone of skeletally immature patients.

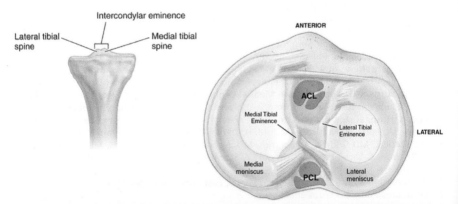

Fig. 1. Drawing (frontal and axial) of the tibial plateau of a right knee. Note the highlighted areas represent the insertion of the posterior and anterior cruciate ligament. The promi-nences in the center of this images note the medial and lateral tibial spine.

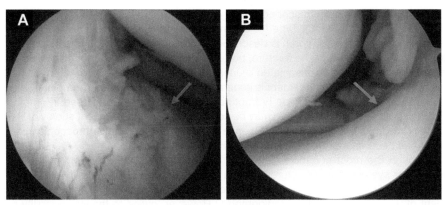

Fig. 2. (*A*) Red arrow points to lateral tibial spine adjacent to ACL tibial insertion. (*B*) Blue arrow points to medial tibial spine just anterior to medial meniscal posterior root.

EPIDEMIOLOGY

TSFs occur at an annual incidence of 3 per 100,000 persons and in 2% to 5% of traumatic knee hemarthroses in adolescents.[6–8] A recent systematic review and several large multicenter studies have reported these injuries to occur in patients with a mean age of 11.0 to 12.4 years with a range from 3.5 to 21.0 years.[9,10] A multicenter collaboration of 471 TSF found that 73% of TSF patients were less than 14 years old and a majority of those were between 12 and 14 years old.[11] TSFs are more common in male individuals than female individuals.[9,10] In a retrospective review of 122 cases of TSFs, females with TSFs were more likely to be younger than males (9.8 vs 11.6 years, $P = .004$), and displaced TSFs were more likely in younger patients (<11.5 years old, $P = .02$).[10] Higher patient body mass index has also been associated with higher grade fracture severity.[11]

Like ACL ruptures, TSFs typically occur during a pivoting, rotational maneuver in a partially flexed knee or via a hyperextension mechanism. Historically, TSFs have been known to occur during a bicycle related injury in children. More recent, large series confirm that bicycle related injury is common (20.4%); however, the most common mechanism of injury is from organized sports (39.9%)[9,10] (**Table 1**) with American football accounting for 53% of injuries in one study.[11]

CLASSIFICATION

Meyers and McKeever[12] were the first to provide a descriptive classification of TSFs. This classification is based on the fracture displacement measured on the lateral

Table 1 Mechanism of injury combining the two largest multicenter epidemiologic series and a systematic review of tibial spine fractures[9–11]	
Organized sports	39.9%
Bicycle	20.4%
Outdoor sports	19.1%
Motor vehicle collision	10.9%
Other	9.7%

radiograph and originally described three types (Type I-III); this was later modified to include a Type IV[13] (**Fig. 3**). Type I is a non- or minimally displaced TSF and can be treated non-operatively. Type II is described as a displaced TSF with an intact hinge in the posterior aspect of the fracture, potentially amenable to nonoperative or operative treatment (based on associated injuries and ability to obtain a satisfactory closed reduction). Operative management is generally considered for Type III completely displaced fractures as well as Type IV fractures (comminuted and/or flipped fragment). Arthroscopic or open approaches may be considered, although a recent survey of Pediatric Orthopedic Society of North America members showed that arthroscopic treatment has become more common than open treatment.[14]

Although the most common method to classify these injuries is the Meyers and McKeever system, many fractures can be difficult to definitively classify. A reliable measure for tibial spine displacement has been the measurement of superior displacement of the TSF on the lateral radiograph.[15] However, owing to the low reliability of other radiographic measures of fracture severity as well as high rates of associated soft-tissue injuries,[15,16] an magnetic resonance imaging (MRI) evaluation and classification may also be useful. Green and colleagues proposed a novel MRI-based classification system, with Grade 1 fractures having ≤2 mm of displacement, Grade 2 fractures showing an intact posterior hinge with greater than 2 mm of anterior lip displacement but ≤2 mm of posterior displacement, and Grade 3 fractures having either greater than 2 mm of posterior displacement, meniscal entrapment, or extension to the weight bearing surface of the medial or lateral tibial plateau with greater than 2 mm of displacement[17] (**Fig. 4**). In the authors' study, this classification system showed fair-to-moderate interrater reliability.

DIAGNOSIS
Physical Examination

Patients who have sustained a TSF typically present with a large knee effusion, difficulty bearing weight, and pain with attempted knee range of motion (ROM). The patient should be placed in a gown or shorts such that both lower extremities can be visualized, and an unimpeded physical examination can be performed.[18] When palpating the knee, one should assess for areas of focal tenderness, paying careful attention to medial or lateral joint line tenderness, which could be associated with concomitant meniscal pathology. If tolerated by the patient, the examiner should assess knee ROM and determine if motion is limited by pain or a mechanical block.

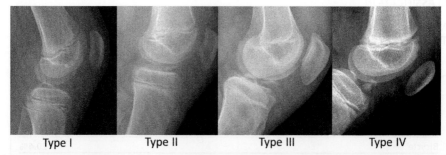

| Type I | Type II | Type III | Type IV |

Fig. 3. Meyers and McKeever radiographic classification for tibial spine fractures based on the lateral radiograph. Type I = non-displaced. Type II = displacement of the anterior lip with an intact posterior hinge. Type III = fracture is completely displaced including with displaced posterior hinge. Type IV = comminuted and/or flipped fragment.

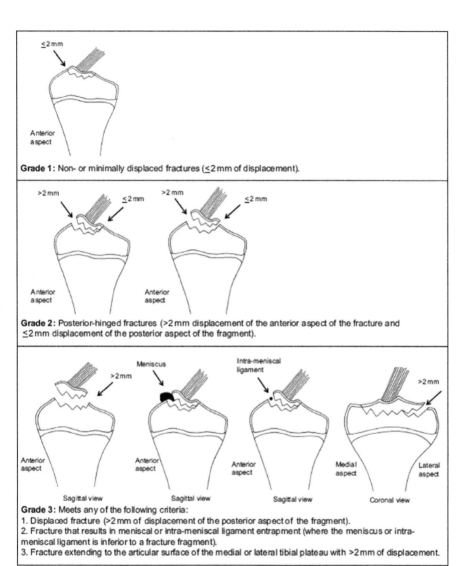

Grade 1: Non- or minimally displaced fractures (≤2 mm of displacement).

Grade 2: Posterior-hinged fractures (>2 mm displacement of the anterior aspect of the fracture and ≤2 mm displacement of the posterior aspect of the fragment).

Grade 3: Meets any of the following criteria:
1. Displaced fracture (>2 mm of displacement of the posterior aspect of the fragment).
2. Fracture that results in meniscal or intra-meniscal ligament entrapment (where the meniscus or intra-meniscal ligament is inferior to a fracture fragment).
3. Fracture extending to the articular surface of the medial or lateral tibial plateau with >2 mm of displacement.

Fig. 4. Green MRI classification of tibial spine fractures. (*Reproduced from*: Green D, Tuca M, Luderowski E, Gausden E, Goodbody C, Konin G. A new, MRI-based classification system for tibial spine fractures changes clinical treatment recommendations when compared to Myers and McKeever. Knee Surg Sports Traumatol Arthrosc. 2019 Jan;27(1):86-92. https://doi.org/10.1007/s00167-018-5039-7. Epub 2018 Jun 30. PMID: 29961096.)

Depending on the fracture severity and magnitude of displacement, the Lachman maneuver may be positive. However, in the acute post-injury setting, patients often show substantial guarding, which may limit the sensitivity of this maneuver. In addition, in the acute setting, patients will often not tolerate knee flexion to 90° for a formal anterior drawer or posterior drawer testing. Further adding to the diagnostic complexity, pain associated with the fracture often limits the specificity of the McMurray test for meniscal tears. Similarly, the assessment of medial or lateral collateral ligament injuries may be limited in because of the pain often associated with the acute fracture. Moderate- to high-grade medial collateral ligament (MCL) or lateral collateral ligament (LCL) tears are frequently discernible on physical examination, though the authors caution that guarding associated with the primary injury may limit the utility of these physical examination maneuvers.

Imaging Studies

Patients should have routine anterior-posterior and lateral radiographs performed of the affected knee. The fracture is nearly always discernible on plain films, though avulsions with only a small fragment of bone attached to the ACL tibial insertion can be difficult to visualize without careful radiographic assessment (**Fig. 5**). It is essential for the treating surgeon to recognize that TSFs often do not occur in isolation, but rather are frequently accompanied by concomitant injuries. The reported rate of concomitant injuries has ranged from 40% to 68.8%.[16,19–21] A recent study by Shimberg and colleagues[22] found that 45% of patients who underwent MRI after sustaining a TSF had a concomitant injury identified with 82% of these injuries requiring further operative management. The authors suggested that concomitant soft tissue and cartilaginous injuries may go undiagnosed in some patients who do not undergo advanced imaging, especially those treated with a closed reduction or a mini open approach (ie, without diagnostic arthroscopy). However, the long-term clinical sequalae of these undiagnosed injuries remains uncertain.

As mentioned above, MRI can also be used to help classify TSFs.[17] In addition to the MRI-based classification system described by Green and colleagues, the investigators in Green's study identified fractures in 6.9% of cases that were not readily apparent on plain radiographs. In 13.1% of cases, raters also increased the grade of the fracture using the MRI-based classification schema compared with the traditional Meyers and McKeever system. The use of advanced imaging to diagnose and classify TSFs remains an area of interest.

NONOPERATIVE TREATMENT

The treatment strategy for TSFs is primarily determined by the degree of bony displacement. Nondisplaced fractures are typically immobilized with the knee in

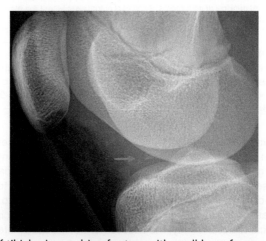

Fig. 5. Example of tibial spine avulsion fracture with small bony fragment.

extension and limited weightbearing.[9,23–26] As noted above, before the decision to proceed with nonoperative treatment, MRI may be performed to confirm the absence of concomitant injuries needing surgical intervention.[16,22,27,28]

Closed Reduction

Recent data suggest that less than half of pediatric orthopedic surgeons perform closed reduction for Meyers and McKeever Type II TSFs.[14] The evolving understanding of soft-tissue entrapment,[16,22,27,29] risk for nonunion and impingement,[30] concomitant injuries,[16,28] and propensity for residual ACL laxity and reinjury[31] may have influenced surgeons to prefer open or arthroscopic reduction and internal fixation over closed reduction in recent years. However, previous research suggests that there remains value in the closed management of a displaced TSF, particularly given the decreased risk of posttreatment arthrofibrosis compared with operative treatment.[24,26,32] Closed reduction of Type II TSFs that results in less than 5 mm of residual anterior displacement leads to good outcomes (as measured by posttreatment Lysholm scores, rates of arthrofibrosis, and visual analog scale pain scores).[32] However, compared with Type II fractures, Type III TSFs may have more concomitant injuries, less intrinsic bony stability, and higher rates of soft-tissue entrapment.[32] Thus, as mentioned previously, surgeons should consider using MRI to evaluate for concomitant injuries and should counsel families about the potential need for additional surgical procedures at the time of treatment for the TSF.[16,28]

Closed Reduction Technique

Ideally, a closed reduction should be performed within 48 h of the injury and with the patient under adequate analgesia/sedation. Aspiration of the hemarthrosis may aid with manipulation of the knee, and intraarticular injection of an analgesic/anesthetic agent may help with post-procedure pain. First, the knee is flexed to 90° to mobilize the tibial spine fragment. As the knee is extended to approximately 30°, a Lachman maneuver is performed, putting tension on the ACL, pulling the tibial spine posteriorly while there is anterior translation of the tibia. This maneuver will promote mobility of any soft tissue (eg, anterior horn of the medial meniscus or the transverse intermeniscal ligament) that is entrapped beneath the fracture fragment to enable reduction of the fragment. Anterior translation is maintained while further extending the knee to 0°. After reduction, lateral fluoroscopic or radiographic imaging with the knee in terminal extension is used to confirm adequacy of the reduction (**Fig. 6**). An MRI can be used to confirm fracture reduction and absence of concomitant injuries, and to evaluate for injury to the substance of the ACL. If an acceptable reduction is obtained, then a long leg cast or knee brace is placed with the knee in extension. Weekly radiographs are recommended to ensure maintenance of reduction. After 3 to 4 weeks of immobilization, the patient should begin ROM exercises with a physical therapist and may initiate weight-bearing with the knee locked in extension for three additional weeks.

OPERATIVE TREATMENT

Various techniques have been described for operative fixation, including screws, sutures, and suture anchors, each offering advantages and disadvantages.[33–41] The goals of surgical management are solid fracture stabilization to allow early restoration of knee ROM, minimization of ACL laxity, and ultimately, bony union to allow return to normal function. Existing research does not indicate a "gold standard" for TSF fixation, with multiple methods of reduction and fixation showing comparable clinical

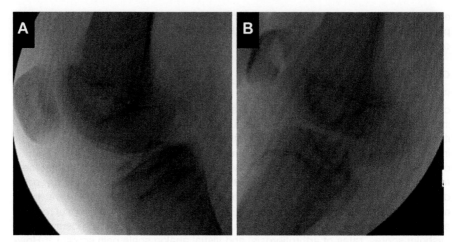

Fig. 6. (*A*) Intraoperative lateral fluoroscopic image of Type II tibial spine fracture before reduction. (*B*) Knee hyperextension maneuver used to reduce Type II tibial spine fracture.

outcomes.[23,25,30,33] Therefore, the approach is dictated by patient, fracture, and concomitant injury characteristics, as well as surgeon preference.

Arthroscopic Techniques

Although open reduction and internal fixation of TSFs have been performed for decades, arthroscopic techniques have advanced considerably.[42,43] The initial step in arthroscopic surgery, after establishing standard AM and anterolateral portals, is evacuation of the hemarthrosis and fracture hematoma (**Fig. 7**A). Standard diagnostic arthroscopy is used to identify the tibial spine avulsion, debride fracture hematoma and early callus, and debride the fracture bed to punctate bleeding bone. This promotes contact between the fragment and its bed to support bony healing and allows for appropriate ACL tension. As an additional consideration, the ACL may undergo some degree of stretch accompanying a TSF. Therefore, even an anatomic reduction of the fracture may result in increased ACL laxity. To correct this, some surgeons consider a more aggressive debridement of the fracture bed, allowing recession of the TSF to allow restoration of appropriate ACL tension with fracture reduction.

If the knee cannot fully extend, this suggests incarcerated tissue at the fracture site, most commonly the anterior horn of the medial meniscus or the intermeniscal ligament.[22,44] To retract these blocks to reduction, an 18-gauge spinal needle can be inserted "outside-in" under the anterior horn of the meniscus (**Fig. 7**B), through which a nonbraided suture can be passed. The suture can then retract the blocking soft-tissue anteriorly (**Fig. 7**C). After removal of any obstacles to reduction, the fracture can be reduced with a combination of knee extension, manipulation with instrumentation (ie, standard ACL tibial guide or a K-wire inserted into the fracture as a joystick), and/or a traction suture (**Fig. 7**D). Use of accessory superolateral, superomedial, or transpatellar portals is recommended for suture and instrumentation management and better visualization during TSF reduction and fixation.[45] After the fracture is reduced, a K-wire can be placed from a superomedial or superolateral entry for temporary fixation of the fracture (see **Fig. 7**D).

Fracture Fixation

Multiple implants have been described for TSF fixation.[23,33,34,38,40,41,43] The most common methods are described below.

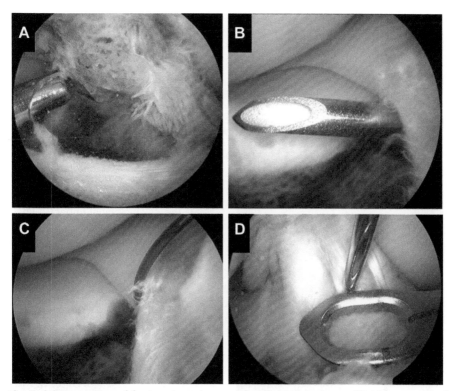

Fig. 7. (*A*) Evacuation of fracture hematoma with arthroscopic shaver. (*B*) 18-gauge spinal needle passed under intermeniscal ligament to facilitate passage of non-braided suture. (*C*) Non-braided suture used to retract intermeniscal ligament from fracture bed. (*D*) Instrumented reduction facilitated by standard ACL guide with provisional K-wire fixation of the tibial spine fracture.

Screw fixation

Screw fixation should only be considered when the fracture fragment is deemed large enough, to avoid comminution during drilling and fixation. After fracture reduction, a superomedial or superolateral portal is created with the knee in 80° to 90° of flexion and two guidewires are placed across the fracture. The reduction is confirmed arthroscopically and fluoroscopically. Screw fixation can also be used via open (as opposed to arthroscopic) methods. Care must be taken not to flex or extend the knee while obtaining the lateral fluoroscopic image to avoid bending the K-wire. Lateral images are needed to avoid placing a screw across the physis in skeletally immature patients. In patients who are closer to skeletal maturity, the physis can be crossed to obtain better screw purchase. Fixation is performed with two partially threaded, self-tapping, cannulated 4.0 mm screws inserted over the guidewires. A washer can be used to distribute compressive forces (**Fig. 8**). If the patient is skeletally immature and the screws cross the proximal tibial physis, the screws should be removed after fracture union. In addition, many surgeons elect to remove screws since they are located intra-articularly, which is a disadvantage of screw fixation.[46]

Suture fixation

One of two approaches for suture stabilization can be used. An arthroscopic suture passer is used to pass sutures and capture the base of the ACL. In one method,

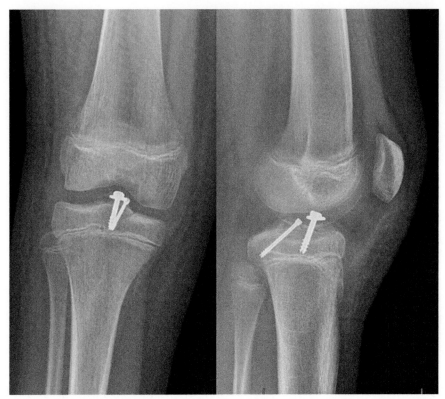

Fig. 8. Cannulated screw fixation with washer. Note that the screws do not cross the physis of this skeletally immature patient.

bone tunnels are drilled through the base of the TSF bed, using an ACL tibial drill guide. These sutures are then shuttled through the bone tunnels and used to reduce the ACL. If the avulsion fracture is a large enough fragment, stabilization with a K-wire may be used before tunnel drilling. With the fracture reduced, a tunnel can be drilled that travels through the avulsion fragment, directly in line with the anterior aspect of the ACL base.[42] Alternatively, bone tunnels can be drilled medial and lateral to the bone fragment, rather than through the bone fragment itself.[34]

When drilling bone tunnels, all-epiphyseal trajectories are technically challenging because of bone tunnel position, suture shuttling, and use of the suture for fracture reduction. However, all-epiphyseal fixation could be considered for young patients to help avoid physeal injury. All-epiphyseal fixation techniques include intraarticular epiphyseal suture anchor fixation and all-epiphyseal bone tunnels with the sutures traversing extra-osseously on the anterior cortex of the tibia, and fixed distal to the tibial physis as described by Allen Anderson for physeal sparing ACL reconstruction.[47] Transphyseal sutures are less technically challenging than all-epiphyseal sutures, but future growth potential should be assessed in skeletally immature patients. The ACL tibial guide is used to pass two to three drill tunnels from the AM aspect of the tibia to the base of the fracture. One must leave an adequate bone bridge at the AM cortex of the tibia to tie the sutures if attempting a suture only construct. The locations where these tunnels exit intraarticularly can be distributed medially and laterally or anteriorly and posteriorly relative to the base of the TSF depending on the fracture pattern and size. Suture passing devices are then passed through the drill tunnels to shuttle the sutures for fixation.

Under direct intraarticular visualization, options to pass the sutures through the tibial drill tunnels include a semirigid plastic tube, metal suture passing devices, and a Hewson suture passer. Suture fixation can be performed with high tensile strength, nonabsorbable suture or a heavy absorbable suture. Absorbable suture can be considered if there is a desire for temporary fixation to minimize the possibility of physeal tethering.

The sutures are tensioned at the AM aspect of the tibia, whereas the fragment is directly visualized to confirm anatomic reduction or slight recession into the fracture bed. The arthroscope is removed, and the knee is brought to 30° of flexion for final tensioning and tying of the sutures. Other methods to secure the sutures to the proximal tibia include tying the sutures over a suture button, screw and post, or fixation with a knotless suture anchor. After fixation, the knee is re-examined for stability using the Lachman maneuver and for ROM to confirm the absence of a block to knee extension and the integrity of the repair.

Final fluoroscopic images can be taken to confirm and document the reduction radiographically. Some degree of anterior lip displacement of the fracture is often seen in lateral radiographs because plastic deformity of the anterior portion of the fracture can occur at the time of injury. Although anterior lip displacement does not affect the structural integrity of the reduction, it is helpful to establish baseline fluoroscopic images for purposes of comparison with postoperative follow-up radiographs.

POSTOPERATIVE REHABILITATION

Although specific rehabilitation protocols vary, the treatment principles are similar and should be based on existing evidence to minimize risk of postoperative complications. Avoiding arthrofibrosis while enabling fracture healing is the focus of early posttreatment rehabilitation. With nonoperative treatment of TSFs, immobilization is typically maintained for 4 to 6 weeks to allow fracture healing, and ROM is initiated immediately afterward.[26,29] Because surgically treated fractures are at higher risk of arthrofibrosis,[32] immobilization after operative treatment should be minimized. If fracture fixation is sufficient, ROM in a hinged knee brace is initiated immediately after surgery. Early motion is often limited to 90° for the first 2 to 4 weeks postoperatively and then increased as tolerated. Limited weight-bearing, with the knee in extension, is usually used for the first 6 weeks to protect the fixation construct. Open chain strengthening exercises are avoided for at least 6 weeks after surgery.[44] Late rehabilitation goals are similar to those after an ACL reconstruction—to allow successful return to activities while avoiding reinjury. Return to sports and other high-intensity activities typically occurs between 3 and 6 months, depending on activity goals and restoration of motion, strength, and functional testing results to 90% or better of the contralateral limb. In general, once the fracture has healed and full ROM is attained, one can consider progressing patients through an ACL reconstruction protocol of one's preference, although the optimal rehabilitation regimen remains an area of research interest.

POSTTREATMENT COMPLICATIONS AND OUTCOMES

Despite advances made in the knowledge and management of TSFs, complications are still common and may occur early or late in the treatment course. Arthrofibrosis is the most common complication after TSF treatment and is defined as a ≥10° extension and/or ≥25° flexion deficit (compared with the contralateral knee) at 3 months posttreatment without other causes, or the need for manipulation under anesthesia or arthroscopic lysis of adhesions.[48–50] Although general knee ROM loss is suboptimal, it is generally agreed that an extension deficit is the least desirable with regard to patient function and restoration of normal gait kinematics. The incidence of arthrofibrosis after TSF has been reported to be between 10% and 60%.[5,21,30,32,51]

Several risk factors have been identified for arthrofibrosis. Although arthrofibrosis most commonly occurs after surgically managed cases, it can also occur after nonoperative management. A recent systematic review reported an overall incidence of 13.7% for knee stiffness after nonoperative treatment of TSF, although the definition of stiffness varied between studies and some studies included adult patients.[52] Prolonged immobilization has been reported by several studies as a major risk factor for arthrofibrosis. One study found that patients who started ROM rehabilitation later than 4 weeks after surgery were 12 times more likely to develop arthrofibrosis.[53] Bram and colleagues[48] found that postoperative cast immobilization was a significant risk factor for arthrofibrosis. Moreover, the authors found that a concomitant ACL injury, a traumatic injury (as opposed to a sport related etiology), and age less than 10 years were additional independent risk factors for arthrofibrosis. Other possible risk factors include injury severity, delay from injury to surgery, operative time, and screw fixation (vs suture fixation), which have been reported inconsistently in smaller case series.[5,30,32,54]

Arthrofibrosis encompasses a range of clinical severities, ranging from minimal stiffness which resolves with rehabilitation, to significant ROM limitation requiring operative management, to development of localized foci of abnormal fibrous tissue, which may be associated with substantial pain and functional deficit. A patient who is not meeting postoperative ROM milestones should prompt the treating physician to consider arthrofibrosis (rather than expected acute postoperative stiffness) as the underlying pathology. Early treatment, in conjunction with physical therapy professionals, aims to break the vicious cycle of fibrosis, pain, and loss of motion, which only intensifies without proper treatment.

Rehabilitation is ideally initiated soon after TSF treatment to regain ROM. Considering the rigid fixation that current surgical techniques provide, ROM can be safely initiated early in the postoperative period (2–4 weeks) in most patients; immobilization longer than 4 weeks is not recommended. Although some degree of stiffness is to be expected immediately posttreatment, if the patient is unable to gain satisfactory ROM with physical therapy and/or has significant pain precluding vigorous rehabilitation, consideration should be given to returning to the operating room for thorough intraarticular evaluation and treatment between 8 and 12 weeks postoperatively. Isolated manipulation under anesthesia is not recommended in skeletally immature patients because of the risk of distal femoral physeal fracture during aggressive manipulation.[51] Instead, an arthroscopic lysis of adhesions and management of other factors that may inhibit ROM (eg, screw impingement, and malunion) is recommended. The results of operative management of arthrofibrosis are generally satisfactory, and most patients will achieve full or at least a functional ROM with proper rehabilitation.[7,48,50,51,53,55]

Hardware-related complications, nonunion and malunion, are less frequent causes of morbidity after TSF treatment. If screw fixation is performed, care should be taken to avoid impingement between the screw head and femoral condyles, which may lead to chondral damage, joint degeneration, and ROM loss. Prominent screws should also be removed once union is achieved if impingement is suspected. Although nonunion is rare in TSF, malunion is more common and may complicate nonoperative treatment of displaced fractures.[31] Malunion of a TSF may mechanically block full knee extension, although the amount of displacement/elevation that is acceptable remains debatable.[33] If symptomatic, the treatment of a TSF malunion is surgical and consists of arthroscopic debridement of the prominent/elevated portion of the tibial spine or a notchplasty to mitigate mechanical impingement. For patients with a delayed presentation following TSF, it is recommended that they be treated similarly to more acute fractures to decrease the rate of longer-term complications. Although data are scarce, one study reported favorable results of arthroscopic treatment of neglected and displaced TSFs presenting 6 to 10 weeks after injury.[56]

Long-term follow-up of TSFs even after healing is achieved is recommended to diagnose and manage late complications. In skeletally immature patients, radiographs at 3, 6, and 12 months post-operatively should be considered to assess for growth arrest. Furthermore, previous studies have shown that at the time of the TSF, the ACL may also be damaged. Traction applied to the ACL causes fiber damage, attenuation of the ligament, and partial ACL tears. Mayo and colleagues[57] reported that 19% of TSFs had visible damage to the ACL on MRI or at the time of arthroscopy that ranged from hyperemia to complete tear. Although the focus of treatment is typically on reduction and fixation of the TSF, long-term knee laxity is important to assess, and patients should be counseled on the possibility of delayed ACL reconstruction because of functional ACL deficiency. Mitchell and colleagues[58] reported that 19% of their TSFs required a formal ACL reconstruction because of laxity at a minimum 2-year follow-up. In addition to ACL injury sustained at the time of TSF, patients are also at an increased risk for a traumatic ACL tear after healing of the fracture. O'Donnell and colleagues[49] reviewed 385 TSF patients and reported that 2.6% of the patients sustained a subsequent ACL tear; however, in a subgroup of patients with at least 2 years of follow-up, the incidence of a subsequent ACL tear was 21.7%. DeFrancesco and colleagues[59] evaluated 876 cases of TSF via an administrative claims database and found a subsequent ACL insufficiency rate of 3.7%. Subsequent ACL reconstructions were performed in 1.7% of cases, most commonly in boys aged 13 to 14 years.

CONTROVERSIES AND FUTURE DIRECTIONS
Classification

Although the Meyers and McKeever classification system is the most widely used schema for classifying TSFs, its utility has been called into question by some authors. Ellis and colleagues[15] examined the reliability of the Meyers and McKeever system among members of the PRiSM (Pediatric Research in Sports Medicine) Tibial Spine Research Interest Group (RIG). Classifying TSFs according to the Meyers and McKeever classification showed only fair agreement ($\kappa = 0.35, 0.33$ [inter]; 0.47 [intra]) with 60% of the rated fractures classified as three different Meyers and McKeever types. In addition, there was only fair agreement among raters regarding the optimal initial treatment (operative reduction/fixation vs closed reduction) of these injuries ($\kappa = 0.33, 0.38$ [inter]; 0.51 [intra]). The measurement of superior displacement on lateral radiographs was the only measure studied that had good inter- and intraobserver reliability. These findings should encourage the development of a more reliable classification system when assessing TSFs.

The Role of Advanced Imaging

Although there is evidence that MRI can aid in the comprehensive diagnosis of other injuries sustained after a TSF,[16,19,22,60] the authors recognize that there are several valid approaches that can be used to make the best diagnostic and treatment decisions following these injuries. For example, if a treating surgeon elects to obtain a preoperative MRI, any identified concomitant pathology can be reviewed with the family as part of the informed consent process. If a closed reduction is considered for definitive treatment of a Type II fracture, an MRI can provide further evidence that other intraarticular pathology is not going undiagnosed. In addition, should any concomitant pathology be identified that would be better treated with an arthroscopic procedure (ie, posterior horn meniscal tear or high-grade ACL tear that may best be treated with primary ACL reconstruction); an arthroscopic rather than open approach may be planned. Finally, in centers with limited "off the shelf" resources, the preoperative identification of concomitant injuries such as a meniscal tear can ensure that necessary implants and instrumentation are available during surgery, and to better estimate expected operative duration.

Nonetheless, several members of the PRiSM Tibial Spine RIG do not routinely obtain preoperative MRIs. During the informed consent process, many tell patients and their families about the high incidence of associated intraarticular pathology that may require additional treatment and perform a diagnostic arthroscopy with careful intraarticular examination in all cases. Their institutions always have any potentially needed equipment and implants readily available. Supporting this approach is the imperfect sensitivity of MRI in the setting of TSFs. For example, Shimberg and colleagues[22] found that, when compared with intraoperative findings, soft-tissue entrapment at the fracture site was only identified in two of nine cases (22%) on MRI, lateral meniscus tears were identified in 62% (37/60) of cases on MRI, and medial meniscal tears were identified in 80% of cases on MRI. The treating surgeon must therefore recognize that concomitant injuries may still exist even with an otherwise negative preoperative MRI. As such, a careful intraarticular examination should be performed at the time of surgery, which may be best approached arthroscopically.

Amount of Acceptable Displacement

The amount and location of fracture displacement that is deemed acceptable for tibial spine avulsion fractures remains unclear. Adams and colleagues[61] assessed the variability of treatment recommendations for Type II fractures among a group of 20 fellowship trained pediatric orthopedic surgeons that had expertise treating TSFs. The authors found that surgeons were 28% more likely to recommend operative treatment with each 1 mm of fracture displacement. Although 64% of surgeons recommended surgical treatment of fractures with $\geq$3.5 mm of displacement, this means that 36% (or greater than one-third) did not. Callanan and colleagues[33] compared outcomes between those who underwent suture versus screw fixation for TSFs. The authors found that although fracture displacement on postoperative imaging was significantly greater in the suture group (5.4 mm vs 3.5 mm; $P = .005$), postoperative fracture displacement did not influence surgical outcomes. The PRiSM Tibial Spine RIG is currently examining the influence of residual displacement of the tibial spine anterior lip on outcomes (Yi-Meng Yen, unpublished data, 2022).

Future Directions

Given the relatively rare nature of pediatric TSFs, multicenter collaboration is important to perform well-powered analyses of these injuries. In addition, a vast majority of the literature published on TSFs use retrospective study designs, which are inherently limited by data heterogeneity and limited patient reported outcome metrics. The PRiSM Tibial Spine RIG is currently enrolling patients in a multicenter, prospective cohort to help confront the limitations of prior literature and to address knowledge gaps regarding the optimal evaluation and treatment of these relatively uncommon injuries.

SUMMARY

TSFs in young patients have a relatively low incidence when compared with other pediatric fractures and sports-related injuries. Initial evaluation consists of early recognition, classification, and identification of concomitant injuries. Definitive treatment depends on the amount of fracture displacement and any associated injuries. Nonoperative treatment with closed reduction and immobilization is generally reserved for minimally displaced fractures. Operative treatment is performed in more displaced fractures or in injuries with concomitant intraarticular pathology. Although open approaches to treatment can be performed, arthroscopy may offer many advantages compared with open treatment; however, this can be technically challenging. When performing operative treatment, anatomic reduction and stable fixation are important to allow early range of motion during postoperative rehabilitation, which may help prevent the development of knee stiffness, which is the most common complication after these injuries.

CLINICS CARE POINTS

- MRI may be considered when evaluating tibial spine avulsion fractures to assess for concomitant injury such as meniscus tear
- Fixation of these injuries can be achieved with either screw, suture, suture anchor, or combined methods
- Long-term follow-up after treatment is important as there may an increased risk for sustaining future ACL tear despite fracture healing

ACKNOWLEDGMENTS

Tibial Spine RIG members (not listed as individual authors): Julien T. Aoyama, Thomas Jefferson University, Peter D. Fabricant, MD, MPH, Hospital for Special Surgery, Daniel W. Green, MD, MS, Hospital for Special Surgery, Benjamin Johnson, PA-C, Texas Scottish Rite Hospital for Children, Scott D. McKay, MD, Texas Children's Hospital, Neeraj M. Patel, MD, MPH, MBS, Lurie Children's Hospital, Brant Sachleben, MD, Arkansas Children's Hospital, Gregory A. Schmale, MD, Seattle Children's Hospital, Jessica L. Traver, MD, The University of Texas Health Science Center, Yi-Meng Yen, MD, PhD, Boston Children's Hospital.

REFERENCES

1. Ziegler CG, Pietrini SD, Westerhaus BD, et al. Arthroscopically pertinent landmarks for tunnel positioning in single-bundle and double-bundle anterior cruciate ligament reconstructions. Am J Sports Med 2011;39(4):743–52.
2. Iriuchishima T, Goto B. Tibial spine location influences tibial tunnel placement in anatomical single-bundle anterior cruciate ligament reconstruction. J Knee Surg 2022;35(3):294–8.
3. Petersen W, Tillmann B. [Anatomy and function of the anterior cruciate ligament]. Orthopade 2002;31(8):710–8.
4. Herring JA. 4th edition. Tachdjian's pediatric orthopaedics: lower extremity injuries, vol. 3. Philadelphia: Saunders Elsevier; 2008.
5. Wiley JJ, Baxter MP. Tibial spine fractures in children. Clin Orthop Relat Res 1990;(255):54–60.

6. Abbasi D, May MM, Wall EJ, et al. MRI findings in adolescent patients with acute traumatic knee hemarthrosis. J Pediatr Orthop 2012;32(8):760–4.

7. Adams AJ, Talathi NS, Gandhi JS, et al. Tibial Spine Fractures in Children: Evaluation, Management, and Future Directions. J Knee Surg 2018;31(5):374–81.

8. Strauss EJ, Kaplan DJ, Weinberg ME, et al. Arthroscopic management of tibial spine avulsion fractures: principles and techniques. J Am Acad Orthop Surg 2018;26(10):360–7.

9. Coyle C, Jagernauth S, Ramachandran M. Tibial eminence fractures in the paediatric population: a systematic review. J Child Orthop 2014;8(2):149–59.

10. Axibal DP, Mitchell JJ, Mayo MH, et al. Epidemiology of Anterior Tibial Spine Fractures in Young Patients: A Retrospective Cohort Study of 122 Cases. J Pediatr Orthop 2019;39(2):e87–90.

11. LaValva SM, Aoyama JT, Adams AJ, et al. The epidemiology of tibial spine fractures in children: a multicenter investigation. Orthop J Sports Med 2020;8(4 suppl3).

12. Meyers MH, McKeever FM. Fracture of the intercondylar eminence of the tibia. J Bone Joint Surg Am 1970;52(8):1677–84.

13. Zaricznyj B. Avulsion fracture of the tibial eminence: treatment by open reduction and pinning. J Bone Joint Surg Am 1977;59(8):1111–4.

14. Jackson TJ, Storey EP, Ganley TJ. Tibial Spine Interest G. The Surgical Management of Tibial Spine Fractures in Children: A Survey of the Pediatric Orthopaedic Society of North America (POSNA). J Pediatr Orthop 2019;39(8):e572–7.

15. Ellis HB, Zynda AJ, Cruz AI Jr, et al. Classification and treatment of pediatric tibial spine fractures: assessing reliability among a tibial spine research interest group. J Pediatr Orthop 2021;41(1):e20–5.

16. Rhodes JT, Cannamela PC, Cruz AI, et al. Incidence of Meniscal Entrapment and Associated Knee Injuries in Tibial Spine Avulsions. J Pediatr Orthop 2018;38(2): e38–42.

17. Green D, Tuca M, Luderowski E, et al. A new, MRI-based classification system for tibial spine fractures changes clinical treatment recommendations when compared to Myers and Mckeever. Knee Surg Sports Traumatol Arthrosc 2019; 27(1):86–92.

18. Beck JJ, Niu EL, Cruz AI Jr, et al. Physical exam for sports medicine knee injuries in pediatric patients: current concepts review. JPOSNA 2021;3(4):1–9.

19. Ishibashi Y, Tsuda E, Sasaki T, et al. Magnetic resonance imaging AIDS in detecting concomitant injuries in patients with tibial spine fractures. Clin Orthop Relat Res 2005;434:207–12.

20. Kendall NS, Hsu SY, Chan KM. Fracture of the tibial spine in adults and children. A review of 31 cases. J Bone Joint Surg Br 1992;74(6):848–52.

21. Lafrance RM, Giordano B, Goldblatt J, et al. Pediatric tibial eminence fractures: evaluation and management. J Am Acad Orthop Surg 2010;18(7):395–405.

22. Shimberg JL, Aoyama JT, Leska TM, et al. Tibial Spine Fractures: How Much Are We Missing Without Pretreatment Advanced Imaging? A Multicenter Study. Am J Sports Med 2020;48(13):3208–13.

23. Bogunovic L, Tarabichi M, Harris D, et al. Treatment of tibial eminence fractures: a systematic review. J knee surg 2015;28(3):255–62.

24. Scrimshire AB, Gawad M, Davies R, et al. Management and outcomes of isolated paediatric tibial spine fractures. Injury 2018;49(2):437–42.

25. Shin YW, Uppstrom TJ, Haskel JD, et al. The tibial eminence fracture in skeletally immature patients. Curr Opin Pediatr 2015;27(1):50–7.

26. Wilfinger C, Castellani C, Raith J, et al. Nonoperative treatment of tibial spine fractures in children-38 patients with a minimum follow-up of 1 year. J Orthop Trauma 2009;23(7):519–24.
27. Archibald-Seiffer N, Jacobs J Jr, Zbojniewicz A, et al. Incarceration of the intermeniscal ligament in tibial eminence injury: a block to closed reduction identified using MRI. Skeletal Radiol 2015;44(5):717–21.
28. Mitchell JJ, Sjostrom R, Mansour AA, et al. Incidence of meniscal injury and chondral pathology in anterior tibial spine fractures of children. J Pediatr Orthop 2015; 35(2):130–5.
29. Kocher MS, Micheli LJ, Gerbino P, et al. Tibial eminence fractures in children: prevalence of meniscal entrapment. Am J Sports Med 2003;31(3):404–7.
30. Gans I, Baldwin KD, Ganley TJ. Treatment and Management Outcomes of Tibial Eminence Fractures in Pediatric Patients: A Systematic Review. Am J Sports Med 2014;42(7):1743–50.
31. Prasad N, Aoyama JT, Ganley TJ, et al. A Comparison of Nonoperative and Operative Treatment of Type 2 Tibial Spine Fractures. Orthop J Sports Med 2021;9(1). 2325967120975410.
32. Edmonds EW, Fornari ED, Dashe J, et al. Results of displaced pediatric tibial spine fractures: a comparison between open, arthroscopic, and closed management. J Pediatr Orthop 2015;35(7):651–6.
33. Callanan M, Allen J, Flutie B, et al. Suture Versus Screw Fixation of Tibial Spine Fractures in Children and Adolescents: A Comparative Study. Orthop J Sports Med 2019;7(11). 2325967119881961.
34. DeFroda SF, Hodax JD, Shah KN, et al. Tibial Eminence Fracture Repair With Double Hewson Suture Passer Technique. Arthrosc Tech 2017;6(4):e1275–9.
35. Fox JC, Saper MG. Arthroscopic Suture Fixation of Comminuted Tibial Eminence Fractures: Hybrid All-Epiphyseal Bone Tunnel and Knotless Anchor Technique. Arthrosc Tech 2019;8(11):e1283–8.
36. Ganley TJ, Brusalis CM. Surgical Reduction and Fixation of Tibial Spine Fractures in Children: Multiple Fixation Strategies. JBJS Essent Surg Tech 2016;6(2):e18.
37. Harouna AD, Cherrabi H, Atarraf K, et al. [Tibial spine fractures in children]. Pan Afr Med J 2017;28:244.
38. Kobayashi S, Harato K, Udagawa K, et al. Arthroscopic Treatment of Tibial Eminence Avulsion Fracture With Suture Tensioning Technique. Arthrosc Tech 2018;7(3):e251–6.
39. Li J, Liu C, Li Z, et al. Arthroscopic Fixation for Tibial Eminence Fractures: Comparison of Double-Row and Transosseous Anchor Knot Fixation Techniques with Suture Anchors. Med Sci monitor 2018;24:7348–56.
40. R R, Jaseel M, Murugan C, et al. Arthroscopic tibial spine fracture fixation: Novel techniques. J orthopaedics 2018;15(2):372–4.
41. Thome AP, O'Donnell R, DeFroda SF, et al. Effect of Skeletal Maturity on Fixation Techniques for Tibial Eminence Fractures. Orthop J Sports Med 2021;9(11). 23259671211049476.
42. Kushare I, Lee RJ, Ellis HB Jr, et al. Tibial Spine Research Interest Group (PRiSM), Mistovich, R.J. Tibial spine fracture management: surgical & technical tips from the tibial spine fracture research interest group. JPOSNA 2020;2(1):1–9.
43. Osti L, Buda M, Soldati F, et al. Arthroscopic treatment of tibial eminence fracture: a systematic review of different fixation methods. Br Med Bull 2016;118(1):73–90.
44. Kushare I, Lee RJ, Ellis HBJ, et al. Tibial spine fracture management - Technical tips and tricks from the tibial spine fracture research interest group. JPOSNA 2020;2(1):1–9.

45. Sekiya H, Takatoku K, Kimura A, et al. Arthroscopic fixation with EndoButton for tibial eminence fractures visualised through a proximal superomedial portal: a surgical technique. J Orthop Surg (Hong Kong) 2016;24(3):417–20.

46. Veselko M, Senekovic V, Tonin M. Simple and safe arthroscopic placement and removal of cannulated screw and washer for fixation of tibial avulsion fracture of the anterior cruciate ligament. Arthroscopy 1996;12(2):259–62.

47. Anderson AF. Transepiphyseal replacement of the anterior cruciate ligament using quadruple hamstring grafts in skeletally immature patients. J Bone Joint Surg Am 2004;86:201–9. A Suppl 1(Pt 2).

48. Bram JT, Aoyama JT, Mistovich RJ, et al. Four Risk Factors for Arthrofibrosis in Tibial Spine Fractures: A National 10-Site Multicenter Study. Am J Sports Med 2020;48(12):2986–93.

49. O'Donnell R, Bokshan S, Brown K, et al. Anterior Cruciate Ligament Tear Following Operative Treatment of Pediatric Tibial Eminence Fractures in a Multicenter Cohort. J Pediatr Orthop 2021;41(5):284–9.

50. Parikh SN, Myer D, Eismann EA. Prevention of arthrofibrosis after arthroscopic screw fixation of tibial spine fracture in children and adolescents. Orthopedics 2014;37(1):e58–65.

51. Vander Have KL, Ganley TJ, Kocher MS, et al. Arthrofibrosis after surgical fixation of tibial eminence fractures in children and adolescents. Am J Sports Med 2010; 38(2):298–301.

52. Zhang K, Catapano M, Carsen S, et al. Management and Complications in Nonoperative Fractures of the Tibial Spine: A Systematic Review. J Pediatr Orthop 2021;41(3):e272–8.

53. Patel NM, Park MJ, Sampson NR, et al. Tibial eminence fractures in children: earlier posttreatment mobilization results in improved outcomes. J Pediatr Orthop 2012;32(2):139–44.

54. Watts CD, Larson AN, Milbrandt TA. Open versus arthroscopic reduction for tibial eminence fracture fixation in children. J Pediatr Orthop 2016;36(5):437–9.

55. Shin CH, Lee DJ, Choi IH, et al. Clinical and radiological outcomes of arthroscopically assisted cannulated screw fixation for tibial eminence fracture in children and adolescents. BMC Musculoskelet Disord 2018;19(1):1–9.

56. Abdelkafy A, Said HG. Neglected ununited tibial eminence fractures in the skeletally immature: arthroscopic management. Int Orthop 2014;38(12):2525–32.

57. Mayo MH, Mitchell JJ, Axibal DP, et al. Anterior cruciate ligament injury at the time of anterior tibial spine fracture in young patients: an observational cohort study. J Pediatr Orthop 2019;39(9):e668–73.

58. Mitchell JJ, Mayo MH, Axibal DP, et al. Delayed anterior cruciate ligament reconstruction in young patients with previous anterior tibial spine fractures. Am J Sports Med 2016;44(8):2047–56.

59. DeFrancesco CJ, Wilson L, Lebrun DG, et al. Pediatric Tibial Spine Fractures: Exploring Case Burden by Age and Sex. Orthop J Sports Med 2021;9(9). 23259671211027237.

60. Shea KG, Grimm NL, Laor T, et al. Bone bruises and meniscal tears on MRI in skeletally immature children with tibial eminence fractures. J Pediatr Orthop 2011;31(2):150–2.

61. Adams AJ, O'Hara NN, Abzug JM, et al. Pediatric Type II Tibial Spine Fractures: Addressing the Treatment Controversy With a Mixed-Effects Model. Orthop J Sports Med 2019;7(8). 2325967119866162.

Using Motion Analysis in the Evaluation, Treatment & Rehabilitation of Pediatric & Adolescent Knee Injuries: A Review of the Literature

Jason Rhodes, MD[a,*], Alex Tagawa, BS[a,b], Andrew McCoy, MD[c],
David Bazett-Jones, PhD, AT, ATC, CSCS[d], Austin Skinner, BS[a,b],
Lise Leveille, MD[e], Corinna Franklin, MD[f],
Ross Chafetz, PT, DPT, PhD, MPH[f,g], Kirsten Tulchin-Francis, PhD[h]

KEYWORDS

• Motion capture • Knee injuries • Pediatric sports injuries • Motion analysis

KEY POINTS

- There is a lack of studies on three-dimensional motion capture and knee injuries in adolescents and children.
- Most studies focus on the biomechanical characteristics of knee injuries, including kinematic and electromyogram data with limited data and protocols for knee injury work-up, treatment, or rehabilitation.
- Future research should identify risk factors, assessing the effectiveness of intervention and development of rehabilitation protocols for knee injuries.

[a] Department of Orthopedics, Children's Hospital Colorado, 13123 East 16th Avenue, Aurora, CO, USA; [b] Children's Hospital Colorado, Musculoskeletal Research Center, 13123 East 16th Avenue, Aurora, CO, USA; [c] Department of Physical Medicine and Rehabilitation, Children's Hospital Colorado, 13123 East 16th Avenue, Aurora, CO, USA; [d] University of Toledo, School of Exercise and Rehabilitation Sciences, 2801 West Bancroft Street, Toledo, OH 43606, USA; [e] Department of Orthopaedics, BC Children's Hospital, 4500 Oak Street, Vancouver British Columbia V6H 3N1, Canada; [f] Department of Orthopedics, Shriners Hospital for Children, 3551 North Broad Street, Philadelphia, PA, USA; [g] Department of Orthopedics, Hahnemann University Hospital, 230 North Broad Street, Philadelphia, PA, USA; [h] Department of Orthopedic Surgery, Nationwide Children's Hospital, 700 Children's Drive, Columbus, OH, USA
* Corresponding author.
E-mail address: jason.rhodes@childrenscolorado.org

Clin Sports Med 41 (2022) 671–685
https://doi.org/10.1016/j.csm.2022.07.001
0278-5919/22/© 2022 Elsevier Inc. All rights reserved.

INTRODUCTION

Knee injuries are common in children and adolescents, with an incidence ranging from 3 to 12 knee injuries per 1000 persons.[1,2] These injuries are largely caused by sports, recreational activities (eg, trampoline use), and falls.[1,2] There has been an increase in the incidence of acute pediatric and adolescent knee injuries in the United States, which will likely continue to increase.[3–6] It is imperative that there be effective tools to understand risk factors of these injuries, to effectively evaluate, treat, and prevent them.

A tool that has been effective in the evaluation of human movement and helpful in steering treatment and rehabilitation protocols within the pediatric and adolescent populations is three-dimensional motion capture (3DMA). 3DMA allows for the quantitative assessment of human movement, in which kinematics and kinetics of different joints and segments of the human body are measured during movements.[7–10] Biomechanical assessments are performed during tasks, such as walking, running, throwing, and kicking.[9,11,12] The data can then be used to determine which individuals are at risk for injury and to create injury prevention protocols,[13–17] and assess the effectiveness of postoperative rehabilitation protocols and other interventions.[18,19] In the cerebral palsy population, motion analysis is used extensively in the work-up and treatment of patients, and contributes to surgical and orthotic decision making, rehabilitation, and has demonstrated treatment cost savings. Its demonstrated success in the neurologically involved patient demonstrates the potential it has for these same evaluations and improvement in neurotypical patients, specifically using motion analysis in sports injury work-up, treatment, and rehabilitation.

Although 3DMA has been extensively used to help with evaluation, treatment, and rehabilitation within the pediatric and adolescent populations, it is rarely used for knee injuries.[16] This review evaluates the literature to determine how 3DMA has been used to improve the evaluation, treatment, and rehabilitation of patellofemoral instability (PFI), intra-articular injuries (eg, multiligament, condylar, meniscus), injury prevention, and anterior knee pain. This review also evaluates the literature on the use of 3DMA in the prevention of knee injuries. These aims allow one to identify which areas are understudied so that practitioners can focus on these areas and better use motion capture in this patient population. There are numerous studies and literature evaluating and presenting results on the use of motion analysis in patients with anterior cruciate ligament injury and treatment. Given the amount of literature on that topic, it is not included in this review because it is too extensive in amount and would be best represented in a separate literature review.

METHODOLOGY

A review of the literature was conducted to synthesize evidence on studies that used 3DMA to evaluate, treat, and rehabilitate pediatric knee injuries: PFI, intra-articular injuries (eg, multiligament, condylar, meniscus), anterior knee pain, and injury prevention. A comprehensive search strategy was devised from the following electronic databases with no date restrictions: MEDLINE via OVID, EMBASE via OVID, and PubMed. Keywords included "gait or kinematic or biomechanical phenomena or whole body kinematics or lower body kinematics or upper body kinematics," "knee or knee injuries or PFI or intra-articular knee injuries or discoid meniscus or posterior cruciate ligament (PCL) or multiligament injuries or patellar tendinopathy or knee pain or chronic knee pain," and "child or children or boy or girl or teen or adolescent or youth or high school or a combination." The initial search was limited to studies published between January 1, 2000 and December 1, 2021 and an updated PubMed search limited to studies published between January 1, 2020 and May 1, 2022. The following sections are a narrative summary of the literature on 3DMA in the evaluation, treatment, and prevention of pediatric and adolescent knee injuries.

PATELLOFEMORAL INSTABILITY

PFI is a disorder where the patella disarticulates from the patellofemoral joint, most commonly in the lateral direction, and is associated with patellofemoral pain (PFP) and injury.[20] The incidence is estimated to be highest among adolescents with an annual incidence of 23.3 per 100,000 per year and specifically 147.7 per 100,000 per year in ages 14 to 18,[21] in which females from ages 10 to 17 years of age have the highest incidence. Anatomic risk factors for lateral PFI include patella alta, trochlear dysplasia, and increased lateral patellar tilt.[22]

Kinematic and kinetic data through gait analysis with 3DMA has arisen as a tool in the context of PFI. Studies focus on the use of kinematics/kinetics and 3DMA for patients with PFI to distinguish the static and dynamic biomechanical factors that may precipitate instability. Most 3DMA system use cameras that detect reflective markers placed on anatomic landmarks. Ground reaction force data are typically obtained force plate system.

Two-dimensional (2D) analysis applied to videos of real-world patellar dislocations found evidence for injury in most noncontact situations with the knee in a flexed, valgus position with a contracted quadriceps.[23] However, 2D video analysis was unable to distinguish the role of hip and ankle movements in the mechanism, which is an aspect that 3DMA is able to assess. In a cross-sectional study with adolescent and young adult participants with PFI, gait deviations and muscle strength parameters have been characterized using 3DMA.[24] For patients with PFI, knee adduction and hip abduction angles were significantly lower in stance phase leading to an adducted hip and valgus knee with additional significant weakness compared with the control group in knee extension, hip abduction, and hip external rotation.[24] A case-control study of 88 adolescent patients with recurrent PFI compared with age-matched control subjects using 3DMA demonstrated significant decrease in knee flexion during the entire gait cycle, especially at midstance during loading response.[25] This study also pointed to decreased hip flexion and increased plantarflexion as compensatory mechanism for preventing instability.[25]

Another prospective case-control preoperative study characterized the "quadriceps avoidance" phenomenon by stratifying patients into a group with small knee extension moment in early stance weight-acceptance and a group with no knee extension moment and compared both with each other and with a control group.[26] With 3D kinematics and MRI imaging correlation, it found a significant difference in patellofemoral contact between the control groups and PFI groups in full knee extension with activated knee extensors such that the lower amount of contact occurred in the group with no knee extension moment.[26] Based on these studies, there are data showing muscle patterns that may be causative or compensatory to patellofemoral instability, but more research is needed to look closer at 3D kinematics and kinetics to determine clinical recommendations for treatment of patellar instability.

PFI is a complex biomechanical problem that is accompanied by interrelated static and dynamic patterns of movement and bony alignment. 3DMA has demonstrated an important role in clarifying mechanisms and informing operative approaches and postoperative outcomes in PFI. However, several gaps exist that could be addressed with future studies. Most studies involving 3DMA evaluating effectiveness of surgical interventions have been performed through the biomechanical manipulation of cadavers[27–29] or the assessment of postoperative outcomes in adults.[30,31] Although the nuances of the skeletally immature patient with PFI have been well described, it would be beneficial to have longitudinal studies evaluating PFI in children as they mature into adolescence, especially after the first PFI event and undergoing a nonsurgical treatment protocol.[29,32] Rehabilitative protocols have been evaluated for PFP[33]; however, there are no prospective randomized controlled trials for protocols specific to PFI.[34,35] Treatment algorithms based on classification of patellofemoral pathology have been proposed and the role of 3DMA considered in those patients that have either failed conservative treatment or have been deemed to be surgical candidates based on imaging.[36] Although there are quality systematic reviews highlighting existing criteria used for return to play following surgical interventions,[37–39] it would be valuable to use 3DMA as a modality for evaluating postoperative outcome but also highlighting lingering pathologic patterns or gait deficits. This may inform future sports-specific injury prevention programs in the child and adolescent athlete and it is hoped lead to better outcomes.

INTRA-ARTICULAR PATHOLOGY

Intra-articular knee injuries can dramatically disrupt this mechanism, causing significant injury and dysfunction to the patient.[40] This review focuses on discoid meniscus injuries, PCL and multiligament injuries, and patellar tendinopathy. Anterior cruciate ligament injuries are not included because there is a large body of literature analyzing the use of 3DMA and anterior cruciate ligament injuries.

Discoid Meniscus

A discoid meniscus is an aberrant morphologic variation of meniscus tissue, resulting in a hypertrophic and discoid-shaped configuration that can become symptomatic.[41] It is estimated that the annual incidence of discoid meniscus is 3.2 per 100,000 person-years. Risk factors include increased meniscus size and thickness, deficient peripheral attachments, and meniscus instability. There is currently limited understanding of the impact of meniscal pathology or atypical morphology, such as discoid meniscus, on gait biomechanics. Harato and colleagues[42] first characterized the kinematics of gait in patients (mean age, 14 years) with discoid lateral meniscus. Despite full range of motion on physical examination, knees with symptomatic discoid lateral meniscus showed a "stiffening strategy" with decreased excursion into full extension in midstance.[42] Asymptomatic discoid meniscus showed less severe involvement in comparison with the normal control subjects but a similar pattern to the symptomatic discoid meniscus. This was hypothesized to be a strategy to avoid snapping of the knee. In the transverse plane, increased external rotation was seen in the symptomatic discoid lateral meniscus.[42] The reason for this is not well understood. Lin and colleagues[43] also found axial differences in patients with meniscal pathology. Using an infrared portable motion capture system, they evaluated kinematic characteristics of patients with symptomatic discoid lateral meniscus in comparison with torn typical lateral meniscus and normal control subjects. Patients with torn discoid or torn typical lateral meniscus had decreased peak knee flexion in swing of 14° to 16°. Knees with lateral discoid meniscus injury showed increased external rotation in compared with healthy knees, which is consistent with the results of the study by Harato and colleagues.[42]

Further studies are needed to better understand the gait adaptations seen with discoid lateral meniscus and clarify the efficacy of surgical management.

Posterior Cruciate Ligament and Multiligament Injuries

PCL and multiligament injuries are trending to increase over time. It is estimated that 3% of all knee injuries are PCL injuries,[44] in which PCL rupture injuries are generally seen in conjunction of other ligament tears.[45] However, it is estimated that the incidence of multiligament injuries is around 0.02% to 0.20% of all orthopedic injuries, in which 27% to 30% of all meniscal tears and cartilage injuries are seen in conjunction with multiligament injuries. Within the current literature, no motion analysis studies have been completed in pediatric or adolescent patients with PCL and/or multiligament knee injuries. Investigations also are limited in the adult population. Varying kinematic patterns in adults have been described with and without ligament reconstruction, including increased knee flexion in early, mid, and late stance phase[46,47] and diminished total knee range of motion through stance and swing phase.[48] Kinetic differences observed include quadriceps avoidance gait pattern with diminished knee extensor moments,[47,48] diminished external rotational moments,[47] and decreased maximum knee valgus moments with greater vertical ground reaction force at midstance.[49] These gait adaptations have been shown to persist up to 3 years[48] and 8 years[47] after multiligament reconstruction. Additional studies are required to better understand gait adaptations in response to PCL and multiligament knee injuries and the impact of ligamentous reconstructions, especially in children and adolescents.

Symmetry in gait adaptation between involved and contralateral limbs was consistently seen resulting in significant differences in kinematics and kinetics only being observed when subjects are compared with normal control subjects.[46–49] Biomechanical adaptation to injury is seen in the involved and uninvolved limb. This is an important reminder that long-term follow-up analyses of patients with PCL and/or multiligament injuries should not use the uninjured contralateral limb as a "normal" control reference.

Motion analysis has an important role in better understanding loads placed on intraarticular structures helping to develop informed rehabilitation protocols. Motion analysis and modeling technologies were applied in combination with in vivo static MRI measurements of PCL length to better understand motion that may put reconstructed ligaments at most risk.[50] PCL length measurements on MRI scans in various degrees of knee flexion showed maximal ligament length around 90° of flexion. Motion capture data showed excellent agreement with largest strain on the ligament seen in dynamic activities using deep knee flexion. Limiting these dynamic motions until graft maturation may improve postoperative outcomes.

Patellar Tendinopathy

Patellar tendinopathy is one of the most common causes of anterior knee pain in jumping athletes, in which it is estimated that 22% of all knee pain in experienced athletes is found to be patellar tendinopathy.[51] Motion analysis studies in adolescents, young adult athletes, and military recruits have helped to understand mechanics and risk factors for patellar tendinopathy.[52–54] Patients with patellar tendinopathy are more likely to squat with a pattern of increased knee valgus collapse throughout the squatting movement.[52] The lower extremity contact angle (LECA) has also been found to be an important variable when considering landing dynamics.[54] LECA is the angle between the ground and the line connecting the center of pressure to the L5S1 marker. LECA encompasses the kinematics of the entire lower extremity and closely correlates with braking impulse. Elite adult male volleyball players with symptomatic patellar tendinopathy demonstrated a significantly more acute LECA compared with the asymptomatic players.[54]

It is difficult to determine if these are biomechanical adaptations to symptoms or are contributing factors to the cause of the condition. Motion analysis studies in asymptomatic athletes suggest that landing mechanics are strongly contributory to disease progressions. Junior pre-elite male basketball players with asymptomatic patellar tendinopathy, in comparison with players without evidence of tendinopathy, are more likely to land with less hip flexion and greater knee flexion at initial contact.[53] Trunk position at initial contact has also been shown to be an important kinematic variable, which is closely associated with hip flexion. Athletes instructed to land with increased trunk flexion had decreased peak patellar tendon force, peak knee extensor moment, and knee pain in comparison with landing with a self-selected trunk position or an extended trunk position.[55]

Identification of biomechanical factors that increase loads across the extensor mechanics at the knee and contribute to the development of symptomatic patellar tendinopathy creates an opportunity for early intervention and development of effective preventative measures. Further studies are needed to assess the efficacy and effectiveness of interventions targeting movement pattern modification in athletes and the duration of their impact.

ANTERIOR KNEE PAIN

Chronic knee pain is a common experience of adolescents.[56] The most common knee conditions in this population are PFP, iliotibial band syndrome, Osgood-Schlatter disease, and Sinding-Larsen–Johansson disease. The prevalence of knee pain in adolescents is 19% to 31%.[57,58] PFP typically represents the largest percentage of this (7.5%–9.7%),[57–59] with variable ranges reported for Sinding-Larsen–Johansson disease (3.1%–9.7%),[57,60] Osgood-Schlatter disease (1.8%–21%),[57,60,61] and iliotibial band syndrome (0.3%).[57] Many of these conditions have been considered self-limiting[62,63]; however, long-term prognosis is not favorable[64] with chronic knee pain proposed to possibly contribute to osteoarthritis later in life.[65]

Motion analysis is commonly used to investigate chronic knee pathologies in adults. This motion analysis work has been so extensive in adults that a pathomechanical model of PFP has been proposed, with biomechanical variables being reported to contribute to the cause and persistence of PFP in adults.[66] However, there has been extremely limited investigation of PFP and other chronic knee conditions in children and adolescents.

Although PFP is commonly called "runner's knee," there are no studies using motion analysis to compare adolescents with and without PFP during running. Adolescents who go on to develop PFP demonstrated altered mechanics. In a study of adolescent female basketball players using 3DMA, increased knee abduction moments during landing were reported in those who later developed PFP.[67] Increased knee abduction kinematics during landing, measured with 2D motion analysis, have also been reported to be predictive of the development of PFP, with 10.6° being identified as the relevant cut point.[68] During the stance phase of stair ambulation, adolescents with PFP demonstrated greater sagittal plane range of motion.[69] Although some studies have included adolescent participants in their analyses,[70–73] their data were not specifically reported separately from adult data. No studies using motion analysis could be found comparing pain-free adolescents with those who have iliotibial band syndrome, Osgood-Schlatter disease, and Sinding-Larsen–Johansson disease.

Understanding the role and utility of motion analysis in the prevention, treatment, and prognosis of anterior knee pain could provide a clinically useful tool. The dearth of literature on this population makes it impossible to discuss biomechanical factors that contribute to chronic anterior knee pain in adolescents.

PREVENTION OF KNEE INJURIES

Motion analysis can also be used as a tool to evaluate risk assessment in individual patients, to develop new training programs aimed at injury prevention, or to improve an athlete's overall sport performance (leading to improved biomechanics, which may limit their injury risk.) The rapid movement of the knee, often accompanied by high forces across the joint, requires dynamic stability and neuromuscular control. Clinical screening movement tests are typically used in controlled settings to assess knee (and hip, ankle/foot, pelvis and/or trunk) position during weightbearing and high-impact landing tasks (eg, drop landing, drop vertical jump, single-limb hopping). Observation and/or 2D video tend to be the default clinical method to assess kinematic position during these tasks and the loading of the knee, although often estimated, is difficult to visualize and quantify. Furthermore, the kinematics and kinetics of sport-specific tasks, either on the field or in the laboratory, are difficult to observe in real time at high-speeds, or capture with video because they rarely occur in a truly planar direction, which makes 2D camera recordings prone to errors. For example, recent data have shown that although there was an association between 2D and 3D trunk and pelvic variables during stepping, landing, and change of direction tasks, the ability of the 2D angles from video to measure the corresponding 3D angles with high degrees of accuracy was limited, leading authors to suggest that 2D measurements should be used cautiously when high levels of agreement or accuracy is required.[74]

Understanding the underlying knee biomechanics during simple tasks is imperative. Previous work in this area has evaluated the sex- and/or age-based differences in knee kinematics/kinetics of running,[75–79] jumping tasks,[80–85] and cutting maneuvers[80,86,87] in children, adolescents, and young adults. Multiple other tasks have been evaluated biomechanically in adolescents using 3DMA including tasks involved in movement screening[88]; directional changes/run-and-cut tasks[89–93]; drop-landing or vertical jump tasks[88,89,94–99]; and sport-specific tasks including soccer kicks,[100] baseball/softball,[101–105] gymnastics,[106] tennis,[107,108] volleyball,[99] and cricket.[109]

Strengthening, training, or injury prevention programs have the potential to reduce injury risk. 3DMA is a useful tool to assess whether these programs are improving biomechanical performance, and whether these changes are adapted long-term by participants. Previous work has shown positive effects of injury prevention programs on knee kinematics and kinetics, most often concentrating on adolescent[90,94–96] or preadolescent girls[89,110] who are most susceptible to knee injuries. Studies evaluating knee-targeted injury prevention programs[80,89,94,110,111] and those evaluating core,[99] plyometric,[96] or balance/postural control[95,96,112] have used a variety of tasks, such as drop landing or drop vertical jump, running, change-of-direction/cutting, or vertical jump height in additional to traditional clinical (strength) or performance measures. Another important consideration when evaluating pediatric and adolescent athletes is that injuries are often sustained during high-intensity training or competitive game situations when the player is fatigued. Several studies have also evaluated the effects of fatigue in children and/or adolescent athletes during tasks, such as single limb squatting,[113] drop vertical jumps,[82] or change of direction.[91]

In the absence of recording an actual injury during in vivo testing of these tasks, cadaveric testing, simulation, statistics, and speculation are used to predict which knee joint positions, impacts, and forces lead to injury. Although there has been a large increase in 3DMA research in knee injury prevention in pediatric sports medicine in the last decade, these studies tend to be cross-sectional in design and sample sizes continue to be small (generally <50 subjects). Future studies should be prospective, multicenter trials aimed at collecting data on large cohorts of preadolescents, including elite youth, recreational, and nonathletes. These trials must include regular follow-up reporting of sport participation, training load, and injuries, and should include periodic, repeated biomechanical testing. This will allow clinicians and researchers to answer many questions on the effectiveness of different injury prevention programs, the impact of sport specialization, differences in sex and age, and begin to truly answer the important questions on how to best reduce knee injury risk in children and adolescents.

DISCUSSION

3DMA is used to evaluate, treat, and rehabilitate knee injuries and improve sports performance with goals for improved results in these injuries and return of young athletes to their full potential. However, there is limited literature to support this and the current work focuses on biomechanical changes, which are primarily reported either in adults or cadavers. This has created a major gap because the pediatric and adolescent populations are heavily understudied. Similar to the adult and cadaver populations, the literature within the pediatric population focuses on biomechanical changes caused by knee injuries. Specifically, knee PFI, discoid meniscus, and patellar tendinopathy have been compared with typically developing healthy control subjects to identify kinematic changes. This is also seen in the literature focused on knee prevention protocols, where the studies focus on the biomechanical mechanism by analyzing specific movements (eg, cutting, drop jump) or a specific sport (eg, soccer, basketball, volleyball). Based on the current knowledge, clinicians have developed strengthening, training, and injury prevention programs and prevention protocols to prevent these specific knee injuries. However, one of the major gaps within the literature is focused around PCL/multiligament knee injuries and anterior knee pain. There are no studies that compare adolescents with/without anterior knee pain during running or that assess PCL and/or multiligament knee injuries in pediatric or adolescent patients. There have been studies that assess the biomechanical differences using 2D assessment; however, no major conclusions can be made about 3DMA. Future studies should be prospective multicenter trials aimed at collecting data on large cohorts. These trials should focus on identifying risk factors of knee injuries, assessing the effectiveness of intervention (surgical and nonsurgical) for knee injuries, and development of return to sport/rehabilitation protocols for these specific knee injuries. Furthermore, these trials must include regular follow-up reporting, mechanism assessment, severity and type of injury, and periodic repeat biomechanical testing. Identification of differences in patterns of motion between adult and children or adolescent populations with knee injuries is crucial. This will allow a comprehensive longitudinal assessment of knee kinematics for children and adolescents who experience knee injuries.

SUMMARY

3DMA can improve evaluation, treatment, and rehabilitation of knee PFI, intra-articular knee injuries (eg, multiligament, condylar, meniscus), and anterior knee pain, because quantitative assessment of the knee improves the understanding of the biomechanical mechanisms. The current body of literature focuses on biomechanical characteristics of certain knee injuries performed primarily in adults. Because of the gaps in the literature, 3DMA is not optimally used in improving knee injury outcomes, leaving much to be desired. Future research investigating knee injuries should focus on identifying risk factors, assessing the effectiveness of surgical and nonsurgical interventions, and developing return to sport/rehabilitation protocols.

DISCLOSURE

Dr J. Rhodes is a consultant for OrthoPediatrics; has research grants with Smith and Nephew; is past president of *Gait and Clinical Movement Analysis Society*; and is an associate editor for Gait and Posture. Dr K. Tulchin-Francis is president of *Gait and Clinical Movement Analysis Society*. There were no financial supports for this article.

REFERENCES

1. Gage BE, McIlvain NM, Collins CL, et al. Epidemiology of 6.6 million knee injuries presenting to United States emergency departments from 1999 through 2008. Acad Emerg Med 2012;19(4):378–85.
2. Ferry T, Bergström U, Hedström EM, et al. Epidemiology of acute knee injuries seen at the emergency department at Umeå University Hospital, Sweden, during 15 years. Knee Surg Sports Traumatol Arthrosc 2014;22(5):1149–55.
3. Shaw L, Finch CF. Trends in pediatric and adolescent anterior cruciate ligament injuries in Victoria, Australia 2005-2015. Int J Environ Res Public Health 2017; 14(6):599.
4. Hsiao M, Owens BD, Burks R, et al. Incidence of acute traumatic patellar dislocation among active-duty United States military service members. Am J Sports Med 2010;38(10):1997–2004.
5. Mayer S, Albright JC, Stoneback JW. Pediatric knee dislocations and physeal fractures about the knee. JAAOS - J Am Acad Orthopaedic Surgeons. 2015; 23(9):571–80.
6. McFarlane KH, Coene RP, Feldman L, et al. Increased incidence of acute patellar dislocations and patellar instability surgical procedures across the United States in paediatric and adolescent patients. J Children's Orthopaedics 2021;15(2):149–56.
7. Feng J, Wick J, Bompiani E, et al. Applications of gait analysis in pediatric orthopaedics. Curr Orthopaedic Pract 2016;27(4):455–64.
8. Carollo JJ, Dennis M. Chapter 16: the assessment of human gait, motion, and motor function. Pediatric rehabilitation: principles and practice, 461. Demos-Medical; 2009. chap 16.
9. Carollo JJ, Matthews DJ Ch. 5 Quantitative assessment of gait: a systematic approach. Pediatr Rehabil Principles Pract 2015;5:78–112.
10. Mirabella O, Raucea A, Fisichella F, et al. A motion capture system for sport training andrehabilitation. Proceedings of the 4th International Conference on Human System Interactions, HSI 2011,19-21 May 2011, 2011. p. 52-59.
11. Ricardo D, Raposo MR, Cruz EB, et al. Effects of ankle foot orthoses on the gait patterns in children with spastic bilateral cerebral palsy: a scoping review. Children (Basel). 2021;8(10). https://doi.org/10.3390/children8100903.
12. Ferrarin M, Rabuffetti M, Bacchini M, et al. Does gait analysis change clinical decision-making in poststroke patients? Results from a pragmatic prospective observational study. Eur J Phys Rehabil Med 2015;51(2):171–84.
13. Yunus MNH, Jaafar MH, Mohamed ASA, et al. Implementation of kinetic and kinematic variables in ergonomic risk assessment using motion capture simulation: a review. Int J Environ Res Public Health 2021;18(16):8342.
14. Johnson WR, Mian A, Donnelly CJ, et al. Predicting athlete ground reaction forces and moments from motion capture. Med Biol Eng Comput 2018;56(10): 1781–92.
15. Pueo B, Jimenez-Olmedo JM. Application of motion capture technology for sport performance analysis. Retos 2017;(32):241–247.
16. Õunpuu S, Pierz K, Rethlefsen SA, et al. Cost savings for single event multilevel surgery in comparison to sequential surgery in ambulatory children with cerebral palsy. Gait Posture 2022;96:53–9.

17. Wren TA, Lening C, Rethlefsen SA, et al. Impact of gait analysis on correction of excessive hip internal rotation in ambulatory children with cerebral palsy: a randomized controlled trial. Dev Med Child Neurol 2013;55(10):919–25.

18. Hayford CF, Pratt E, Cashman JP, et al. Effectiveness of global optimisation and direct kinematics in predicting surgical outcome in children with cerebral palsy. Life (Basel) 2021;(12):11. https://doi.org/10.3390/life11121306.

19. Chang FM, Rhodes JT, Flynn KM, et al. The role of gait analysis in treating gait abnormalities in cerebral palsy. The Orthop Clin North America 2010;41(4): 489–506.

20. Wolfe S, Varacallo M, Thomas JD, et al. Patellar instability. [Updated 2022 May 8]. In: StatPearls [Internet]. Treasure Island (FL): StatPearls Publishing; 2022. Available at: https://www.ncbi.nlm.nih.gov/books/NBK482427/.

21. Sanders TL, Pareek A, Hewett TE, et al. Incidence of first-time lateral patellar dislocation: a 21-year population-based study. Sports Health 2018;10(2): 146–51.

22. Dejour H, Walch G, Nove-Josserand L, et al. Factors of patellar instability: an anatomic radiographic study. Knee Surg Sports Traumatol Arthrosc 1994;2(1): 19–26.

23. Dewan V, Webb MSL, Prakash D, et al. Patella dislocation: an online systematic video analysis of the mechanism of injury. Knee Surg Relat Res 2020;32.

24. Lucas KCH, Jacobs C, Lattermann C, et al. Gait deviations and muscle strength deficits in subjects with patellar instability. Knee 2020;27(4):1285–90.

25. Camathias C, Ammann E, Meier RL, et al. Recurrent patellar dislocations in adolescents result in decreased knee flexion during the entire gait cycle. Knee Surg Sports Traumatol Arthrosc 2020;28(7):2053–66.

26. Clark DA, Simpson DL, Eldridge J, et al. Patellar instability and quadriceps avoidance affect walking knee moments. Knee 2016;23(1):78–84.

27. Philippot R, Boyer B, Testa R, et al. Study of patellar kinematics after reconstruction of the medial patellofemoral ligament. Clin Biomech (Bristol, Avon) 2012; 27(1):22–6.

28. Grantham WJ, Aman ZS, Brady AW, et al. Medial patellotibial ligament reconstruction improves patella tracking when combined with medial patellofemoral reconstruction: an in vitro kinematic study. Arthroscopy 2020;36(9):2501–9.

29. Redler LH, Meyers KN, Brady JM, et al. Anisometry of medial patellofemoral ligament reconstruction in the setting of increased tibial tubercle-trochlear groove distance and patella alta. Arthroscopy 2018;34(2):502–10.

30. Carnesecchi O, Philippot R, Boyer B, et al. Recovery of gait pattern after medial patellofemoral ligament reconstruction for objective patellar instability. Knee Surg Sports Traumatol Arthrosc 2016;24(1):123–8.

31. Asaeda M, Deie M, Fujita N, et al. Knee biomechanics during walking in recurrent lateral patellar dislocation are normalized by 1 year after medial patellofemoral ligament reconstruction. Knee Surg Sports Traumatol Arthrosc 2016; 24(10):3254–61.

32. Schlichte LM, Sidharthan S, Green DW, et al. Pediatric management of recurrent patellar instability. Sports Med Arthrosc Rev 2019;27(4):171–80.

33. Collins NJ, Barton CJ, van Middelkoop M, et al. 2018 Consensus statement on exercise therapy and physical interventions (orthoses, taping and manual therapy) to treat patellofemoral pain: recommendations from the 5th International Patellofemoral Pain Research Retreat, Gold Coast, Australia, 2017. Br J Sports Med 2018;52(18):1170–8.

34. Crossley K, Bennell K, Green S, et al. Physical therapy for patellofemoral pain: a randomized, double-blinded, placebo-controlled trial. Am J Sports Med 2002; 30(6):857–65.
35. McConnell J. Rehabilitation and nonoperative treatment of patellar instability. Sports Med Arthrosc Rev 2007;15(2):95–104.
36. Dejour DH, Mesnard G, Giovannetti de Sanctis E. Updated treatment guidelines for patellar instability: "un menu à la carte". J Exp Orthopaedics 2021;8(1):109.
37. Glattke KE, Tummala SV, Chhabra A. Anterior cruciate ligament reconstruction recovery and rehabilitation: a systematic review. J Bone Joint Surg Am 2022; 104(8):739–54.
38. Roe C, Jacobs C, Hoch J, et al. Test batteries after primary anterior cruciate ligament reconstruction: a systematic review. Sports Health 2022;14(2):205–15.
39. Marom N, Xiang W, Wolfe I, et al. High variability and lack of standardization in the evaluation of return to sport after ACL reconstruction: a systematic review. Knee Surg Sports Traumatol Arthrosc 2022;30(4):1369–79.
40. McKinney B, Cherney S, Penna J. Intra-articular knee injuries in patients with knee extensor mechanism ruptures. Knee Surg Sports Traumatol Arthrosc 2008;16(7):633–8.
41. Sabbag OD, Hevesi M, Sanders TL, et al. Incidence and treatment trends of symptomatic discoid lateral menisci: an 18-year population-based study. Orthop J Sports Med 2018;6(9). 2325967118797886-2325967118797886.
42. Harato K, Sakurai A, Kudo Y, et al. Three-dimensional knee kinematics in patients with a discoid lateral meniscus during gait. Knee 2016;23(4):622–6.
43. Lin Z, Huang W, Ma L, et al. Kinematic features in patients with lateral discoid meniscus injury during walking. Scientific Rep 2018;8(1):5053.
44. Naraghi A, White LM. MR imaging of cruciate ligaments. Magn Reson Imaging Clin N Am 2014;22(4):557–80.
45. Pache S, Aman ZS, Kennedy M, et al. Posterior cruciate ligament: current concepts review. Arch Bone Jt Surg 2018;6(1):8–18.
46. Tibone JE, Antich TJ, Perry J, et al. Functional analysis of untreated and reconstructed posterior cruciate ligament injuries. Am J Sports Med 1988;16(3): 217–23.
47. Brisson NM, Agres AN, Jung TM, et al. Gait adaptations at 8 years after reconstruction of unilateral isolated and combined posterior cruciate ligament injuries. Am J Sports Med 2021;49(9):2416–25.
48. Hart JM, Blanchard BF, Hart JA, et al. Multiple ligament knee reconstruction clinical follow-up and gait analysis. Knee Surg Sports Traumatol Arthrosc 2009; 17(3):277–85.
49. Fontboté CA, Sell TC, Laudner KG, et al. Neuromuscular and biomechanical adaptations of patients with isolated deficiency of the posterior cruciate ligament. Am J Sports Med 2005;33(7):982–9.
50. Charbonnier C, Duthon VB, Chagué S, et al. In vivo static and dynamic lengthening measurements of the posterior cruciate ligament at high knee flexion angles. Int J Comput Assist Radiol Surg 2020;15(3):555–64.
51. Florit D, Pedret C, Casals M, et al. Incidence of tendinopathy in team sports in a multidisciplinary sports club over 8 seasons. J Sports Sci Med 2019;18(4): 780–8.
52. Barker-Davies RM, Roberts A, Watson J, et al. Kinematic and kinetic differences between military patients with patellar tendinopathy and asymptomatic controls during single leg squats. Clin Biomech (Bristol, Avon) 2019;62:127–35.

53. Mann KJ, Edwards S, Drinkwater EJ, et al. A lower limb assessment tool for athletes at risk of developing patellar tendinopathy. Med Sci Sports Exerc 2013; 45(3):527–33.

54. Kulig K, Joiner DG, Chang YJ. Landing limb posture in volleyball athletes with patellar tendinopathy: a pilot study. Int J Sports Med 2015;36(5):400–6.

55. Scattone Silva R, Purdam CR, Fearon AM, et al. Effects of altering trunk position during landings on patellar tendon force and pain. Med Sci Sports Exerc 2017; 49(12):2517–27.

56. Bazett-Jones DM, Rathleff MS, Holden S. Associations between number of pain sites and sleep, sports participation, and quality of life: a cross-sectional survey of 1021 youth from the Midwestern United States. BMC Pediatr 2019;19(1):201.

57. Barber Foss KD, Myer GD, Chen SS, et al. Expected prevalence from the differential diagnosis of anterior knee pain in adolescent female athletes during pre-participation screening. J athletic Train 2012;47(5):519–24.

58. Molgaard C, Rathleff MS, Simonsen O. Patellofemoral pain syndrome and its association with hip, ankle, and foot function in 16-to 18-year-old high school students a single-blind case-control study. J Am Podiatric Med Assoc 2011;101(3): 215–22.

59. Smith BE, Selfe J, Thacker D, et al. Incidence and prevalence of patellofemoral pain: a systematic review and meta-analysis. Meta-Analysis Support and AuthorAnonymous, Research Support, Non-U.S. Gov't Review. PLoS ONE [Electronic Resource] 2018;13(1):e0190892.

60. Foss KDB, Myer GD, Hewett TE. Epidemiology of basketball, soccer, and volleyball injuries in middle-school female athletes. Physician Sportsmed 2014;42(2): 146–53.

61. Kujala UM, Kvist M, Heinonen O. Osgood-Schlatter's disease in adolescent athletes. Retrospective study of incidence and duration. Am J Sports Med 1985; 13(4):236–41.

62. Van Dijk CN, Van Der Tempel WM. Patellofemoral pain syndrome. Editorial. BMJ 2008;337(7677):1006–7.

63. Utting MR, Davies G, Newman JH. Is anterior knee pain a predisposing factor to patellofemoral osteoarthritis? Knee 2005;12(5):362–5.

64. Nimon G, Murray D, Sandow M, et al. Natural history of anterior knee pain: a 14-to 20-year follow-up of nonoperative management. J Pediatr Orthop 1998;18(1): 118–22.

65. Crossley KM. Is patellofemoral osteoarthritis a common sequela of patellofemoral pain? Br J Sports Med 2014;48(6):409–10.

66. Powers CM, Witvrouw E, Davis IS, et al. Evidence-based framework for a pathomechanical model of patellofemoral pain: 2017 patellofemoral pain consensus statement from the 4th International Patellofemoral Pain Research Retreat, Manchester, UK: part 3. Br J Sports Med 2017;51(24):1713–23.

67. Myer GD, Ford KR, Barber Foss KD, et al. The incidence and potential pathomechanics of patellofemoral pain in female athletes. Clin Biomech (Bristol, Avon) 2010;25(7):700–7.

68. Holden S, Boreham C, Doherty C, et al. Two-dimensional knee valgus displacement as a predictor of patellofemoral pain in adolescent females. Scandinavian journal of medicine & science in sports 2017;27(2):188–94.

69. Rathleff MS, Samani A, Olesen JL, et al. Neuromuscular activity and knee kinematics in adolescents with patellofemoral pain. Med Sci Sports Exerc 2013; 45(9):1730–9.

70. Powers CM, Landel R, Perry J. Timing and intensity of vastus muscle activity during functional activities in subjects with and without patellofemoral pain. Research Support, Non-U.S. Gov't. Phys Ther 1996;76(9):946–55 [discussion: 956–67].
71. Powers CM, Perry J, Hsu A, et al. Are patellofemoral pain and quadriceps femoris muscle torque associated with locomotor function?... including commentary by McClay IS and author response. Phys Ther 1997;77(10):1063–78.
72. Powers CM, Chen PY, Reischl SF, et al. Comparison of foot pronation and lower extremity rotation in persons with and without patellofemoral pain. Comparative Study. Foot Ankle Int 2002;23(7):634–40.
73. Messier SP, Davis SE, Curl WW, et al. Etiologic factors associated with patellofemoral pain in runners. Article. Med Sci Sports Exerc 1991;23(9):1008–15.
74. Straub RK, Powers CM. Utility of 2D video analysis for assessing frontal plane trunk and pelvis motion during stepping, landing, and change in direction tasks: a validity study. Int J Sports Phys Ther 2022;17(2):139–47.
75. Ferber R, Davis IM, Williams DS 3rd. Gender differences in lower extremity mechanics during running. Clin Biomech (Bristol, Avon) 2003;18(4):350–7.
76. Nigg BM, Baltich J, Maurer C, et al. Shoe midsole hardness, sex and age effects on lower extremity kinematics during running. J Biomech 2012;45(9):1692–7.
77. Brindle RA, Milner CE, Zhang S, et al. Changing step width alters lower extremity biomechanics during running. Gait Posture 2014;39(1):124–8.
78. Taylor-Haas JA, Long JT, Garcia MC, et al. The influence of maturation and sex on pelvis and hip kinematics in youth distance runners. J Sci Med Sport 2022; 25(3):272–8.
79. Silvernail JF, Boyer K, Rohr E, et al. Running mechanics and variability with aging. Med Sci Sports Exerc 2015;47(10):2175–80.
80. Thompson-Kolesar JA, Gatewood CT, Tran AA, et al. Age influences biomechanical changes after participation in an anterior cruciate ligament injury prevention program. Am J Sports Med 2018;46(3):598–606.
81. Lazaridis SN, Bassa EI, Patikas D, et al. Biomechanical comparison in different jumping tasks between untrained boys and men. Pediatr Exerc Sci 2013;25(1): 101–13.
82. Briem K, Jónsdóttir KV, Árnason Á, et al. Effects of sex and fatigue on biomechanical measures during the drop-jump task in children. Orthop J Sports Med Jan 2017;5(1). 2325967116679640.
83. Hewett TE, Myer GD, Kiefer AW, et al. Longitudinal increases in knee abduction moments in females during adolescent growth. Med Sci Sports Exerc 2015; 47(12):2579–85.
84. DiStefano LJ, Martinez JC, Crowley E, et al. Maturation and sex differences in neuromuscular characteristics of youth athletes. J Strength Cond Res 2015; 29(9):2465–73.
85. Lazaridis S, Bassa E, Patikas D, et al. Neuromuscular differences between prepubescents boys and adult men during drop jump. Eur J Appl Physiol 2010; 110(1):67–74.
86. Petrovic M, Sigurðsson HB, Sigurðsson HJ, et al. Effect of sex on anterior cruciate ligament injury-related biomechanics during the cutting maneuver in preadolescent athletes. Orthop J Sports Med 2020;8(7):2325967120936980.
87. Landry SC, McKean KA, Hubley-Kozey CL, et al. Neuromuscular and lower limb biomechanical differences exist between male and female elite adolescent soccer players during an unanticipated run and crosscut maneuver. Am J Sports Med 2007;35(11):1901–11.

88. Whatman C, Hume P, Hing W. Kinematics during lower extremity functional screening tests in young athletes: are they reliable and valid? Phys Ther Sport 2013;14(2):87–93.

89. Thompson JA, Tran AA, Gatewood CT, et al. Biomechanical effects of an injury prevention program in preadolescent female soccer athletes. Am J Sports Med 2017;45(2):294–301.

90. Zebis MK, Andersen LL, Brandt M, et al. Effects of evidence-based prevention training on neuromuscular and biomechanical risk factors for ACL injury in adolescent female athletes: a randomised controlled trial. Br J Sports Med 2016;50(9):552–7.

91. Hosseini E, Daneshjoo A, Sahebozamani M, et al. The effects of fatigue on knee kinematics during unanticipated change of direction in adolescent girl athletes: a comparison between dominant and non-dominant legs. Sports Biomech 2021;1–10.

92. Garcia MC, Lennon A, Bazett-Jones DM, et al. Influence of hamstring flexibility on running kinematics in adolescent long-distance runners. Gait Posture 2022; 93:107–12.

93. Sigurðsson HB, Karlsson J, Snyder-Mackler L, et al. Kinematics observed during ACL injury are associated with large early peak knee abduction moments during a change of direction task in healthy adolescents. J Orthop Res 2021; 39(10):2281–90.

94. Pfile KR, Hart JM, Herman DC, et al. Different exercise training interventions and drop-landing biomechanics in high school female athletes. J athletic Train 2013; 48(4):450–62.

95. Giustino V, Messina G, Patti A, et al. Effects of a postural exercise program on vertical jump height in young female volleyball players with knee valgus. Int J Environ Res Public Health 2022;(7):19. https://doi.org/10.3390/ijerph19073953.

96. Myer GD, Ford KR, Brent JL, et al. The effects of plyometric vs. dynamic stabilization and balance training on power, balance, and landing force in female athletes. J Strength Cond Res 2006;20(2):345–53.

97. Sigward SM, Havens KL, Powers CM. Knee separation distance and lower extremity kinematics during a drop land: implications for clinical screening. J athletic Train 2011;46(5):471–5.

98. Christoforidou A, Patikas DA, Bassa E, et al. Landing from different heights: biomechanical and neuromuscular strategies in trained gymnasts and untrained prepubescent girls. J Electromyogr Kinesiol 2017;32:1–8.

99. Tsai YJ, Chia CC, Lee PY, et al. Landing kinematics, sports performance, and isokinetic strength in adolescent male volleyball athletes: influence of core training. J Sport Rehabil 2020;29(1):65–72.

100. Clagg SE, Warnock A, Thomas JS. Kinetic analyses of maximal effort soccer kicks in female collegiate athletes. Sports Biomech Jun 2009;8(2):141–53.

101. Milewski MD, Õunpuu S, Solomito M, et al. Adolescent baseball pitching technique: lower extremity biomechanical analysis. J Appl Biomech 2012;28(5): 491–501.

102. Kung SM, Shultz SP, Kontaxis A, et al. Changes in lower extremity kinematics and temporal parameters of adolescent baseball pitchers during an extended pitching bout. Am J Sports Med 2017;45(5):1179–86.

103. Fava AW, Downs Talmage JL, Plummer HA, et al. Drive-leg kinematics during the windup and pushoff is associated with pitching kinetics at later phases of the pitch. Am J Sports Med Apr 2022;50(5):1409–15.

104. Friesen KB, Shaw RE, Shannon DM, et al. Single-leg squat compensations are associated with softball pitching pathomechanics in adolescent softball pitchers. Orthop J Sports Med 2021;9(3). 2325967121990920.

105. Wasserberger K, Barfield J, Anz A, et al. Using the single leg squat as an assessment of stride leg knee mechanics in adolescent baseball pitchers. J Sci Med Sport 2019;22(11):1254–9.

106. Rutkowska-Kucharska A, Szpala A, Jaroszczuk S, et al. Muscle coactivation during stability exercises in rhythmic gymnastics: a two-case study. Appl Bionics Biomech 2018;2018. https://doi.org/10.1155/2018/8260402. 8260402.

107. Herbaut A, Chavet P, Roux M, et al. The influence of shoe drop on the kinematics and kinetics of children tennis players. *Eur J Sport Sci* Nov 2016;16(8):1121–9.

108. Fett J, Oberschelp N, Vuong JL, et al. Kinematic characteristics of the tennis serve from the ad and deuce court service positions in elite junior players. PLoS One 2021;16(7). e0252650.

109. Schaefer A, O'Dwyer N, Ferdinands RED, et al. Consistency of kinematic and kinetic patterns during a prolonged spell of cricket fast bowling: an exploratory laboratory study. *J Sports Sci* Mar 2018;36(6):679–90.

110. Parsons JL, Carswell J, Nwoba IM, et al. Athlete perceptions and physical performance effects of the fifa 11 + program in 9-11 year-old female soccer players: a cluster randomized trial. Int J Sports Phys Ther 2019;14(5):740–52.

111. Yang C, Yao W, Garrett WE, et al. Effects of an intervention program on lower extremity biomechanics in stop-jump and side-cutting tasks. Am J Sports Med 2018;46(12):3014–22.

112. Lin CW, You YL, Chen YA, et al. Effect of integrated training on balance and ankle reposition sense in ballet dancers. Int J Environ Res Public Health 2021;(23):18. https://doi.org/10.3390/ijerph182312751.

113. García-Luna MA, Cortell-Tormo JM, García-Jaén M, et al. Acute effects of ACL injury-prevention warm-up and soccer-specific fatigue protocol on dynamic knee valgus in youth male soccer players. Int J Environ Res Public Health 2020;(15):17. https://doi.org/10.3390/ijerph17155608.

Rehabilitation After Pediatric and Adolescent Knee Injuries

Joseph T. Molony Jr, PT, MS. SCS, CSCS[a],*,
Elliot M. Greenberg, PT, DPT, PhD[b], Adam P. Weaver, PT, DPT[c],
Mimi Racicot, PT, DPT, SCS[d], Donna Merkel, PT, DPT, SCS, CSCS[e],
Christin Zwolski, PT, DPT, PhD[f]

KEYWORDS

- Young athlete • Youth sports • Rehabilitation • Pediatric • Adolescent • Knee

KEY POINTS

- More details are now available for decision making regarding return to play, with a continuum consisting of return to participation, return to sports and eventually return to performance.
- Ideal functional mechanics, such as symmetric weight-bearing with double leg tasks, neutral knee alignment, and hip strategy are of great importance in the rehabilitation of young athletes.
- While there is limited evidence available regarding the rehabilitation of JOCD, up-to-date recommendations are provided in this article
- Blood flow restriction therapy (BFRT/BFR) is gaining popularity in the treatment of the young athlete's knee.

INTRODUCTION

According to epidemiology studies, most of the youth sports injuries presenting to primary care, athletic trainers, and emergency departments impact the musculoskeletal

[a] Young Athlete Program, Department of Pediatric Rehabilitation, HSS | Hospital for Special Surgery, 535 East 70th Street, New York, NY 10021, USA; [b] Children's Hospital of Philadelphia Sports Medicine and Performance Center, Bucks County, 500 West Butler Ave. Chalfont, PA 18914, USA; [c] Connecticut Children's, 399 Farmington Avenue, Farmington, CT 06032, USA; [d] Rehabilitation & Sports, Department of Rehabilitation, Seattle Children's Hospital, 4800 Sand Point Way Northeast, Seattle, WA 98105, USA; [e] Main Line Health System, Collegeville, 599 Arcola Rd, Collegeville, PA 19426, USA; [f] Division of Occupational Therapy & Physical Therapy, Cincinnati Children's Hospital Medical Center, 2800 Winslow Avenue, Cincinnati, OH 45206, USA
* Corresponding author.
E-mail address: molonyj@hss.edu
Twitter: egreenberg01 (E.M.G.); @adampweaver (A.P.W.)

Clin Sports Med 41 (2022) 687–705
https://doi.org/10.1016/j.csm.2022.05.007
0278-5919/22/© 2022 Elsevier Inc. All rights reserved.

system.[1] Effective rehabilitation of knee injuries ensures a timely return to sports participation and minimizes the negative physical, psychological, and social consequences of becoming injured. The following article provides rehabilitation and return to play strategies for postsurgical and nonsurgical injuries of the young athlete's knee.

CHONDRAL INJURIES

There is a limited body of evidence available to specifically guide operative or nonoperative rehabilitation for patients with Juvenile Osteochondritis Dissecans (JOCD). Nevertheless, principles of general knee rehabilitation with regards to impairment resolution, progressive resistance exercises, neuromuscular training, and gradual advancement of external loading demands can be applied to this population.[2,3] Communication with the referring orthopedic provider is important as lesion-specific characteristics, such as location, size and stability may require specific adaptations to the rehabilitation program.[4,5]

Both operative and nonoperative rehabilitation have shared principles that involve protecting the healing articular cartilage, addressing local impairments (eg, effusion, decreased range of motion, weakness), addressing remote impairments or neuromuscular control deficits that may alter knee or lower limb loading patterns (eg, hip strength, ankle mobility, core strength), and progressive functional loading to meet patient goals of returning to desired activities.

During nonoperative rehabilitation, the protection of healing tissue usually consists of reduced joint loading initially, typically involving a period of non–weight-bearing, modified weight-bearing, or reduced activity. At times a knee immobilizer or valgus unloader brace may be prescribed to further limit the loading of lesions in specific areas.[4] Patient-specific factors such as age, lesion size, location, and stability will dictate the extent and duration of these restrictions, but typically a duration of 6 to 8 weeks can be expected.[3,4] During this time, rehabilitation should focus on limiting any secondary impairments in motion, strength, and flexibility throughout the lower extremity which may result from reduced activity levels, while also addressing any preexisting impairments in hip and core strength, as well as neuromuscular control. Exercise selection can be diverse and specifically tailored to each patient, based on individual presentation and weight-bearing restrictions. Patient education regarding adherence to limited weight-bearing status during functional tasks is important during this time. Proper education in the use of crutches and activity restrictions will optimize the healing environment. In addition, education regarding rehabilitation progression and recovery expectations is important, to help ensure patient/parent expectations match reality and facilitate a good therapeutic alliance.

Once weight-bearing and/or immobilization restrictions have been lifted, rehabilitation can progress to focus on restoring normal gait mechanics, resolution of any deficits in isolated muscle strength, and continued focus on neuromuscular control to resolve any impairments in frontal or sagittal plane knee control, which may contribute to excessive shear or compressive forces on articular cartilage. Exercise prescription should include both open and closed chain exercises, as these will help address isolated strength deficits and improve dynamic limb control. Balance and proprioception exercises should be progressed to appropriately challenge the patient; however, the clinician should always be mindful to ensure proper body and limb control is maintained during these activities. The goal of this phase of rehabilitation is to establish a solid foundation of strength, normalized functional movement patterns, and load tolerance to allow the patient to safely progress to impact and sports-specific training. It is imperative to continually monitor the patient's knee for effusion, pain, mechanical symptoms, or changes in ROM, which may signal the knee is not adapting well to increased demands. Transient effusion that lasts for less than 48 hours can be addressed by icing, compression, and decreasing exercise loads. A persistent effusion, mechanical symptoms/clicking/locking, or loss of ROM should be discussed with the referring physician immediately as this may signal lesion progression or failure of conservative management.

To progress rehabilitation to include impact activities (eg, jogging, light plyometrics, agility exercises), the patient should demonstrate 5/5 strength in quadriceps, high-quality limb control during closed chain exercises, and be tolerating the current joint loads without issue. If available, more precise measures of quadriceps strength using handheld dynamometry or isokinetic dynamometer should be used, with a limb symmetry index of at least 75%-80% required to advance to impact activities. In addition, communication with the orthopedic provider is necessary to verify that adequate radiographic healing has been established. Abnormalities in dynamic limb control seen earlier in rehabilitation may return when advancing to impact activities. Strategies favoring implicit learning, external cuing, visual feedback, and task progression to include cognitive demands should be used to optimize neuromuscular control within this phase.[6] The criteria to begin the return to sports progression are similar to those published for anterior cruciate ligament rehabilitation and should include at least 85% to 90% limb symmetry in strength and functional testing.[3,7]

Postoperative rehabilitation shares similar overarching principles with regard to providing a protected environment for healing and tissue remodeling, while using time-based and objective criteria, with consistent monitoring of patient responses to help guide the progression of rehabilitation.[7] Many articular cartilage restoration procedures exist and differences in surgical procedure, lesion location, size, and rate of healing will dictate specific time-frames required to progress through the various phases of rehabilitation. Weight-bearing restrictions typically last between 4 and 6 weeks for transarticular drilling procedures, fixation of unstable lesions, and microfracture, while a longer duration of 8 to 10 weeks may be required for cell-based procedures such as autologous chondrocyte implantation (ACI/MACI), particulated juvenile cartilage, bone marrow aspirate concentrate (BMAC), and so forth. Typically, some type of hinged knee brace will be recommended for protection and locking the brace in extension is an excellent way of maintaining or helping regain full knee extension, which is of utmost importance. Range of motion exercises through flexion and extension helps prevent stiffness, decrease pain and effusion, while also providing an improved environment for healing and nutrient exchange at the surgical site. While ROM should be emphasized early and often, flexion motion limitations may be imposed early depending on procedure type and lesion location. Aggressive stretching/ROM should be avoided, and instead, a low load long duration approach should be taken. Quadriceps muscle weakness due to activation failure and disuse atrophy is a major concern and should be addressed early using neuromuscular electrical stimulation and active exercises. Proximal and distal strengthening exercises should also be initiated at this time, while ensuring maintenance of any weight-bearing or ROM restrictions.

Once the patient has achieved appropriate time from surgery and demonstrates adequate ROM and quadriceps control for safe ambulation, their rehabilitation can progress to focus on more advanced closed chain exercises, such as single-leg squats, lunges, and balance activities. As with nonoperative care, a heavy emphasis on symmetric loading, limb alignment, and neuromuscular control is essential while incorporating more dynamic exercises into the rehabilitation regimen. Isolated muscle strengthening should continue to address ongoing localized strength deficits. Similar objective criteria outlined earlier can be used for progressing the athlete to impact activities. Time frames for return to sports progression will vary significantly depending on individual healing factors and type of procedure. Athletes undergoing transarticular drilling procedures or microfracture typically can return to sports around 4 to 6 months, while those undergoing more complex cellular procedures may have a more prolonged recovery, perhaps not returning to sports until 12 months postoperatively.[2]

LIGAMENT INJURIES

High-quality rehabilitation of ligamentous knee injuries in pediatric and adolescent athletes is essential to optimize return to daily activities and allow safe return to sports. At the start of rehabilitation, the clinician should consider numerous factors including age, activity level, athletic history, the patient's future athletic plans, graft type, and concomitant pathologies. There should also be complete knowledge of the patient's general health, injury history, and comorbidities.

Graft selection will dictate clinical decision making in the early phases of rehabilitation after ACLR and each has rehabilitation implications. Bone-patellar tendon-bone (BPTB/BTB) and hamstring tendon autografts are the most widely used, with quadriceps tendon (QT) autografts growing in popularity. Drawbacks of BPTB/BTB include delayed quadriceps strength recovery and anterior knee pain. Proponents of hamstring tendon autograft note decreased anterior knee pain and improved knee extensor strength. In the skeletally immature population, the iliotibial band (ITB) is widely used for its physeal sparing benefits.[8] Challenges persist in this young age group for the management of pain and home exercise program adherence. Quadriceps tendon knee extension strength recovery seems to be comparable to other graft types in adults,[9] but it is still unknown in the pediatric population.

Meniscus tears with ACL injury are recognized as the most common concomitant injury in adolescent athletes.[10] There has been a recent trend toward meniscal repair in this population due to poor long-term outcomes after partial meniscectomy.[11] Meniscus tear type and location will impact the range of motion and weight-bearing limitations postoperatively, but newer evidence has suggested that early weight-bearing and unrestricted range of motion has no impact on outcomes.[12–14] Meniscus root tears must also be considered during rehabilitation as these tears require a limited range of motion and weight-bearing, and require a more cautious rehabilitation approach.[15]

While less common, special considerations should be made for medial and lateral collateral ligament injuries. In isolation, most are managed nonoperatively and with bracing. Of note, Salter-Harris fractures of the distal femur are associated with the same valgus trauma to the knee that causes MCL injuries in this population. Multiligament injuries in the knee often involve the posterolateral corner and have a significant impact on rehabilitation. In these injuries, care must be taken to protect all damaged structures in the early phases of rehabilitation and communication with the surgeon regarding the details of the surgery is essential.

Arthrofibrosis after ACLR is a common complication and is defined as a loss of either extension or flexion motion.[16,17] Cyclops lesions, or anterior arthrofibrosis, are defined as the formation of scar tissue located anteriorly to the graft after ACLR. The incidence is reported between 1% and 9.8%,[18] and has been reported more commonly with the use of QT grafts.[19–21] Symptoms include progressive loss of terminal knee extension as scar tissue forms in femoral notch. Knee extension deficits beyond 3 weeks after ACLR are a risk factor for cyclops lesions.[18,22]

Rehabilitation following ligamentous injury with or without surgical intervention is common in the field of physical therapy. Refer to **Table 1** for special considerations and up-to-date concepts for each phase.

PATELLAR INSTABILITY

There are numerous factors, both static and dynamic, that contribute to the stability of the patellofemoral joint. Clinical evaluation includes history and physical examination. Historically relevant information includes the age of the patient at first dislocation, number of episodes of instability, and family history of patellar instability and/or hypermobility. The description of the injury includes the mechanism of injury, position of the limb when injured, direction of the dislocation, and whether relocation was spontaneous or manual. Evidence suggests that skeletally immature patients who have a primary patellar dislocation at a younger age have a greater chance of developing chronic instability and recurrent dislocations. Each subsequent dislocation can increase the chances of additional dislocations and potential cartilage damage.[40–42]

Physical examination of the acute injury includes the assessment of pain and effusion, tenderness along the medial patella, and/or and Basset sign (tenderness of the attachment of the MPFL on the medial femoral condyle). General ROM, quadriceps atrophy, hypermobility (Beighton score) including the presence of knee hyperextension should be assessed.[43] Comprehensive examination should also include meniscal pathology, assessment of ACL and MCL, and presence of any neurologic symptoms. Rotational alignment of the lower extremity, including femoral anteversion, tibial torsion, knee valgus, and protonation should be noted. Physical findings should be compared with the contralateral limb.[44] Additional comprehensive assessment, if tolerated, includes patellar glides at full extension and early flexion, an Apprehension test at 30° of flexion, and J sign with active knee flexion and extension.[45,46]

If the patient is less acute and without restrictions on weight-bearing, a standing assessment can be completed. Standing alignment and dynamic gait should be observed. Specific attention should be directed at rotational components of hip, knee, and foot with weight-bearing. Additional functional testing (if tolerated) includes single-leg stance, partial squat, and step downs (within pain-free range) to assess hip and quadriceps strength and core control.

Nonoperative or conservative management of patellar instability is standard practice for a first-time primary dislocation without osteochondral fracture.[47–51] Although systematic studies show there is no consensus on the initial management of acute dislocation in children,[52,53] traditional nonoperative management includes a period of immobilization (1–4 weeks) followed by the initiation of ROM and functional rehabilitation.[54] Nonoperative treatment focuses on decreasing the risk factors that can contribute to patellar instability. Local risk factors for instability include general ligamentous laxity, and/or specific laxity of the medial retinaculum, medial patellofemoral ligament (MPFL) injury, weakness of the abductors and external rotators of the hip, and weakness or atrophy of the Quadriceps (VMO),[55] Tight lateral structures including the ITB complex can also be a factor. Deficits of proximal muscular strength and decreased neuromuscular control can result in abnormal lower extremity kinematics, increasing the mechanical risk factors of excessive hip internal rotation and knee valgus.

There is general agreement on the following the principals of rehabilitation:

- Ambulatory aide should be used until normal gait is possible, control of effusion and early return of ROM is the initial primary focus, followed by the return of muscle strength and functional rehabilitation.
- Nonoperative treatment is directed both at the recovery of the injury as well as addressing strength and flexibility deficits, and neuromuscular control of the lower extremity including proximal hip, and core strength.

Table 1
Postoperative rehabilitation of pediatric and adolescent knee ligament injuries: special considerations and up-to-date concepts

Phases	Goals	Restrictions and Considerations	Rehabilitation Exercises	Criteria for Progression to Next Phase
I Weeks 1–4	• Protect graft • Reduce pain and swelling • Progress to WBAT/wean off crutches	• Braced for weeks 1–2 locked in extension for ambulation and for sleep until pain is minimal and quadriceps control is sufficient • Crutches until minimal swelling and full active terminal knee extension in weight-bearing • Concomitant pathologies: altered weight-bearing and ROM restrictions per surgeon • The impact of reflex inhibition and arthrogenic muscle inhibition on ROM and quadriceps strength calls for the aggressive management of pain and swelling.[23]	• Active, active assistive and passive ROM • Low intensity, long duration electrical stimulation can help reduce swelling by increasing venous return[24,25] • Quadriceps and hamstring isometrics[26–28] • Straight leg raises • Open-chain hip strengthening • Early implementation of blood flow restriction training (BFRT/BFR) will allow for the reduction of quadriceps atrophy[29,30]	• Minimal knee swelling • Full weight bearing • Active terminal knee extension • Straight leg raises without extension lag
II Weeks 6–12	• Reduce Pain/Swelling • Quadriceps Control	• Monitor for quad avoidance patterns including: offloading involved extremity, increased trunk flexion, decreased knee flexion • No cutting, pivoting	• High-intensity NMES with active quadriceps isometrics at 60° of knee flexion[31] • Single and double leg hip dominant (deadlift) and knee dominant (squat) • Sensorimotor training • Neuromuscular reeducation	• Full range of motion, minimal swelling and no pain • Knee extension limb symmetry index of ≥70% via handheld/isokinetic dynamometer[33] Functional testing demonstrates high-quality movement: hip

Phase	Goals	Assessment	Interventions	Criteria for Progression
				strategy, symmetry, good depth, and neutral alignment of lower extremity, hip/pelvis, and trunk
III Weeks 12–24	• Prepare to return to run • Symmetric limb strength, power, and endurance	• Fitting of RTS brace • Patient-Reported Outcomes: ACL-RSI/Pedi IKDC (IKDC for 18 and older): low scores are predictive of poor function and reinjury[34–37]	• Cross-training: stationary bike, elliptical, walking program (No swelling) • Integration of visual feedback, external focus of attention to encourage motor learning[32] • Progression of hip and knee dominant movement patterns with emphasis on improving muscular power and endurance. • Initiate plyometric and jump training with progression to lateral cutting and jumping progressions • Initiation and completion of criterion-based running program[38] • Integration of neurocognitive challenges in conjunction with training[39]	• Full knee ROM/No swelling/ No lasting pain • Symmetry, proper alignment, high-quality movement strategies, and force attenuation with impact tasks • Isometric/Isokinetic knee extension limb symmetry ≥ 85% (at 300, 180,° and 60°/ sec if equipment available)
IV Months 6–9	• Return to participation	• No Restrictions	• Hip and knee dominant movement patterns with emphasis on power and rate of force development. • Progression of plyometric training and agility with emphasis on cutting movements at 45° and 90° • Sport-specific skill training in collaboration with a coach and medical training staff.	• Criteria for Progression to Return to Play – refer to Return to Playtesting and Decision-Making section of this article

- Physical therapy to restore strength, range of motion, and function following MPFL reconstruction with or without tibial tubercle osteotomy (TTO) or hemiepiphysiodesis improves patient outcomes.

Published rehabilitation protocols for MPFL reconstruction are variable, but typically include a phased progression of the range of motion, weight-bearing (usually with bracing), strength and stability and return to full activity. Of the published protocols reviewed many did not specify PROM limitations; however, most recommend limiting PROM to 0 to 90°, with a goal of full ROM between 6 and 8 weeks. This was consistent with or without TTO.[47]

Immediately postoperatively, partial weight-bearing with crutches is allowed during the first 2 weeks. During weeks 2 to 6, weaning off crutches, normalizing gait, and progressing weight-bearing as tolerated are implemented with the goal of full weight-bearing without assistive devices by week 6. Most MPFL reconstruction protocols specify bracing postoperatively. Recommendation for wearing a knee brace is generally 6 weeks; however, some recommended a timeframe of 3 to 9 weeks without TTO, and 5 to 9 weeks with TTO.

The strength and dynamic stability phase are initiated when full ROM, full weight-bearing, strength, and neuromuscular control allow for normal gait, usually beginning at 6 to 8 weeks. During this phase, closed chain weight-bearing activities are progressed. Proximal hip and core strength and neuromuscular control are emphasized as rehabilitation progresses into light plyometrics and jogging at 12 to 16 weeks.[56]

The final stage of rehabilitation is the return to full activity. There is significant variability in timing and recommendation regarding return to sport (RTS) following MPFL surgery. Many protocols specify a timeframe ranging from 4 to 6 months for both isolated MPFL surgery and MPFL with TTO. However, most did not specify specific RTS testing guidelines or criteria.[57,58] Studies have shown that quadriceps weakness negatively affects function and performance.[59] There is limited information regarding RTS after MPFL surgery. Studies looking at RTS following MPFL reconstruction demonstrate that patients who underwent MPFL surgery showed significant deficits of isometric knee extension strength and functional testing and may need prolonged rehabilitation beyond 7 months.[60–63] Review of current practices indicates a need to standardize rehabilitation protocols and standardize return to sports testing criteria.

OVERUSE INJURIES

Tensile forces across apophyses and tight tissue structures associated with times of rapid growth increase the risk of overuse injuries in the young athlete's knee. The assessment, treatment and return to play decision process begins with a comprehensive history.[64] In addition to past medical history, questions regarding injury history, menstrual function, sleep, nutrition, and hydration assist with the overall assessment of the health and wellness of the young athlete. Sport-specific questions include sports, positions, number of teams, hours of practice and hours of competition per week, level of play, and sport specialization. Important training information includes intensity of training, distances, training surfaces, training and competition shoes, strength and conditioning with teams and on own, as well as any changes in training over the last 1 to 3 months.

In the young athlete's knee, biomechanical malalignment, either structural or functional, tight tissue structures, muscle imbalances, weakness throughout the kinetic chain, and poor technique during skill execution are often contributory factors to overuse injuries. Initial functional examination includes all the following as able based on pain production: gait with shoes on and off, single-leg balance, bilateral squats with an overhead dowel, single-leg squats, heel walks, toe walks, duck walks, core stability, impact/plyometrics, running and agility. Beyond a typical knee examination, palpation specific to the young athlete includes growth plates, inferior patellar pole, and the tibial tubercle.

Osgood–Schlatter Disease (OSD), Sinding-Larsen–Johansson (SLJ), and patellofemoral pain represent the most common causes of anterior knee pain in the young athlete, often requiring a multifactorial approach that addresses all potentially causative factors of the injury. Treatment of anterior knee pain includes addressing impairments of flexibility, strength, and functional mechanics throughout the lower extremity, hip/pelvis, and trunk. Interventions include static and dynamic stretching of hamstrings and other tight tissues, gradual strength training avoiding painful activities, straight leg raises in all planes, body weight resistance functional movements progressing from bilateral to unilateral exercises adding external resistance as able, neuromuscular control with good alignment using visual feedback and manual contact and/or taping for the facilitation of improved hip, knee and foot alignment, and eventual progression to functional drills. Muscular imbalances at the hip and pelvis region need to be addressed including loosening of tight soft tissues and strengthening hip abductors, extensors, and rotators. Cross-training via pain-free nonimpact activities such as biking, elliptical, and swimming, is important to keep athletes active and minimize deconditioning. Patellofemoral bracing, knee sleeves, and dynamic tape maybe used for symptom relief or patellar stability in the short term; however, the recommendation for using a knee brace is based on each athlete's injury presentation as widespread use is not substantiated in the literature. The effectiveness of custom or over-the-counter shoe inserts to reduce foot protonation and improve biomechanical alignment remains inconclusive. If an athlete is unable to achieve pain-free sports participation, mild pain of 2 or less out of 10 on the visual analog scale that dissipates afterward, preferably on the same day and certainly by the next day, may be acceptable if agreed on by the medical team.

STRENGTH AND CONDITIONING IN REHABILITATION

A common question is whether it is safe for youth to perform strength and conditioning. Not only are these activities safe, but they are also recommended, for health and wellness as well as injury prevention. Review studies have identified that these activities improve strength and functional performance as well as reduce injuries.[65,66] Position statements from the National Strength and Conditioning Association (NSCA) and the American Academy of Pediatrics (AAP) describe the guidelines for strength and conditioning in this population. The central tenants are that there should be a warmup and cool down, strengthening should be performed with adult supervision ensuring safety and proper technique, initially exercises should be learned with no load, and 1 to 3 sets of higher repetitions (eg, 6–15) should be performed 2 to 3 times per week. With adult supervision strengthening can be safely performed by children, pre-adolescents, and adolescents.[67,68]

Strength and conditioning of the young athlete during rehabilitation is multifaceted. A foundational component is the SAID principle: Specific Adaptations to Imposed Demands.[69] Muscles and the cardiovascular system need to be trained at a demand level sufficient to require adaptation—too little, and no adaptation will occur. Adaptations are also specific—an athlete whose sport is largely anaerobic should be exposed to anerobic exercises, and muscles such as the quadriceps which have a great need for eccentric capacity need to be trained with eccentrics.

Further considerations include open-chain exercises to target specific muscles, such as knee extension for the quadriceps, and closed chain exercises to emphasize functional movement patterns such as single-leg squats. Loading is also a key factor—the accumulated load based on intensity, sets, repetitions, and overlapping exercises, such as leg press and squats, all contribute to the total load. Rest is another factor in loading, particularly when looking at total load across a week of rehabilitation. Common identifiers of overloading are pain and/or swelling in the knee. As rehabilitation progresses to preparation for return to participation, impact activities of running, cutting, jumping and agility/footwork need to be specific to the demands of the athlete's sport.

A common modality used in strengthening, particularly of the quadriceps, is Neuromuscular Electrical Stimulation (NMES). While it can be helpful in facilitating muscle recruitment, it may not be well-tolerated in the younger population due to muscular discomfort. Biofeedback is also a useful modality for muscle recruitment and has the added benefit of being well-tolerated.

Blood flow restriction therapy (BFRT/BFR) is gaining popularity in the rehabilitation of the young athlete's knee. It is not a new technique, making its debut in the 1990s and having been researched over the years. BFRT has been demonstrated to improve strength with low resistance exercises, making it attractive in the rehabilitation setting immediately after an injury and in the early postoperative phase once sutures are removed and the incision is fully healed with no signs of infection. A systematic review and meta-analysis by Hughes and colleagues found that low load BFRT generated greater strength gains than low load training without BFRT.[70] This is relevant to rehabilitation as patients often are unable to tolerate high loads due to pain or structural risk. In a prospective study by Korkmaz and colleagues, knee extension strength after a 6 weeks of training program with BFRT was statistically higher than resistance training without BFRT, despite that the BFRT training load was 30% of one rep max (1RM) versus 80% of 1RM in the traditional resistance group.[71] The typical lower extremity BFRT parameters are 80% arterial blood flow occlusion/100% venous return occlusion with a low load exercise, such as straight leg raises in the early phase of rehabilitation, performing 30 initial repetitions, followed by 3 sets of 15, with 30 seconds rest between each set. Multiple exercises can be performed in a given session, and over time more advanced exercises can be performed, such as squatting and leg press. 30% of 1RM is a typical load/resistance level. BFRT can be performed 2 to 3 times per week for many weeks.[72]

RETURN TO PLAYTESTING AND DECISION-MAKING

Following a pediatric or adolescent knee injury, the process of safe return to play (RTP) should be viewed as a continuum: first, a graded return to participation, followed by a return to the preinjury sport, and finally, a return to preinjury performance (**Fig. 1**).[73] The clinical decision-making throughout this continuum requires careful consideration of the young athlete's physical and psychological readiness, in addition to a sufficient allowance of healing time. The key domains for RTP assessments, in addition to age- and activity-relevant RTP criteria, are shown in **Table 2** and described later in discussion.

As deficits in muscle performance are a common outcome of knee injuries among youth, restoration of preinjury strength should be a key consideration of the rehabilitation process. Attainment of at least 90% limb symmetry index (LSI) has been recommended for knee and hip musculature before clearance to sports participation.[74] However, emerging research indicates that measures of sufficiency, or absolute

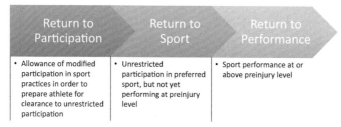

Fig. 1. Return to play continuum following knee injury.

muscle performance, may serve as more appropriate targets for this population. Use of preinjury measures of strength (estimated preinjury capacity)[75] or established normative values[76] are recommended for comparison to involved limb strength at the time of RTP. For surgical patients, estimated preinjury capacity of the uninvolved limb is measured preoperatively to calculate a within-patient target for involved limb strength.[75] Comparing a young athlete's functional strength performance to that of age- and sex-matched healthy athletes may also serve as a more suitable means of assessing strength after injury.[76]

In addition to strength, the functional performance of the injured knee must be restored for safe RTP. For young athletes returning to cutting/pivoting sports such as soccer or basketball, measures that allow for both quantitative and qualitative assessment of performance are warranted to assess readiness to participate. Examples of valid and reliable functional performance measures include single-limb hop tests,[77] 10-s tuck jump assessment,[78] drop vertical jump,[79] and the Vail Sport Test.[80] Furthermore, for youth in particular, proper execution of fundamental movements such as athletic stance, squat, hinge, and landing (double and single limb) is critical for the reduction of future injury risk. Qualitative assessments, such as the Landing Error Scoring System (LESS) can identify risky movement patterns that require further intervention.[79]

Traditionally, a heavy emphasis is placed on the restoration of physical function following knee injury. Yet, a young athlete's psychological response to knee injury and/or subsequent surgery may be a better indicator of readiness to RTP.[81] Negative psychological responses to severe sports-related injury are common and include anger, depression, anxiety, lack of confidence, and fear, the most cited reason for not returning to activity.[81–84] Furthermore, these responses may negatively affect the rehabilitation process, return to sport, and heighten the risk of new injury.[81,85,86] Psychological assessments appropriate for use following knee injury among youth include the Anterior Cruciate Ligament-Return to Sport after Injury (ACL-RSI) scale,[87] Athletic Identity Measurement Scale,[88] Tampa Scale of Kinesiophobia (TSK-11),[89,90] and the Knee Self-Efficacy Scale (K-SES).[91] Young athletes who present with a negative psychological response to knee injury or RTP are good candidates for referral to a sports psychologist.

Similarly, the assessment of a patient's perception of his or her function serves as an important indicator of both physical and psychological readiness for RTP. Traditional knee-related patient-reported outcomes measures, such as the International Knee Documentation Committee Subjective Knee Evaluation Form (IKDC),[92] which also comes in a pediatric form for ages 17 and under, and the Knee injury and Osteoarthritis Outcome Score (KOOS),[93] have been modified and validated for use among youth.[94,95] The aid of novel measurements of the patient experience, such as functional recovery, have provided further insight into the interpretation of patient-

Table 2
Recommended criteria for progression through a return to play continuum

	Return to Participation	Return to Sports	Return to Performance
		Recommended Criteria to Enter Each Phase	
Strength	• ≥90% LSI for main LE muscle groups • ≥90% quadriceps sufficiency	• ≥95% LSI for main LE muscle groups • ≥95% quadriceps sufficiency	• 95%–100% LSI for main LE muscle groups • ≥100% quadriceps sufficiency
Functional performance	• ≥90% LSI on SL hop tests	• ≥95% LSI on SL hop tests	• 95%–100% LSI on SL hop tests
Psychological response	• ACL-RSI score ≥77 • TSK-11 score <17	• ACL-RSI score ≥77 • TSK-11 score <17	• No decline in psychological response scores
Patient-reported function	• Score in 90th percentile of Pedi-IKDC or KOOS-Child subscales -or- • Met at least 3 of 5 KOOS subscale FR targets	• Score in 95th percentile of Pedi-IKDC or KOOS-Child subscales -or- • Met all KOOS subscale FR targets: Symptoms, Pain, ADLs, Sport, QoL	• Met all KOOS subscale FR targets: Symptoms, Pain, ADLs, Sport, QoL
Movement quality	• Mastery of fundamental movement skills (eg, athletic stance, squat, hinge) • ≤5 errors on 10-s tuck jump assessment • Score of ≤1 on lateral step-down test	• ≤2 errors on 10-s tuck jump assessment • LESS score ≤4 for drop-landing task	• ≤1 error on 10-s tuck jump assessment (0 errors preferred) • Good sport-specific neuromuscular control (cutting, pivoting, deceleration; with and without the ball, stick, racquet, and so forth)
Performance	• No onset of symptoms during rehabilitation or home workout sessions	• Completion of at least 2–4 wk of restricted practice (~10 sport exposures) without onset of symptoms • Additional inclusion of at least 3–5 "scrimmage" exposures is preferred	• Self-reported return to preinjury performance or higher • Improvement on any performance measure tested prior to injury

Abbreviations: ACL-RSI, anterior cruciate ligament return to injury after sport questionnaire; ADLs, activities of daily living; FR, functional recovery; KOOS, knee injury and osteoarthritis outcome score questionnaire; KOOS-Child, knee injury and osteoarthritis outcome score child questionnaire; LE, lower extremity; LESS, landing error scoring system; LSI, limb symmetry index; Pedi-IKDC, Pedi International Knee Documentation Committee; QoL, quality of life; sec, second; SL, single limb; TSK-11, Tampa Scale of Kinesiophobia.

ACL-RSI: McPherson 2019. TSK-11: Paterno 2018. Pedi-IKDC: van der Velden 2019. KOOS-Child: van der Velden 2019. KOOS FR: Ithurburn (in press). Tuck Jump: Myer 2008. Lateral step-down (Piva 2006). LESS (Padua 2009).

reported outcome measure scores.[96] Based on the data from young healthy athletes, established target scores for the KOOS subscales can be used to determine the achievement of functional recovery among youth following knee injury.[97]

For young patients, adequate healing time for the restoration of baseline joint health and function will vary depending on the type and severity of knee injury. This amount of time can range from 1 week for a knee joint contusion,[98] to 18+ months for nonsurgical management of osteochondritis dissecans.[99] For example, research has indicated that young patients should delay RTP for at least 9 months following ACL reconstruction to reduce risk of second ACL injury.[100] However, emerging evidence also suggests the full restoration of joint function may not occur for up to 2 years following intra-articular knee surgery.[101] The importance of using both time and objective readiness criteria is imperative for safe reintegration to sports, as well as long-term health and physical activity participation among this population.

CLINICS CARE POINTS

- During rehabilitation of a post operative JOCD lesion, knowing the specifics of the lesion, such as location and size, insures the prevention of damage to the surgical site.
- Since arthrofibrosis is a possible complication following ACLR it is important to emphasize early restoration of ROM.
- Taking a comprehensive history for a young athlete with an overuse knee injury is important for identifying and addressing root causes, otherwise the injury will likely return after a period of rest, strength and conditioning.
- Utilization of the SAID principle optimizes strength and conditioning decision making in rehabilitation.
- The use of pediatric specific patient reported outcome measures such as the Pedi-IKDC, as well as psychological readiness tools such as the ACL-RSI, is a key component of effective return to play decision making.

DISCLOSURE

The authors have nothing to disclose.

REFERENCES

1. Patel D, Yamasaki A, Brown K. Epidemiology of sports related musculoskeletal injuries in young athletes in United States. Transl Pediatr 2017;160–6.
2. Schmitt LC, Quatman CE, Paterno MV, et al. Functional outcomes after surgical management of articular cartilage lesions in the knee: a systematic literature review to guide postoperative rehabilitation. J Orthop Sports Phys Ther 2014;44. 565-A510.
3. Campbell AB, Pineda M, Harris JD, et al. Return to sport after articular cartilage repair in athletes' knees: a systematic review. Arthroscopy 2016;32:651–668 e651.
4. Benjaminse A, Gokeler A, Dowling AV, et al. Optimization of the anterior cruciate ligament injury prevention paradigm: novel feedback techniques to enhance motor learning and reduce injury risk. J Orthop Sports Phys Ther 2015;45: 170–82.
5. Cruz AI Jr, Shea KG, Ganley TJ. Pediatric Knee Osteochondritis Dissecans Lesions. Orthop Clin North Am 2016;47:763–75.

6. Kocher MS, Tucker R, Ganley TJ, et al. Management of osteochondritis disse-cans of the knee: current concepts review. Am J Sports Med 2006;34:1181–91.

7. Logerstedt DS, Scalzitti DA, Bennell KL, et al. Knee pain and mobility impair-ments: meniscal and articular cartilage lesions revision 2018. J Orthop Sports Phys Ther 2018;48:A1–50.

8. Frank JS, Gambacorta PL. Anterior cruciate ligament injuries in the skeletally immature athlete: diagnosis and management. J Am Acad Orthop Surg 2013; 21(2):78–87.

9. Lee JK, Lee S, Lee MC. Outcomes of anatomic anterior cruciate ligament recon-struction: bone-quadriceps tendon graft versus double-bundle hamstring tendon graft. Am J Sports Med 2016;44(9):2323–9.

10. McConkey MO, Bonasia DE, Amendola A. Pediatric anterior cruciate ligament reconstruction. Curr Rev Musculoskelet Med 2011;4(2):37–44.

11. Mosich GM, Lieu V, Ebramzadeh E, et al. Operative treatment of isolated meniscus injuries in adolescent patients: a meta-analysis and review. Sports Health: A Multidisciplinary Approach 2018;10(4):311–6.

12. Lind M, Nielsen T, Faunø P, et al. Free rehabilitation is safe after isolated meniscus repair. Am J Sports Med 2013;41(12):2753–8.

13. Dai W, Leng X, Wang J, et al. Second-look arthroscopic evaluation of healing rates after arthroscopic repair of meniscal tears: a systematic review and meta-analysis. Orthopaedic J Sports Med 2021;9(10). 232596712110382.

14. O'Donnell K, Freedman KB, Tjoumakaris FP. Rehabilitation protocols after iso-lated meniscal repair: a systematic review. Am J Sports Med 2017;45(7): 1687–97.

15. LaPrade RF, LaPrade CM, James EW. Recent advances in posterior meniscal root repair techniques. J Am Acad Orthop Surg 2015;23(2):71–6.

16. Ekhtiari S, Horner NS, De Sa D, et al. Arthrofibrosis after ACL reconstruction is best treated in a step-wise approach with early recognition and intervention: a systematic review. Knee Surg Sports Traumatol Arthrosc 2017;25(12):3929–37.

17. Rushdi I, Sharifudin S, Shukur A. Arthrofibrosis following anterior cruciate liga-ment reconstruction. Malaysian Orthopaedic J 2019;13(3):34–8.

18. Kambhampati SBS, Gollamudi S, Shanmugasundaram S, et al. Cyclops lesions of the knee: a narrative review of the literature. Orthopaedic J Sports Med 2020; 8(8). 232596712094567.

19. Sonnery-Cottet B, Lavoie F, Ogassawara R, et al. Clinical and operative charac-teristics of cyclops syndrome after double-bundle anterior cruciate ligament reconstruction. Arthroscopy 2010;26(11):1483–8.

20. Schmucker M, Haraszuk J, Holmich P, et al. Graft failure, revision ACLR, and re-operation rates after ACLR with quadriceps tendon versus hamstring tendon au-tografts: a registry study with review of 475 patients. Am J Sports Med 2021; 49(8):2136–43.

21. Hunnicutt JL, Slone HS, Xerogeanes JW. Implications for early postoperative care after quadriceps tendon autograft for anterior cruciate ligament reconstruc-tion: a technical note. J Athletic Train 2020;55(6):623–7.

22. Delaloye J-R, Murar J, Vieira TD, et al. Knee extension deficit in the early post-operative period predisposes to cyclops syndrome after anterior cruciate liga-ment reconstruction: a risk factor analysis in 3633 patients from the SANTI study group database. Am J Sports Med 2020;48(3):565–72.

23. Rice DA, McNair PJ. Quadriceps arthrogenic muscle inhibition: neural mecha-nisms and treatment perspectives. Semin Arthritis Rheum 2010;40(3):250–66.

24. Snyder AR, Perotti AL, Lam KC, et al. The influence of high-voltage electrical stimulation on edema formation after acute injury: a systematic review. J Sport Rehabil 2010;19(4):436–51.

25. Blum K, Ho C-K, Chen ALC, et al. The H-Wave® device induces NO-dependent augmented microcirculation and angiogenesis, providing both analgesia and tissue healing in sports injuries. Phys Sportsmed 2008;36(1):103–14.

26. Escamilla RF, Macleod TD, Wilk KE, et al. ACL strain and tensile forces for weight bearing and non—weight-bearing exercises after ACL reconstruction: a guide to exercise selection. J Orthop Sports Phys Ther 2012;42(3):208–20.

27. Perriman A, Leahy E, Semciw AI. The effect of open- versus closed-kinetic-chain exercises on anterior tibial laxity, strength, and function following anterior cruciate ligament reconstruction: a systematic review and meta-analysis. J Orthop Sports Phys Ther 2018;48(7):552–66.

28. Noehren B, Snyder-Mackler L. Who's afraid of the big bad wolf? Open-chain exercises after anterior cruciate ligament reconstruction. J Orthop Sports Phys Ther 2020;50(9):473–5.

29. Hughes L. Blood flow restriction training in rehabilitation following anterior cruciate ligament reconstructive surgery: a review. Tech Orthop 2018;33(2):106–13.

30. Hughes L, Rosenblatt B, Haddad F, et al. Comparing the effectiveness of blood flow restriction and traditional heavy load resistance training in the post-surgery rehabilitation of anterior cruciate ligament reconstruction patients: a UK National Health Service randomised controlled trial. Sports Med 2019;49(11):1787–805.

31. Fitzgerald GK, Irrgang JJ. A modified neuromuscular electrical stimulation protocol for quadriceps strength training following anterior cruciate ligament reconstruction. J Orthop Sports Phys Ther 2003;33(9):492–501.

32. Gokeler A, Benjaminse A, Hewett TE, et al. Feedback techniques to target functional deficits following anterior cruciate ligament reconstruction: implications for motor control and reduction of second injury risk. Sports Med 2013;43(11):1065–74.

33. Kline PW, Johnson DL, Ireland ML, et al. Clinical predictors of knee mechanics at return to sport after ACL reconstruction. Med Sci Sports Exerc 2016;48(5):790–5.

34. McPherson AL, Feller JA, Hewett TE, et al. Psychological readiness to return to sport is associated with second anterior cruciate ligament injuries. Am J Sports Med 2019;47(4):857–62.

35. McPherson AL, Feller JA, Hewett TE, et al. Smaller change in psychological readiness to return to sport is associated with second anterior cruciate ligament injury among younger patients. Am J Sports Med 2019;47(5):1209–15.

36. Webster KE, Feller JA. Clinical tests can be used to screen for second anterior cruciate ligament injury in younger patients who return to sport. Orthop J Sports Med 2019;7(8). 2325967119863003.

37. Lynch AD, Logerstedt DS, Grindem H, et al. Consensus criteria for defining 'successful outcome' after ACL injury and reconstruction: a Delaware-Oslo ACL cohort investigation. Br J Sports Med 2015;49(5):335–42.

38. Lorenz D, Domzalski S. Criteria-based return to sprinting progression following lower extremity injury. Int J Sports Phys Ther 2020;15(2):326–32.

39. Walker JM, Brunst CL, Chaput M, et al. Integrating neurocognitive challenges into injury prevention training: A clinical commentary. Phys Ther Sport 2021;51:8–16.

40. Khormaee S, Kramer DE, Yen Y, et al. Evaluation and management of patellar instability in pediatric and adolescent athletes. Sports Health 2015;7(2):115–23.

41. Fithian DC, Paxton EW, Stone ML, et al. Epidemiology and natural history of acute patellar dislocation. Am J Sports Med 2004;32:1114–21.
42. Palmu S, Kallio PE, Donell ST, et al. Acute patellar dislocation in children and adolescents: a randomized clinical trial. J Bone Joint Surg Am 2008;90:463–70.
43. Bassett FH. Acute dislocation of the patella, osteochondral fractures, and injuries to the extensor mechanism of the knee. Amer Acad Orth Surg Instr Course Lect 1976;25:40–9.
44. Post WR, Fithian DC. Patellofemoral Instability: A consensus statement from the AOSSM/PFF patellofemoral instability workshop. Orthop J Sports Med 2018; 6(1). 2325967117750352.
45. Ahmad CS, McCarthy M, Gomez JA, et al. The moving patellar apprehension test for lateral patellar instability. Am J Sports Med 2009;37:791–6.
46. Smith TO, Davies L, O'Driscoll M-L, et al. An evaluation of the clinical tests and outcome measures used to assess patellar instability. Knee 2008;15:255–62.
47. Reed G, Coda BS, Sana G, et al. Online rehabilitation protocols for medial patellofemoral ligament reconstruction with and without tibial tubercle osteotomy are variable among institutions. Arthrosc Sports Med Rehabil 2021;3(Issue 2): e305–13.
48. Manske RC, Prohaska D. Rehabilitation following medial patellofemoral ligament reconstruction for patellar instability. Int J Sports Phys Ther 2017;12:494–511.
49. Sillanpää PJ, Mattila VM, Mäenpää H, et al. Treatment with and without initial stabilizing surgery for primary traumatic patellar dislocation. A prospective randomized study. J Bone Joint Surg Am 2009;91:263–73.
50. Greenberg EM, Greenberg ET, Ganley TJ, et al. Strength and functional performance recovery after anterior cruciate ligament reconstruction in preadolescent athletes. Sports Health 2014;6(4):309–12.
51. Anand BS, Ho S, Kambhampati S. Recent advances and future trends in patellofemoral instability. J Arthrosc Surg Sport Med 2020;1(1):110–7.
52. Jain NP, Khan N, Fithian DC. A treatment algorithm for primary patellar dislocations. Sports Health 2011;3(2):170–4.
53. Desio SM, Burks RT, Bachus KN. Soft tissue restraints to lateral patellar translation in the human knee. Am J Sports Med 1998;26:59–65.
54. Sillanpää PJ, Maenpaa H, Arendt EA. Treatment of lateral patella dislocation in the skeletally immature athlete. Oper Tech Sports Med 2010;18(2):83–92.
55. Smith TO, Donell S, Song F, et al. Surgical versus nonsurgical interventions for treating patellar dislocation. Cochrane Databse Syst, John Wiley and Sons LTD; 2015.
56. Saper MG, Fantozzi P, Bompadre V, et al. Return-to-sport testing after medial patellofemoral ligament reconstruction in adolescent athletes. Orthop J Sports Med 2019;7(3):1–7.
57. Harrison RK, Magnussen RA, Flanigan DC. Avoiding complications in patellofemoral surgery. Sports Med Arthrosc Rev 2013;21(2):121–8.
58. Chatterji R, White AE, Hadley CJ, et al. Return-to-play guidelines after patellar instability surgery requiring bony realignment: A systematic review. Orthop J Sports Med 2020;8(12). 2325967120966134.
59. Schmitt LC, Paterno MV, Hewett TE. The impact of quadriceps femoris strength asymmetry on functional performance at return to sport following anterior cruciate ligament reconstruction. J Orthop Sports Phys Ther 2012;42(9):750–9.
60. Krych AJ, O'Malley MP, Johnson NR, et al. Functional testing and return to sport following stabilization surgery for recurrent lateral patellar instability in competitive athletes. Knee Surg Sports Traumatol Arthrosc 2018;26(3):711–8.

61. Xergia SA, Pappas E, Zampeli F, et al. Asymmetries in functional hop tests, lower extremity kinematics, and isokinetic strength persist 6 to 9 months following anterior cruciate ligament reconstruction. J Orthop Sports Phys Ther 2013;43(3):154–62.

62. Zwolski C, Schmitt LC, Quatman-Yates C, et al. The influence of quadriceps strength asymmetry on patient-reported function at time of return to sport after anterior cruciate ligament reconstruction. Am J Sports Med 2015;43(9):2242–9.

63. Zwolski C, Schmitt LC, Thomas S, et al. The utility of limb symmetry indices in return-to-sport assessment in patients with bilateral anterior cruciate ligament reconstruction. Am J Sports Med 2016;44(8):2030–8.

64. Sweeney E, Rodenberg R, MacDonald J. Overuse knee pain in the pediatric and adolescent athlete. Am Coll Sports Med Curr Sports Med Rep 2020;19(11): 479–85.

65. Zwolski C, Quatman-Yates C, Paterno MV. Resistance training in youth: laying the foundation for injury prevention and physical literacy. Sports Health 2017; 9(5):436–43.

66. McQuilliam SJ, Clark DR, Erskine RM, et al. Free-weight resistance training in youth athletes: a narrative review. Sports Med 2020;50(9):1567–80.

67. Faigenbaum, Avery D, Kraemer WJ, et al. Youth resistance training: updated position statement paper from the National Strength and Conditioning Association. J Strength Conditioning Res 2009;23(5):S60–79.

68. McCambridge TM, Stricker PR. Strength training by children and adolescents. American Academy of Pediatrics Council on Sports Medicine and Fitness. Pediatrics 2008;121(4):835–40.

69. Sands W, Wurth J, Hewit J. Basics of strength and conditioning. Colorado Springs, Colorado: The National Strength and Conditioning Association (NSCA); 2012.

70. Hughes L, Paton B, Rosenblatt B, et al. Blood flow restriction training in clinical musculoskeletal rehabilitation: a systematic review and meta-analysis. Br J Sports Med 2017;51(13):1003–11.

71. Korkmaz E, Donmez G, Uzuner K, et al. Effects of blood flow restriction training on muscle strength and architecture. J Strength Cond Res 2020. https://doi.org/10.1519/JSC.0000000000003612.

72. Vanwye W, Weatherholt A, Mikesky A. Blood flow restriction training: implementation into clinical practice. Int J Exerc Sci 2017;10(5):649–54.

73. Ardern CL, Glasgow P, Schneiders A, et al. 2016 Consensus statement on return to sport from the First World Congress in Sports Physical Therapy, Bern. Br J Sports Med 2016;50(14):853–64.

74. Adams D, Logerstedt DS, Hunter-Giordano A, et al. Current concepts for anterior cruciate ligament reconstruction: a criterion-based rehabilitation progression. J Orthop Sports Phys Ther 2012;42(7):601–14.

75. Wellsandt E, Failla MJ, Snyder-Mackler L. Limb symmetry indexes can overestimate knee runction after anterior cruciate ligament injury. J Orthop Sports Phys Ther 2017;47(5):334–8.

76. Magill JR, Myers HS, Lentz TA, et al. Establishing age- and sex-specific norms for pediatric return-to-sports physical performance testing. Orthop J Sports Med 2021;9(8). 23259671211023100.

77. Noyes FR, Barber SD, Mangine RE. Abnormal lower limb symmetry determined by function hop tests after anterior cruciate ligament rupture. Am J Sports Med 1991;19(5):513–8.

78. Myer GD, Ford KR, Hewett TE. Tuck jump assessment for reducing anterior cruciate ligament injury risk. Athl Ther Today J Sports Health Care Prof 2008;13(5): 39–44.
79. Padua DA, Marshall SW, Boling MC, et al. The Landing Error Scoring System (LESS) is a valid and reliable clinical assessment tool of jump landing biomechanics: The JUMP-ACL Study. Am J Sports Med 2009;37(10):1996–2002.
80. Garrison JC, Shanley E, Thigpen C, et al. The reliability of the vail sport test ™ as a measure of physical performance following anterior cruciate ligament reconstruction. Int J Sports Phys Ther 2012;7(1):20–30.
81. Nwachukwu BU, Adjei J, Rauck RC, et al. How much do psychological factors affect lack of return to play after anterior cruciate ligament reconstruction? A systematic review. Orthop J Sports Med 2019;7(5). 2325967119845313.
82. Ardern CL, Taylor NF, Feller JA, et al. A systematic review of the psychological factors associated with returning to sport following injury. Br J Sports Med 2013; 47(17):1120–6.
83. Putukian M. The psychological response to injury and illness. In: Hong E, Rao AL, editors. Mental health in the athlete: modern perspectives and novel challenges for the sports medicine provider. Gewerbestrasse, Switzerland: Springer International Publishing; 2020. p. 95–101.
84. Wiese-bjornstal DM, Smith AM, Shaffer SM, et al. An integrated model of response to sport injury: Psychological and sociological dynamics. J Appl Sport Psychol 1998;10(1):46–69.
85. Fältström A, Hägglund M, Magnusson H, et al. Predictors for additional anterior cruciate ligament reconstruction: data from the Swedish national ACL register. Knee Surg Sports Traumatol Arthrosc 2016;24(3):885–94.
86. Ivarsson A, Tranaeus U, Johnson U, et al. Negative psychological responses of injury and rehabilitation adherence effects on return to play in competitive athletes: a systematic review and meta-analysis. Open Access J Sports Med 2017;8:27–32.
87. Webster KE, Feller JA, Lambros C. Development and preliminary validation of a scale to measure the psychological impact of returning to sport following anterior cruciate ligament reconstruction surgery. Phys Ther Sport Off J Assoc Chart Physiother Sports Med 2008;9(1):9–15.
88. Padaki AS, Noticewala MS, Levine WN, et al. Prevalence of posttraumatic stress disorder symptoms among young athletes after anterior cruciate ligament rupture. Orthop J Sports Med 2018;6(7). 2325967118787159.
89. Paterno MV, Flynn K, Thomas S, et al. Self-reported fear predicts functional performance and second ACL injury after ACL reconstruction and return to sport: a pilot study. Sports Health 2018;10(3):228–33.
90. Trigsted SM, Cook DB, Pickett KA, et al. Greater fear of reinjury is related to stiffened jump-landing biomechanics and muscle activation in women after ACL reconstruction. Knee Surg Sports Traumatol Arthrosc 2018;26(12):3682–9.
91. Thomeé P, Währborg P, Börjesson M, et al. A new instrument for measuring self-efficacy in patients with an anterior cruciate ligament injury. Scand J Med Sci Sports 2006;16(3):181–7.
92. Irrgang JJ, Anderson AF, Boland AL, et al. Development and validation of the international knee documentation committee subjective knee form. Am J Sports Med 2001;29(5):600–13.
93. Roos EM, Roos HP, Lohmander LS, et al. Knee Injury and Osteoarthritis Outcome Score (KOOS)–development of a self-administered outcome measure. J Orthop Sports Phys Ther 1998;28(2):88–96.

94. Nasreddine AY, Nelson SE, Connell P, et al. The Pediatric International Knee Documentation Committee (Pedi-IKDC) Subjective Knee Evaluation Form. Orthop J Sports Med 2015;3(7 suppl2). 2325967115S00109.

95. Örtqvist M, Roos EM, Broström EW, et al. Development of the Knee Injury and Osteoarthritis Outcome Score for children (KOOS-Child): comprehensibility and content validity. Acta Orthop 2012;83(6):666–73.

96. Barenius B, Forssblad M, Engström B, et al. Functional recovery after anterior cruciate ligament reconstruction, a study of health-related quality of life based on the Swedish National Knee Ligament Register. Knee Surg Sports Traumatol Arthrosc 2013;21(4):914–27.

97. Ithurburn MP, Barenius B, Thomas S, et al. Few young athletes meet newly derived age- and activity-relevant functional recovery targets after ACL reconstruction. Knee Surg Sports Traumatol Arthrosc 2022;30(10):3268–76.

98. Materne O, Chamari K, Farooq A, et al. Injury incidence and burden in a youth elite football academy: a four-season prospective study of 551 players aged from under 9 to under 19 years. Br J Sports Med 2021;55(9):493–500.

99. Yang JS, Bogunovic L, Wright RW. Nonoperative treatment of osteochondritis dissecans of the knee. Clin Sports Med 2014;33(2):295–304.

100. Beischer S, Gustavsson L, Senorski EH, et al. Young athletes who return to sport before 9 months after anterior cruciate ligament reconstruction have a rate of new injury 7 times that of those who delay return. J Orthop Sports Phys Ther 2020;50(2):83–90.

101. Nagelli CV, Hewett TE. Should return to sport be delayed until 2 years after anterior cruciate ligament reconstruction? Biological and functional considerations. Sports Med Auckl NZ 2017;47(2):221–32.

Stress Injuries of the Knee

Emily Kraus, MD[a],*, Katherine Rizzone, MD, MPH[b], Mahala Walker, BS[c],
Naomi Brown, MD[d], Japsimran Kaur, BS[e], Danielle Magrini, DO[f], Jayden Glover, BS[g],
Eric Nussbaum, ATC[h]

KEYWORDS

- Bone stress injury • Apophysitis • Physeal stress injury • Bipartite patella
- Osgood–Schlatter disease

KEY POINTS

- Apophyseal injuries of the knee occur at the insertion of the patellar tendon at the tibial tubercle (Osgood–Schlatter disease, OSD) or at the inferior pole of the patella (Sinding-Larsen–Johansson disease, SLJ).
- Primary periphyseal stress injuries of the proximal tibia and distal femur develop from repetitive submaximal stress that causes microtrauma to some components of the epiphyseal–physeal–metaphyseal complex.
- Bipartite patellae result from an abnormal fibrocartilaginous connection between patellar ossification centers instead of bone and can be symptomatic in athletes involved in activities such as jumping, running, squatting, and kneeling or trauma.
- Distal femur and proximal tibia BSIs of the metaphysis are less common than other BSIs, but should be considered in athletes involved in running and jumping activities who present with vague knee pain of insidious onset.
- Most of the stress injuries of the knee resolve with relative rest but will occasionally need surgical intervention in more severe cases.

[a] Division of Physical Medicine and Rehabilitation, Department of Orthopedic Surgery, Stanford University, Center for Academic Medicine, Pediatric Orthopaedic Surgery, MC 5658, 453 Quarry Road, Stanford, CA 94304, USA; [b] Division of Orthopaedics and Pediatrics, University of Rochester Medical Center, RUR601 Elmwood Avenue, Box 665, Rochester, NY 14642, USA; [c] University of Kentucky College of Medicine, 800 Rose Street MN 150, Lexington, KY, 40506, USA; [d] Department of Pediatrics, Perelman School of Medicine, University of Pennsylvania, Sports Medicine and Performance Center, Children's Hospital of Philadelphia, 3401 Civic Center Blvd. Philadelphia, PA, 19104, USA; [e] University of Rochester School of Medicine and Dentistry, 601 Elmwood Ave, Rochester, NY 14642, USA; [f] Division of Pediatric Sports Medicine, Swedish Medical Center, 1101 Madison St., Suite 800 Seattle, WA, 98104, USA; [g] Lake Erie College of Osteopathic Medicine, 5000 Lakewood Ranch Blvd, Bradenton, FL 34211, USA; [h] Department of Orthopaedic Surgery, Rutgers, Robert Wood Johnson Medical School, One Robert Wood Johnson Place, New Brunswick, NJ, 08903-0019, USA
* Corresponding author.
E-mail address: ekraus@stanford.edu

Clin Sports Med 41 (2022) 707–727
https://doi.org/10.1016/j.csm.2022.05.008
0278-5919/22/© 2022 Elsevier Inc. All rights reserved.

sportsmed.theclinics.com

INTRODUCTION

Stress injuries to the bone and physis of the knee are common in the active adolescent patient and can be separated into bone stress injuries (BSIs) and chronic physeal stress injuries. Bone stress injuries (BSIs) occur in bone tissue resulting from prolonged repetitive loading. When the stress and repair mechanisms of the body become overwhelmed by microinjury, the body's mechanisms that are designed to reabsorb, repair and remodel to mechanical stress fail, leading to a BSI.[1] The degree of bone stress can range from periostitis to periosteal, endosteal and bone tissue edema, to partial or complete stress fracture. stress reactions or bone stress injuries are often used interchangeable; however, stress reaction typically denotes a less severe stage than stress fracture.[2]

Maximal rates of bone mineral accrual occur after peak height velocity by 6 to 12 months, resulting in relatively undermineralized bone and increased BSI risk in adolescence.[3–5] Further, the physis is more susceptible to injury during these periods of rapid growth.[5] Chronic physeal injuries are another form of overuse injury developing from repetitive loading. Risk factors for BSI include overtraining, biomechanical inefficiency, female gender, low bone density, poor diet, and menstrual disturbances.[6,7] The most common location of a BSI in athletes under the age of 20 in the leg, accounting for 40.3% of all BSI in a study of 389 high school athletes.[1,2]

Overuse injuries to the bone and physis of the knee can lead to significant time loss from sport and, in rare cases, premature growth arrest or chronic bone deformity. Early and accurate identification of injury is paramount to optimal management. The most common bone stress injuries of the knee will be reviewed, including epidemiology, pathophysiology, clinical findings, diagnosis, and management.

Apophyseal Stress Injuries of the Knee

Background

The apophysis is a secondary ossification center and site of attachment for a muscle-tendon unit. Apophysitis of the knee occurs at the insertion of the patellar tendon at the tibial tubercle (Osgood–Schlatter disease, OSD) or at the inferior pole of the patella (Sinding-Larsen–Johansson disease, SLJ).[8,9] Although the exact spectrum of pathophysiology is still unclear, there are some agreed on components. The apophysis is reported as the "weakest link" compared with the bone, the myotendinous structures, and surrounding ligamentous and fibrocartilage.[8] The apophysis is susceptible to stress and injury. Repetitive microtraumas, possibly with small microtears to the tendon, thickening of the tendon, fragmentation, and bony ossicles at the tendinous insertion points are all part of the structural changes seen.[10] Commonly, these conditions occur during periods of rapid growth when young athletes undergo peak height velocity.[8,11] It is postulated that the leading cause for traction and apophyseal tension at the knee is a relative weakness of hamstrings and quadriceps along with a disproportional elongation of the femur compared with the growth of the knee extensor mechanism.[12] This results in femoral growth that exceeds the growth contributed to the anterior knee structures.[13]

Athletes involved in running and jumping sports seem to be particularly prone to knee apophysitis.[9] Athletic exposures per week, intensity of play, and number of rest days likely all factor into symptom provocation. Early sport specialization (ESS) becomes an important factor to consider while evaluating children with possible apophysitis.[8,12,14]

Osgood–Schlatter disease

Epidemiology and pathophysiology OSD is commonly seen in men aged 12 to 15 year old[12,15] and in women between 8 and 12 years of age.[15] Twenty to 30% of patients with OSD experience symptoms bilaterally.[14,16] OSD has historically shown greater incidence in males,[12,17] however, with increasing participation of women in sport, the sexual dimorphism is declining.[17,18]

Assessing patients for traction apophysitis should entail an appraisal of the intrinsic and extrinsic risk factors for that individual. Intrinsic factors to consider are age, sex, peak height velocity, pubertal status, and muscular tightness.[19] Posterior tibial slope (PTS) may also be an intrinsic factor, but further studies are needed.[20] Extrinsic factors for overuse conditions include but are not limited to, sport(s) played, ESS, hours of participation in a week, number of rest days each week and time off from sport each year.[21]

Adolescents participating in sports whereby the main activities involve sprinting, jumping, squatting, and kicking are at increased risk for developing OSD.[12,14,22,23] These movements are commonly seen in sports such as soccer, basketball, gymnastics, and volleyball.[14,24] Eccentric lengthening of the quadriceps musculature places repetitive stress onto the patellar tendon and tibial tubercle apophysis,[22,23] precipitating symptoms of OSD. Athletes who specialize early in a single sport have been shown to have a four-fold increase in relative risk of developing OSD[25] and a 2.25 greater odds of developing an overuse condition in general.[26]

Adolescents with a greater PTS may be at increased risk for OSD. In a retrospective review of 258 knees, patients with OSD had a slightly increased PTS when compared with individuals with anterior knee pain but no diagnosis of OSD.[27] Another series of 251 knees similarly demonstrated that patients with OSD had a greater PTS when compared with control patients.[20] It is not fully known if and why increased PTS may be associated with OSD but studies are underway. A proposed theory suggests an association between increased PTS and an imbalance between anterior and posterior forces on the tibial tubercle,[27] leading to OSD and possibly tibial tubercle fractures.[20,27]

Clinical findings The diagnosis of OSD is primarily clinical.[9] Classically, patients present with insidious onset of pain, mainly provoked by activity and localized to the tibial tubercle.[8,9,12,28] In addition to pain, a subset of patients may demonstrate mild soft tissue swelling around the tibial tubercle[8,12] and possible thickening of the patellar tendon.[18] Pain may be particularly pronounced with impact activities or direct pressure such as kneeling.[8,9] Pain often subsides following the cessation of activity.[9] Physical examination is notable for pain reproduced with active and passive flexion of the knee.[9] Keep in mind that when evaluating the knee, it is equally important to examine the hip, helping clarify that pain is not emanating from a referral pattern.

Diagnostic imaging Although imaging is not mandatory for the diagnosis, it may be used to verify that other sources of pathology or fracture are not part of the chief complaint.[8] X-ray is usually the first-line imaging modality. Take note of the tibial tubercle apophysis, seen best on the lateral view (**Fig. 1**). The apophysis may be widened and/or fragmented;[12] however, a "normal" appearing apophysis does not exclude the diagnosis.[9] Radiographic features may not always correlate with clinical presentation.

Advanced imaging such as ultrasound (US) and magnetic resonance imaging (MRI) may also be incorporated into the evaluation of a patient. US is particularly useful for a variety of reasons; it's readily available, noninvasive, and can allow providers rapid visualization of the soft tissues and apophysis. Thickening of the distal patellar tendon, widening of the nonossified cartilage, and potential fragmentation of the tibial tuberosity have all been noted (**Fig. 2**).[29] Color mode can demonstrate increased blood flow or neovascularization to the apophysis and distal tendon.[8,11] MRI is also helpful in

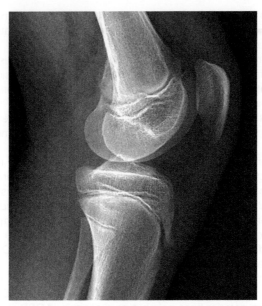

Fig. 1. Lateral radiograph demonstrating OSD. (*Courtesy of* Danielle Magrini, MD, Seattle, WA.)

patients with an atypical presentation[28] or when trying to exclude other pathology such as osteochondritis dissecans (OCD), or other osseous destructive lesions such as infection or tumor.[30–32] In early stages of OSD, MRI will likely demonstrate edema surrounding the tibial tuberosity. Partial tears in the tendinous attachment to the apophysis or avulsion of bone and/or cartilage may be evident in progressive or recalcitrant forms of OSD.[25]

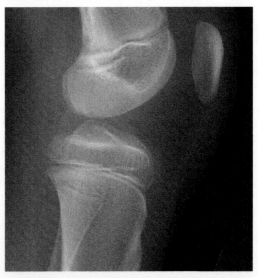

Fig. 2. Longitudinal US of OSD. (*From* Czyrny Z. Osgood-Schlatter disease in ultrasound diagnostics – a pictorial essay. Med Ultrason.:14.)

Management The mainstay of treatment involves relative rest, activity modification, stretching and icing.[8,18,33,34] Activity modification is dictated by the patient's pain level.[34] Patients can be encouraged to continue with sports participation if activity-related pain subsides with rest.[34] Playing through moderate pain when mechanics or gait is altered is not recommended. Adjunctive treatments can also include strengthening programs, oral or topical nonsteroidal antiinflammatory drugs (NSAIDs) or acetaminophen and bracing, commonly a cho-pat strap, which is thought to redirect tensile forces.[34,35] Strength and flexibility training, in particular, may prevent recurrence of OSD.[11,12] Cross-training with lower impact activity such as biking or swimming may also provide cardiovascular training without directly exacerbating symptoms.[8] It is important to realize that OSD is often self-limiting; the overwhelming most of the patients will experience symptom resolution following skeletal maturity.[15,17,18]

Ultrasound-guided prolotherapy is still under evaluation but preliminary work demonstrates promise as a treatment modality for those suffering from OSD.[36] A randomized clinical trial of 54 patients found that those who received dextrose injections were significantly more likely to return to sport at 3 months and be asymptomatic at 1 year when compared with those treated with the mainstream, standard of care treatment plan.[36] Unfortunately, the proposed effectiveness of dextrose injections is not consistent across studies. A randomized controlled trial comparing dextrose injections to saline injections in 49 knees from 38 patients with OSD found no significant difference in patient symptoms at any time point during the study protocol.[37] Even though the trial's findings showed no statistical significance, both the dextrose and the saline group had decreased symptoms 4 weeks post the first injection, suggesting that hyperosmolar dextrose may still be a possible treatment option.

Surgical intervention is rarely indicated but may be considered for skeletally mature patients who do not experience symptom resolution within 12 to 24 months of conservative treatment.[12] Surgical intervention can involve ossicle excision, tibial tubercleplasty, or longitudinal excision of the patellar tendon.[12,28,33] Surgical intervention can decrease pain and improve knee function.[38,39] In a study by Pihlajamaki and colleagues, 178 military recruits underwent surgery for unresolved issues from OSD over a 13-year period, at an occurrence of 42 per 100,000 recruits.[13] The median age at the time of surgery was 20 years, but a majority had symptoms since the age of 15 years. Ninety-three percent presented with ossicles on radiographic imaging. While most operative OSD cases are uncomplicated with excellent long-term success, surgery is rarely needed except in certain situations such as pain, dysfunction with kneeling, prolonged activity restrictions, or whereby conservative treatments have failed.[13]

Tibial tubercle avulsion fractures, although uncommon, make up 0.4% to 2.7% of all physeal injuries[20] are may be a complication of Osgood–Schlatter's disease. This acute injury is a major reason why medical providers provide anticipatory guidance to patients about slowing or stopping play when pain is increasing and mechanics are altered. Recent studies have looked at those who have succumbed to a tibial tubercle avulsion and found that most of these patients had increased posterior tibial slope angles (PTSA) suggesting a relationship.[40] Tibial tubercle fractures are categorized by the Ogden classification system. Sheppard and colleagues expanded on results from Watanabe and colleagues and found that those patients who had an Ogden classified fracture also had an increased PTSA compared with controls.

Sinding-Larsen–Johansson disease

Epidemiology and pathophysiology Sinding-Larsen–Johansson disease (SLJ) shares many features with OSD. It results from a traction injury to the inferior pole of the patella.[2] SLJ is most commonly seen in adolescent athletes who are 10 to 12 year old.[41] Much like OSD, SLJ can be attributed to impact-type activities namely, running and jumping.[12] SLJ is a noninflammatory extensor-mechanism traction injury.[12]

Clinical findings Diagnosis of SLJ is also made clinically. Patients present with anterior knee pain,[8,9] exacerbated by running, jumping, and climbing,[12] with focal tenderness and possible swelling of the inferior patellar pole.[8,9] It is not uncommon for patients to exhibit tenderness both at the inferior patellar pole and the tibial tubercle concomitantly.[12]

Diagnostic imaging Radiographic imaging is again not necessary for diagnosis but may be obtained if concerned for other pathology. X-rays may be unremarkable or demonstrate fragmentation/calcification[42] or slight widening of the apophysis at the inferior patellar pole (**Fig. 3**).[9,12] Radiographs are also useful for excluding other more significant pathology such as a patellar sleeve avulsion injury.[12]

Advanced imaging is not usually indicated but may be used in the appropriate clinical setting. Osseous fragmentation can also be seen on MRI[9]; both US and MRI can demonstrate swelling within and thickening of the proximal patellar tendon as well as infrapatellar bursitis.[9,42] Occasionally a patellar sleeve fracture may also be in the differential diagnosis and MRI can be very helpful in distinguishing this pathology from SLJ alone.

Management Treatment principles are similar to those used in OSD. Relative rest and activity modification is the mainstay of treatment.[8,12] Patients are encouraged to

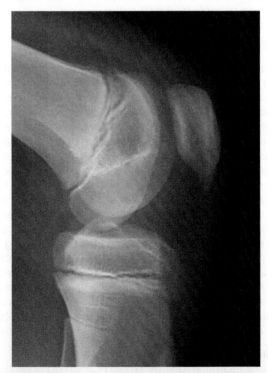

Fig. 3. Lateral radiograph demonstrating mild fragmentation seen in SLJ. (*Courtesy of* Danielle Magrini, MD, Seattle, WA.)

stay active but are advised to take breaks from activities that increase pain.[12] Patellar counterforce (cho-pat) straps may also be used to alleviate pain during activity.[8] Icing, a short course of NSAIDs or acetaminophen, and stretching focused on the hamstrings, quadriceps, and heel cord are also efficacious for symptom relief.[29] If a home exercise program does not provide adequate relief, physical therapy, and cross-training can be used to improve flexibility, strength and improve overall mechanics.

Symptom resolution typically occurs within 12 to 24 months of treatment initiation.[9,42] Symptom resolution is associated with skeletal maturity and apophyseal fusion.[9,42] If conservative treatment and skeletal maturity do not result in symptom resolution, and a synchondrosis results in pain, surgical intervention and excision of the fragment, can be considered.[43]

Stress Injuries of the Patella

The bipartite patella

The patella is the largest sesamoid bone in the human body, promoting the extension of the quadriceps via the patella ligament moment arm and acting as a protective mechanism for the quadriceps tendon from friction.[44,45] Normal development is the initiation of ossification by 3 to 5 years of age, with the fusion of ossification centers over the first decade of life. Bipartite patellae are caused by a nonunion created by an abnormal fibrocartilaginous connection between patellar ossification centers instead of bone (first described by Gruber in 1883).[44,46] Nondevelopmental-related patellar nonunion pathophysiology has also been noted and includes traumatic injury, anomalous tendinous traction, and vascular insufficiency.[46]

Epidemiology and classification. Bipartite patellae are estimated to exist in 1% to 2% of the population with bilateral presentation in 43% of those cases.[47,48] This pathology is most commonly classified using the Saupe classification system which categorized bipartite patella into 3 types based on the location of the accessory fragment placement as seen in **Fig. 4**.[44,49] In Type 1 (5% of patients), the accessory fragment is inferior to the patella. In Type 2 (20% of patients), the accessory fragment is located in the lateral aspect of the patella. Type 3 is the most common type of bipartite patella, seen in 75% of bipartite cases, with the accessory fragment located at the superolateral aspect of the patella.[44,49]

Despite the Saupe classification being the most widely accepted system, it has also been noted that it does not include other aspects of the bipartite patella, including etiology, or the less common tripartite patella (**Fig. 5**) and medial bipartite patella.[44] Oohashi and colleagues have proposed a different classification system accounting for both location and number of fragments.[47]

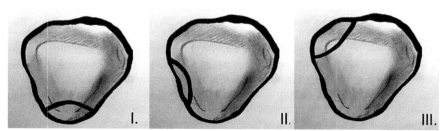

Fig. 4. Bipartite patella Saupe classification types 1, 2, and 3. (*Adapted from* Atesok K, Doral NM, Lowe J, Finsterbush A. Symptomatic Bipartite Patella: Treatment Alternatives. JAAOS - J Am Acad Orthop Surg. 2008;16(8):455-461.)

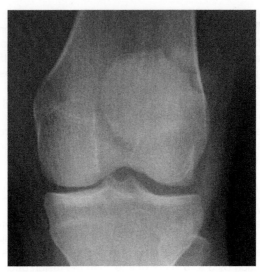

Fig. 5. Tripartite patella provided by Dr. Dominique Stevens MD, Northwestern University Health Service/Northwestern Medicine.

Most of the bipartite patellae are likely asymptomatic with most being found incidentally on radiographs.[44,50] In a systematic review of 22 studies, only 2% of affected individuals presented symptomatically (mean age 15.7 ± 4.4 years), commonly as a result of overuse inciting stress injury from sports and/or activities that involve jumping, running, squatting, and kneeling or trauma.[44] Epidemiologically, the most frequently affected populations are adolescents, specifically young adult men. There is currently no reported anatomic or physiologic reason to explain this age and gender predominance.[47,51,52]

Clinical findings. The most common presentation of bone stress injuries (BSI) in bipartite patellae is anterior knee pain with activity.[44,53] Physical examination may demonstrate tenderness superficial to the location of the accessory fragment, accessory prominence on palpation, enlarged appearance of the patella, effusion, hematoma, or decreased quadriceps engagement.[54]

Diagnostic imaging. Although bipartite patella can be diagnosed by anteroposterior radiograph as demonstrated in **Fig. 6**, various other imaging positions may be beneficial for diagnosis.

Ishikawa and colleagues report more robust displacement via Skyline view (**Fig. 7**) at 60° and 90° of knee flexion in each of 9 symptomatic young athletes under evaluation.[52]

Magnetic resonance imaging (MRI) is the gold standard to diagnose BSI of a bipartite patella as sall clear / 6-septandard x-ray films will not demonstrate the bony edema of bone stress injury although a robust callus reaction to the pathology could be observed on plain film radiography (**Fig. 8**) MRI can also demonstrate the extent of the synchondrosis, in addition to allowing for the measurement of fragment height and fragment-patella distance.[55] Radha suggests that pathology may be created by forces exerted on the patella by the patellar and quadriceps tendons in addition to forces from the medial patellofemoral ligament during activity, leading to pain and bony edema in the nonunited areas.[56] An analysis of the MRI's of 25 asymptomatic patients

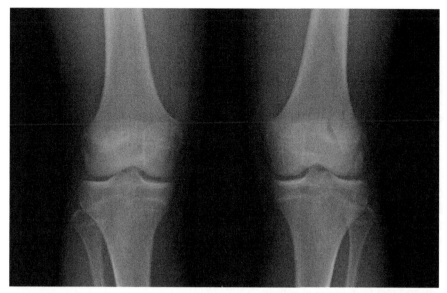

Fig. 6. AP radiograph of bipartite patella provided by Dr. Stephanie MacDonald DO, University of Rochester Medical Center.

with bipartite patellae, may highlight that bony edema correlates with symptomatology, as the images showed no bony fluid around the fragment.[57] Bone scintigraphy can also be a diagnostic tool of the bipartite patella as it can highlight areas of active bony pathology but is less specific as compared with MRI.[58]

Management. Symptoms can hinder the activity of daily living in addition to athletic activity. Nonoperative and operative management options exist, with nonoperative treatment being first line.[53] Most of patients recover with conservative treatment, which includes immobilization via bracing or tape, nonsteroidal antiinflammatories,

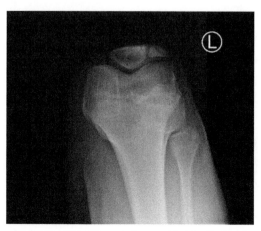

Fig. 7. Skyline view of left knee bipartite patella provided by Dr. Stephanie MacDonald DO, University of Rochester Medical Center.

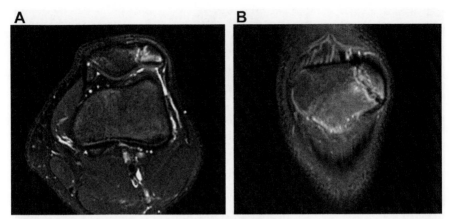

Fig. 8. Skyline (*A*) and AP (*B*) MRI views of bipartite patella provided by Dr. Katherine Rizzone, MD MPH, University of Rochester Medical Center.

cryotherapy (ice), physical therapy with isometric exercises involving quadricep extension, and rest from physical activity.[44,50,54,59,60]

If first-line treatment is ineffective, Marya and colleagues demonstrated that bupivacaine and methylprednisolone injections are helpful for symptomatic bilateral bipartite patella in a 20-year-old patient.[60] Low-intensity pulsed US is another potential management option as demonstrated in two 13-year-old males following 2 months of treatment.[61] Newer nonoperative outpatient techniques have also demonstrated potential, including US-guided injection (1% lidocaine (2 mL) and triamcinolone acetonide (5 mg)) and the "pie crust" technique for the lengthening of capsular tendon

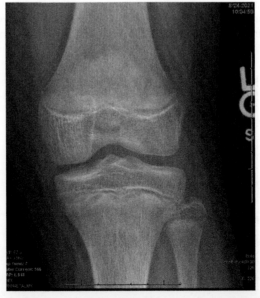

Fig. 9. AP radiograph of the left knee demonstrating distal femoral periphyseal stress injury with irregularity at the medial physis in a 13-year-old male football athlete.

structures detailed by Nakase and colleagues in 15 knees with an average age of 13 years, no complications were reported following return to activity.[62]

Surgical intervention is an option with persistent symptomology and has been shown to be efficacious in return to activity, but the literature is limited.[44,49,63] Surgical options include arthroscopic excision, surgical excision, combined arthroscopic and surgical excision, tension band wiring, open reduction internal fixation (ORIF), and soft tissue release.

A 2021 retrospective study of 266 patients with symptomatic bipartite patella found the operative treatment was performed in 10% of patients (which included isolated fragment excision, fragment excision with lateral release, isolated lateral release, fragment screw fixation, and synchondrosis drilling). Surgical patients had significantly longer symptom presentation before their initial hospital visit (21.5 vs 7 months, respectively) were older (15.4 vs 12.4 years in the nonoperative group), were more often women (59.3%), and were all competitive athletes (100% vs 85%) as compared with those treated nonoperatively. Following surgery, athletes had a mean 2.2-month recovery before returning to sport, compared with 1.9 months in the nonoperative cohort. Persistent symptoms were observed in 15% of surgical patients postoperatively.[49] A cohort of 127 surgically managed knees open fragment excision (66.9%), arthroscopic fragment excision (3.9%), vastus lateralis release (13.3%), lateral retinacular release (12.5%), and ORIF (3.1%) in patients with symptomatic bipartite patella of a mean age of 28.7 years showed that 84.1% of the patients reported total resolution of pain postoperatively, and 98.3% of patients were able to achieve a return to activity levels equivalent to preoperative state. There was an 11% complication rate (delayed wound healing, synovitis, wound infection, effusion, arthritis).[63] Each proposed surgical procedure demonstrated success and low complication rate, but there is currently no definitive gold-standard approach.[63]

Stress injuries of the patella
Patella BSI are rare, and since 2018 have been reported less than 15 times in the literature.[64] Clinically, patients report pain with activity. Due to the similarity in anterior knee pain between patellar BSI and congenital bipartite patella, it is important to accurately distinguish the diagnosis. Radiograph, bone scan, and MRI can all be used to diagnose patella BSI. Management is dependent on the extent and severity of the fracture. Less severe BSI treatment may involve decreased activity or immobilization, while displaced fractures require surgical reduction and internal fixation or excision.[65]

Stress Injuries of the Proximal Tibia and Distal Femur

Proximal tibia
Epidemiology and pathophysiology. The most common site of lower extremity (LE) BSI is the tibia, comprising half of all BSIs in both children and adults.[66] Tibial BSI occur in active individuals, most frequently in those involved in running and jumping activities.[66,67] While tibial BSIs have been extensively described in the literature, BSIs of the proximal tibial metaphysis are less frequently reported.[68]

Predisposition to proximal tibial BSI includes biomechanical pathology of the LE, such as limb malalignment, cavus deformity, or hyperpronation of the foot. Additional risk factors include training conditions such as changes in footwear, running biomechanics, dietary limitations, running surface, and training regimens that increase LE load including the incorporation of hill running.[68–70] The literature suggest these risk factors exist in addition to low energy availability, amenorrhea, low bone mass, low Body Mass Index (BMI), low cortical bone strength, low cortical area, and low muscle cross-sectional area (MCSA).[71–73]

Clinical findings. Presentation is often insidious knee pain that worsens on impact-associated activity and resolves with rest.[69] Other symptoms may include tenderness about the area of injury, with or without swelling.[67,69,74,75] Following a thorough history and physical examination, imaging plays a key diagnostic role in this injury. Plain films or musculoskeletal US may capture the callus of a proximal tibia BSI, but MRI is the definitive gold standard for diagnosis.[68,69,76,77]

Management. Nonoperative and operative management options are used, depending on the extent of injury. Nonoperatively, rest, nonweight bearing status, and analgesic therapy can be an effective mode of treatment.[67,74] Four patients with BSIs of the posteromedial aspect of the tibia in the location of the popliteal-soleal line were described by Daffner and colleagues Ages of cases ranged from 11 to 21 and all patients were men with some history of activity or running. Each patient was treated via rest from activity.[74]

Operative therapies have been reported in the literature but are more commonly used in adult patients with bone comorbidities such as osteoporosis, rheumatoid arthritis, extended use of corticosteroids and methotrexate, varus gonarthrosis, valgus gonarthrosis, pyrophosphate arthropathy, rheumatoid arthritis, osteoporosis, and Paget disease.[67,75]

Distal femur
Epidemiology. BSIs in the distal femur are rare, and their prevalence in the general public, adult athlete, or young athlete populations is unknown.[68,78] However, in an Israeli study of military recruits, 9.2% of diagnosed BSIs were of the distal femur.[68]

Clinical findings and diagnostic imaging. Vague knee pain is the most common presenting symptom of BSI in the distal femur, and an accurate and timely diagnosis is necessary to avoid potential complications, including complete or displaced fracture-necessitating further treatment.[68,79,80] Other presenting symptoms include mild patellar crepitus, suprapatellar swelling, and pain with varus and valgus stress.[79] As in the previously discussed BSIs, MRI is the gold standard for diagnosis.[68]

Management. With the paucity of reported evidence, treatment guidance is limited. As in other BSIs of the LEs, rest and nonweight bearing status are first-line management choices.[78] Additional workup to explore other biomechanical, metabolic, or anatomic risk factors for BSI previously mentioned for other locations may also be warranted.

Periphyseal Stress Injuries

Distal femur and proximal tibia
Epidemiology and pathophysiology. While much is known about bone stress injuries, research is more limited regarding primary periphyseal stress injuries in the knee. In children and adolescents, overuse injuries typically involve some or all components of the epiphyseal–physeal–metaphyseal (EPM) complex found on the ends of long bones.[6] Primary periphyseal stress injuries (PPSIs) often develop in the same way BSIs develop, that is, repetitive submaximal stress that causes microtrauma to some component of the EPM complex.[6]

Primary periphyseal stress injuries in the distal femur and proximal tibia are often caused by high impact, repetitive loading actions that cause compression and shearing valgus or varus biomechanical forces.[6] In a 2021 systematic review by Caine and colleagues, the nature and extent of PPSIs affecting the EPM complex was reviewed. A variety of high-impact repetitive youth sports activities had an increase incidence of PPSIs (**Table 1**). PPSIs of the knee are thought to result from microtrauma to components of the EPM complex, typically seen in repetitive submaximal stress.[6,81,82]

An important distinction between an overuse injury and PPSI is that a PPSI results from prolonged repetitive loading rather than from an increase in recent activity.[82] The physis of long bones is cartilaginous and ossifies last, making it weaker than surrounding bone.[83] The physis first closes centrally and then proceeds to close peripherally.[81,84] The central area of the physis is most susceptible to trauma due to decreased elasticity and the earlier closure compared with the periphery.[81] Between ages 12 and 15 years, the physes about the knee begin to close, and concurrently, adolescents experience a rapid growth spurt. This puts the physis at risk for stress and injury.[81,82]

Widening of the physis is the most common diagnostic feature of PPSI seen on imaging.[6] The widening physis begins in the metaphysis due to disrupted blood supply to the metaphysis.[6] The repetitive loading seen in a metaphyseal stress injury alters the perfusion of the metaphysis, ultimately interfering with apoptosis of the hypertrophied chondrocytes and preventing the ossification of chondrocytes in the zone of provisional calcification.[6,82,85] Germinal and proliferative zone growth continue to widen the physis in the hypertrophic zone due to the accumulation of chondrocytes that cannot calcify.[6,82] Although the widening physis may mimic a fracture, no fracture is present on MRI imaging.[6] Microtrauma at the distal femur and proximal tibia can disrupt normal endochondral ossification and even lead to permanent growth disturbances.[85]

Fortunately, once perfusion has been restored, the widening of the growth plate within the hypertrophic zone is reversible; therefore, the epiphyseal and metaphyseal blood supplies are unaltered. Unfortunately, many metaphyseal stress injuries are undiagnosed or not treated appropriately, which can ultimately lead to BSI in the EPM complex.[6] These injuries commonly produce a Salter–Harris type fracture pattern, but the hallmark is a slow progression of clinical symptoms.[6]

Clinical findings. Clinical presentation of PPSI often presents with vague, progressively worsening knee pain, often not associated with mechanical symptoms or history of knee trauma.[6,81,86] Physical examination with suspected periphyseal stress injury often yields point tenderness, joint line tenderness on palpation, knee stiffness, tenderness in the infrapatellar region or isolated tenderness on various locations of the knee.[81,86] The physical examination is usually negative for swelling, atrophy, motion limitations, and all special tests.[86] For some, the physical examination is nonspecific, thus further imaging is warranted for accurate diagnosis.[6,81,82]

Table 1
Sports with highest risk for physeal stress injuries about the knee[6]

Distal Femur Stress Injury	Proximal Tibia Stress Injury
Baseball	Baseball
Figure skating	Basketball
Gymnastics	Cheerleading
Basketball	Dance
Football	Gymnastics
Soccer	Long-distance running
Softball	Rugby
Tennis	Soccer
	Softball
	Tennis

Diagnostic imaging. Physeal imaging commonly consists of radiographs, computed tomography (CT), and MRI. Radiographs are typically the first-line imaging approach for a PPSI.[87] Physeal injuries can demonstrate physeal widening, epiphyseal displacement, periphyseal osteopenia, indistinctness of the epiphyseal and metaphyseal sides of the physis and fragmentation on the radiograph; however, the complex nature of the physis makes it challenging to diagnose with a 2D image.[6,87] Often, initial radiographic imaging of PPSI are normal and a heightened awareness is necessary to order advanced imaging, such as CT and MRI.[82] Contralateral radiographs can also be helpful in detecting subtle physeal changes.[87–89] Common PPSI findings on CT include areas of periphyseal widening and osseous bridging.[90] CTs provide minimal additional information compared with a radiograph and the large amount of radiation required to obtain a CT may be harmful to adolescent patients.[87] MRI is considered the gold standard for diagnosing BSIs due to the increased view of soft tissue and multiplanar images compared with CT and radiographs.[87,91] Physeal injuries are depicted on MRI with subtle physeal widening and irregularities and edema along the physis (**Fig. 10**). metaphyseal intrusions of physeal cartilage and extension of hypertrophic chondrocytes into the metaphysis.[87,92,93] On MRI, cartilage signal intensities of apparent physeal widening are evident due to long column formation of hypertrophic cartilage.[93] Reevaluation of periphyseal stress injuries is commonly monitored through repeat imaging with radiograph, MRI and/or CT.

Management. Treatment for periphyseal stress injuries of the knee is generally conservative, although it depends on the severity and location.[6,83] Management typically consists of strict rest, immobilization in some situations, and slow return to activity.[6] Immobilization is recommended if patients have pain with ADLs or cannot be compliant with activity restrictions, typically with crutches, knee immobilizers or long leg cast.(15)[6] Cross-training that does not stress the knee is often recommended to keep the athlete active but allow for healing.[82] It is imperative to recognize physeal widening on MRIs, as impact activity and physical therapy should be avoided until physeal changes resolve.(15) Return to sport may take anywhere from 4 to 20 weeks, depending on the severity of injury and patient's compliance to relative rest.[6] Surgery is rarely indicated, but may be performed if conservative measures are unsuccessful

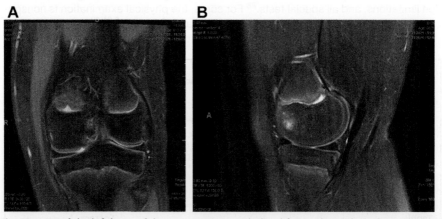

Fig. 10. MRI of the left knee of the same patient with distal femoral periphyseal stress injury showing physeal widening involving the posterior medial physis without edema, coronal (*A*) and sagittal (*B*) views.

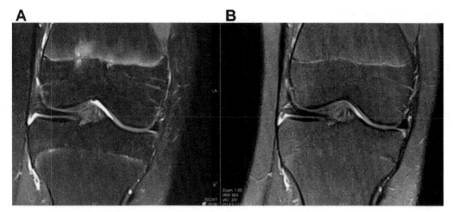

Fig. 11. MRI coronal images taken 5 months apart (initial: *A*; follow-up: *B*) in a 14-year-old female basketball athlete with FOPE.

and repeat imaging suggests surgical intervention, for the correction of knee deformity due to PPSI or if skeletal growth disruption occurs.[6] Although the literature is limited on monitoring for growth arrest in PPSI, the recommendation for general physeal injuries is the documentation of normal growth for at least 6 months.[94,95]

Focal periphyseal edema
Focal periphyseal edema (FOPE) is characterized by a focal bone marrow edema pattern centered at the physis of the distal femur, proximal tibia or proximal fibula and extending to the neighboring metaphysis and epiphysis in a "starburst" pattern.[84,86] It is unknown whether this finding is physiologic and related to normal physeal closure, or if FOPE is a painful phenomenon that is related to mechanical stress placed on the physis during physeal closure.[81] Most patients with FOPE have spontaneous resolution once the physis closes, suggesting that FOPE may be a physiologic process that is exacerbated by small microtrauma from impact activity.[81,84] On MRI, FOPE presents as bone marrow edema pattern on either side of the site of coalition (**Fig. 11**).[84] FOPE is typically treated conservatively with reduced weight bearing and rest.[81,84,86]

SUMMARY

Clinicians should include stress injuries of the knee in the differential for all active adolescent patients presenting with vague, insidious onset knee pain. A focused work-up with appropriate imaging to rule out bone-related pathology is recommended. Patients who specialize in a single sport, or are involved in weekly physical activity > age, travel teams, or year-round competition should be considered high risk for injury. Evaluation should also consider contralateral involvement in the pediatric population. Treatment options for most BSI's and physeal stress injuries are usually conservative including activity modification, relative rest, and addressing risk factors. In some severe or chronic cases, patients may require surgical intervention. However, the consequences of missed diagnosis could result in frank fracture, the need for surgical intervention, or arrested bone growth which could result in a limb length discrepancy. For the active adolescent, the consequences of quitting sports and embracing a sedentary lifestyle due to chronic undiagnosed injury are significant.

CLINICS CARE POINTS

- Bone stress injuries (BSI) are a common medical condition that often occur in bone tissue resulting from prolonged, repetitive loading.

- Chronic physeal stress injuries are another form of overuse injury that can develop from repetitive loading to the apophysis or epiphysis with increased susceptibility observed during periods of rapid growth.

- Apophyseal injuries of the knee occur at the insertion of the patellar tendon at the tibial tubercle (Osgood–Schlatter disease, OSD) or at the inferior pole of the patella (Sinding-Larsen–Johansson disease, SLJ).

- Primary periphyseal stress injuries of the proximal tibia and distal femur develop from repetitive submaximal stress that causes microtrauma to the epiphyseal–physeal–metaphyseal complex.

- Bipartite patellae result from an abnormal fibrocartilaginous connection between patellar ossification centers instead of bone and can be symptomatic in athletes involved in activities such as jumping, running, squatting, and kneeling or trauma.

- Distal femur and proximal tibia BSIs of the metaphysis are less common than other BSIs, but should be considered in athletes involved in running and jumping activities who present with vague knee pain of insidious onset.

- Most of the stress injuries of the knee resolve with relative rest but will occasionally need surgical intervention in more severe cases.

- Early and accurate identification of stress injuries of the knee is paramount for both optimal management and to avoid long-term consequences.

DISCLOSURE

The authors certify that they have no affiliations with or involvement in any organization or entity with any financial interest (such as honoraria; educational grants; participation in speakers' bureaus; membership, employment, consultancies, stock ownership, or other equity interest; and expert testimony or patent-licensing arrangements), or nonfinancial interest (such as personal or professional relationships, affiliations, knowledge or beliefs) in the subject matter or materials discussed in this article.

REFERENCES

1. Gaeta M, Mileto A, Ascenti G, et al. Bone stress injuries of the leg in athletes. Radiol Med (Torino) 2013;118(6):1034–44.
2. Beck B, Drysdale L. Risk Factors, Diagnosis and Management of Bone Stress Injuries in Adolescent Athletes: A Narrative Review. Sports Basel Switz 2021;9(4). https://doi.org/10.3390/sports9040052.
3. Bachrach LK. Acquisition of optimal bone mass in childhood and adolescence. Trends Endocrinol Metab TEM 2001;12(1):22–8.
4. Maggioli C, Stagi S. Bone modeling, remodeling, and skeletal health in children and adolescents: mineral accrual, assessment and treatment. Ann Pediatr Endocrinol Metab 2017;22(1):1–5.
5. Caine D, DiFiori J, Maffulli N. Physeal injuries in children's and youth sports: reasons for concern? Br J Sports Med 2006;40(9):749–60.
6. Caine D, Meyers R, Nguyen J, et al. Primary Periphyseal Stress Injuries in Young Athletes: A Systematic Review. Sports Med Auckl NZ 2021. https://doi.org/10.1007/s40279-021-01511-z.

7. De Souza MJ, Nattiv A, Joy E, et al. 2014 Female Athlete Triad Coalition Consensus Statement on Treatment and Return to Play of the Female Athlete Triad: 1st International Conference held in San Francisco, California, May 2012 and 2nd International Conference held in Indianapolis, Indiana, May 2013. Br J Sports Med 2014;48(4):289.
8. Achar S, Yamanaka J. Apophysitis and Osteochondrosis: Common Causes of Pain in Growing Bones. Am Fam Physician 2019;99(10):10.
9. Kuwabara A, Kraus E, Fredericson M. Narrative Review — Knee Pain in the Pediatric Athlete. Curr Rev Musculoskelet Med 2021;14(3):239–45.
10. Gowda N. Simultaneous Bilateral Tibial Tubercle Avulsion Fracture in a case of Pre-Existing Osgood-Schlatter Disease (OSD). J Orthop Case Rep 2012;2(1):4.
11. Yanagisawa S, Osawa T, Saito K, et al. Assessment of Osgood-Schlatter Disease and the Skeletal Maturation of the Distal Attachment of the Patellar Tendon in Preadolescent Males. Orthop J Sports Med 2014;2(7). 232596711454208.
12. Gerbino PG. Adolescent Anterior Knee Pain. Oper Tech Sports Med 2006;14(3): 203–11.
13. Pihlajamäki HK, Mattila VM, Parviainen M, et al. Long-term outcome after surgical treatment of unresolved Osgood-Schlatter disease in young men. J Bone Joint Surg Am 2009;91(10):2350–8.
14. Wall EJ. Osgood-schlatter disease: practical treatment for a self-limiting condition. Phys Sportsmed 1998;26(3):29–34.
15. Launay F. Sports-related overuse injuries in children. Orthop Traumatol Surg Res 2015;101(1):S139–47.
16. Circi E, Atalay Y, Beyzadeoglu T. Treatment of Osgood–Schlatter disease: review of the literature. Musculoskelet Surg 2017;101(3):195–200.
17. Domingues M. Osgood Schlatter's disease - A burst in young football players. Montenegrin J Sports Sci Med 2013;2:23–7.
18. Ladenhauf HN, Seitlinger G, Green DW. Osgood–Schlatter disease: a 2020 update of a common knee condition in children. Curr Opin Pediatr 2020;32(1): 107–12.
19. Riederer M, Jayanthi N. AMSSM Sports Medicine Topics: Apophysitis. SportsMedToday. Available at: https://www.sportsmedtoday.com/apophysitis-va-117.htm. Accessed December 3, 2021.
20. Sheppard ED, Ramamurti P, Stake S, et al. Posterior Tibial Slope is Increased in Patients With Tibial Tubercle Fractures and Osgood-Schlatter Disease. J Pediatr Orthop 2021;41(6):e411–6.
21. Bell DR, Post EG, Biese K, et al. Sport Specialization and Risk of Overuse Injuries: A Systematic Review With Meta-analysis. Pediatrics 2018;142(3):e20180657.
22. Itoh G, Ishii H, Kato H, et al. Risk assessment of the onset of Osgood–Schlatter disease using kinetic analysis of various motions in sports. PLoS One 2018; 13(1):e0190503.
23. Chang GH, Paz DA, Dwek JR, et al. Lower extremity overuse injuries in pediatric athletes: clinical presentation, imaging findings, and treatment. Clin Imaging 2013;37(5):836–46.
24. de Lucena GL, dos Santos Gomes C, Guerra RO. Prevalence and Associated Factors of Osgood-Schlatter Syndrome in a Population-Based Sample of Brazilian Adolescents. Am J Sports Med 2011;39(2):415–20.
25. Hall R, Foss KB, Hewett TE, et al. Sport Specialization's Association With an Increased Risk of Developing Anterior Knee Pain in Adolescent Female Athletes. J Sport Rehabil 2015;24(1):31–5.

26. Jayanthi NA, LaBella CR, Fischer D, et al. Sports-Specialized Intensive Training and the Risk of Injury in Young Athletes: A Clinical Case-Control Study. Am J Sports Med 2015;43(4):794–801.
27. Green DW, Aitchison AH, Sidharthan S, et al. Knee Radiographs Demonstrate Small but Statistically Significant Increase in Posterior Tibial Slope in Patient with Osgood-Schlatter Disease. Orthop J Sports Med 2021;9(7_suppl3). 2325967121S0012.
28. Gholve PA, Scher DM, Khakharia S, et al. Osgood Schlatter syndrome. Curr Opin Pediatr 2007;19(1):44–50.
29. Jacobson JA. Fundamentals of musculoskeletal ultrasound. 3rd edition. Philadelphia, PA: Elsevier; 2018.
30. Buldu H, Bilen FE, Eralp L, Kocaoglu M. Bilateral Brodie's abscess at the proximal tibia. Singapore Med J 2012;53(8):e159.
31. Jamshidi K, Mirkazemi M, Izanloo A, et al. Benign bone tumours of tibial tuberosity clinically mimicking Osgood-Schlatter disease: a case series. Int Orthop 2019; 43(11):2563–8.
32. Hirano A, Fukubayashi T, Ishii T, et al. Magnetic resonance imaging of Osgood-Schlatter disease: the course of the disease. Skeletal Radiol 2002;31(6):334–42.
33. Weiss JM, Jordan SS, Andersen JS, et al. Surgical Treatment of Unresolved Osgood-Schlatter Disease: Ossicle Resection With Tibial Tubercleplasty. J Pediatr Orthop 2007;27(7):844–7.
34. Smith JM, Varacallo M. Osgood Schlatter Disease. In: StatPearls. StatPearls Publishing; 2021. Available at: http://www.ncbi.nlm.nih.gov/books/NBK441995/. Accessed September 9, 2021.
35. Vaishya R, Azizi AT, Agarwal AK, et al. Apophysitis of the Tibial Tuberosity (Osgood-Schlatter Disease): A Review. Cureus 2016. https://doi.org/10.7759/cureus.780.
36. Topol GA, Podesta LA, Reeves KD, et al. Hyperosmolar Dextrose Injection for Recalcitrant Osgood-Schlatter Disease. PEDIATRICS 2011;128(5):e1121–8.
37. Nakase J, Goshima K, Numata H, et al. Precise risk factors for Osgood–Schlatter disease. Arch Orthop Trauma Surg 2015;135(9):1277–81.
38. Pagenstert G, Wurm M, Gehmert S, et al. Reduction Osteotomy of the Prominent Tibial Tubercle After Osgood-Schlatter Disease. Arthrosc J Arthrosc Relat Surg 2017;33(8):1551–7.
39. Nierenberg G, Falah M, Keren Y, et al. Surgical treatment of residual osgood-schlatter disease in young adults: role of the mobile osseous fragment. Orthopedics 2011;34(3):176.
40. Watanabe H, Majima T, Takahashi K, et al. Posterior tibial slope angle is associated with flexion-type Salter–Harris II and Watson–Jones type IV fractures of the proximal tibia. Knee Surg Sports Traumatol Arthrosc 2019;27(9):2994–3000.
41. Yen YM. Assessment and Treatment of Knee Pain in the Child and Adolescent Athlete. Pediatr Clin North Am 2014;61(6):1155–73.
42. Valentino M, Quiligotti C, Ruggirello M. Sinding-Larsen-Johansson syndrome: A case report. J Ultrasound 2012;15(2):127–9.
43. Kajetanek C, Thaunat M, Guimaraes T, et al. Arthroscopic treatment of painful Sinding-Larsen-Johansson syndrome in a professional handball player. Orthop Traumatol Surg Res 2016;102(5):677–80.
44. McMahon SE, LeRoux JA, Smith TO, et al. The management of the painful bipartite patella: a systematic review. Knee Surg Sports Traumatol Arthrosc 2016; 24(9):2798–805.

45. Cox CF, Sinkler MA, Hubbard JB. Anatomy, Bony Pelvis and Lower Limb, Knee Patella. In: StatPearls. StatPearls Publishing. 2021. Available at: http://www.ncbi.nlm.nih.gov/books/NBK519534/. Accessed November 30, 2021.

46. Felli L, Fiore M, Biglieni L. Arthroscopic treatment of symptomatic bipartite patella. Knee Surg Sports Traumatol Arthrosc 2011;19(3):398–9.

47. Oohashi Y, Koshino T, Oohashi Y. Clinical features and classification of bipartite or tripartite patella. Knee Surg Sports Traumatol Arthrosc 2010;18(11):1465–9.

48. Anderson SJ. Overuse Knee Injuries in Young Athletes. Phys Sportsmed 1991; 19(12):69–80.

49. Kallini J, Micheli LJ, Miller PE, et al. Operative Treatment of Bipartite Patella in Pediatric and Adolescent Athletes: A Retrospective Comparison With a Nonoperatively Treated Cohort. Orthop J Sports Med 2021;9(1). 2325967120967125.

50. Sweeney E, Rodenberg R, MacDonald J. Overuse Knee Pain in the Pediatric and Adolescent Athlete. Curr Sports Med Rep 2020;19(11):479–85.

51. Weckström M, Parviainen M, Pihlajamäki HK. Excision of Painful Bipartite Patella: Good Long-term Outcome in Young Adults. Clin Orthop 2008;466(11):2848–55.

52. Ishikawa H, Sakurai A, Hirata S, et al. Painful Bipartite Patella in Young Athletes The Diagnostic Value of Skyline Views Taken in Squatting Position and the Results of Surgical Excision. Clin Orthop Relat Res 1994;305:223–8.

53. Matic GT, Flanigan DC. Return to activity among athletes with a symptomatic bipartite patella: a systematic review. The Knee 2015;22(4):280–5.

54. Atesok K, Doral NM, Lowe J, et al. Symptomatic Bipartite Patella: Treatment Alternatives. J Am Acad Orthop Surg 2008;16(8):455–61.

55. Akdag T, Guldogan ES, Coskun H, et al. Magnetic resonance imaging for diagnosis of bipartite patella: usefulness and relationship with symptoms. Pol J Radiol 2019;84:e491–7.

56. Radha S, Shenouda M, Konan S, et al. Successful Treatment of Painful Synchondrosis of Bipartite Patella after Direct Trauma by Operative Fixation: A Series of Six Cases. Open Orthop J 2017;11:390–6.

57. O'Brien J, Murphy C, Halpenny D, et al. Magnetic resonance imaging features of asymptomatic bipartite patella. Eur J Radiol 2011;78(3):425–9.

58. Iossifidis A, Brueton RN, Nunan TO. Bone-scintigraphy in painful bipartite patella. Eur J Nucl Med 1995;22(10):1212–3.

59. Wong CK. Bipartite patella in a young athlete. J Orthop Sports Phys Ther 2009; 39(7):560.

60. Marya KM, Yadav V, Devagan A, et al. Painful bilateral bipartite patellae–case report. Indian J Med Sci 2003;57(2):66–7.

61. Kumahashi N, Uchio Y, Iwasa J, et al. Bone union of painful bipartite patella after treatment with low-intensity pulsed ultrasound: report of two cases. The Knee 2008;15(1):50–3.

62. Nakase J, Oshima T, Takata Y, et al. Ultrasound-guided injection and the pie crust technique for the treatment of symptomatic bipartite patella. J Med Ultrason 2001 2019;46(4):497–502.

63. Efficacy of Surgical Interventions for a Bipartite Patella | Orthopedics. Available at: https://journals.healio.com/doi/abs/10.3928/01477447-20140825-07. Accessed September 4, 2021.

64. Baker S, Seales J, Newcomer S, et al. A Case Report: Bilateral Patella Stress Fractures in a Collegiate Gymnast. J Orthop Case Rep 2018;8(4):45–8.

65. Crane TP, Spalding TJW. The Management of Patella Stress Fractures and the Symptomatic Bipartite Patella. Oper Tech Sports Med 2009;17(2):100–5.

66. Sanderlin BW, Raspa RF. Common Stress Fractures. Am Fam Physician 2003; 68(8):1527–32.
67. Demir B, Gursu S, Oke R, et al. Proximal tibia stress fracture caused by severe arthrosis of the knee with varus deformity. Am J Orthop Belle Mead NJ 2009; 38(9):457–9.
68. Drabicki RR, Greer WJ, DeMeo PJ. Stress fractures around the knee. Clin Sports Med 2006;25(1):105–15, ix.
69. Fredericson M, Bergman AG, Hoffman KL, et al. Tibial stress reaction in runners. Correlation of clinical symptoms and scintigraphy with a new magnetic resonance imaging grading system. Am J Sports Med 1995;23(4):472–81.
70. Meardon SA, Willson JD, Gries SR, et al. Bone stress in runners with tibial stress fracture. Clin Biomech Bristol Avon 2015;30(9):895–902.
71. Ihle R, Loucks AB. Dose-response relationships between energy availability and bone turnover in young exercising women. J Bone Miner Res 2004;19(8): 1231–40.
72. Barrack MT, Gibbs JC, De Souza MJ, et al. Higher incidence of bone stress injuries with increasing female athlete triad-related risk factors: a prospective multisite study of exercising girls and women. Am J Sports Med 2014;42(4):949–58.
73. Popp KL, Hughes JM, Smock AJ, et al. Bone geometry, strength, and muscle size in runners with a history of stress fracture. Med Sci Sports Exerc 2009;41(12): 2145–50.
74. Daffner RH, Martinez S, Gehweiler JA, et al. Stress fractures of the proximal tibia in runners. Radiology 1982;142(1):63–5.
75. Tan T, Ho W. Sequential Proximal Tibial Stress Fractures associated with Prolonged usage of Methotrexate and Corticosteroids: A Case Report. Malays Orthop J 2015;9(3):65–7.
76. Niva MH, Kiuru MJ, Haataja R, et al. Bone stress injuries causing exercise-induced knee pain. Am J Sports Med 2006;34(1):78–83.
77. Romani WA, Perrin DH, Dussault RG, et al. Identification of tibial stress fractures using therapeutic continuous ultrasound. J Orthop Sports Phys Ther 2000;30(8): 444–52.
78. Meaney JE, Carty H. Femoral stress fractures in children. Skeletal Radiol 1992; 21(3):173–6.
79. Schmidt-Brudvig TJ. Distal femoral stress fracture in military basic trainees: a report of three cases. J Orthop Sports Phys Ther 1985;7(1):20–2.
80. DeFranco MJ, Recht M, Schils J, et al. Stress fractures of the femur in athletes. Clin Sports Med 2006;25(1):89–103, ix.
81. Beckmann N, Spence S. Unusual Presentations of Focal Periphyseal Edema Zones: A Report of Bilateral Symmetric Presentation and Partial Physeal Closure. Case Rep Radiol 2015;465018.
82. Difiori JP. Overuse injury of the physis: a "growing" problem. Clin J Sport Med 2010;20(5):336–7.
83. Caine D, Meyers R, Nguyen J, Schöffl V, Maffuli N. Primary Periphyseal Stress Injuries in Young Athletes: A Systematic Review. Sports Med 2022;52(4):741–72.
84. Zbojniewicz AM, Laor T. Focal Periphyseal Edema (FOPE) zone on MRI of the adolescent knee: a potentially painful manifestation of physiologic physeal fusion? AJR Am J Roentgenol 2011;197(4):998–1004.
85. Dempewolf M, Kwan K, Sherman B, et al. Youth Kicker's Knee: Lateral Distal Femoral Hemiphyseal Arrest Secondary to Chronic Repetitive Microtrauma. J Am Acad Orthop Surg Glob Res Rev 2019;3(8):e079.

86. Giles E, Nicholson A, Sharkey MS, et al. Focal Periphyseal Edema: Are We Over-treating Physiologic Adolescent Knee Pain? J Am Acad Orthop Surg Glob Res Rev 2018;2(4):e047.
87. Jawetz ST, Shah PH, Potter HG. Imaging of physeal injury: overuse. Sports Health 2015;7(2):142–53.
88. Nguyen JC, Sheehan SE, Davis KW, et al. Sports and the Growing Musculoskeletal System: Sports Imaging Series. Radiology 2017;284(1):25–42.
89. Alison M, Azoulay R, Tilea B, et al. Imaging strategies in paediatric musculoskeletal trauma. Pediatr Radiol 2009;39(Suppl 3):414–21.
90. Nguyen JC, Markhardt BK, Merrow AC, et al. Imaging of Pediatric Growth Plate Disturbances. Radiogr Rev Publ Radiol Soc N Am Inc 2017;37(6):1791–812.
91. Beck BR, Bergman AG, Miner M, et al. Tibial stress injury: relationship of radiographic, nuclear medicine bone scanning, MR imaging, and CT Severity grades to clinical severity and time to healing. Radiology 2012;263(3):811–8.
92. Nanni M, Butt S, Mansour R, et al. Stress-induced Salter-Harris I growth plate injury of the proximal tibia: first report. Skeletal Radiol 2005;34(7):405–10.
93. Laor T, Wall EJ, Vu LP. Physeal widening in the knee due to stress injury in child athletes. AJR Am J Roentgenol 2006;186(5):1260–4.
94. Birch JG, Makarov MA, Jackson TJ, et al. Comparison of Anderson-Green Growth-Remaining Graphs and White-Menelaus Predictions of Growth Remaining in the Distal Femoral and Proximal Tibial Physes. J Bone Joint Surg Am 2019;101(11):1016–22.
95. Dabash S, Prabhakar G, Potter E, et al. Management of growth arrest: Current practice and future directions. J Clin Orthop Trauma 2018;9(Suppl 1):S58–66.

Discoid Meniscus

Emily L. Niu, MD[a],*, Rushyuan Jay Lee, MD[b], Elaine Joughin, MD[c],
Craig J. Finlayson, MD[d], Benton E. Heyworth, MD[e]

KEYWORDS

- Discoid • Meniscus • Pediatric • Knee • Congenital variant

KEY POINTS

- Discoid meniscus is a spectrum of abnormality but generally possess the key features of wider and thicker meniscal tissue with altered collagen makeup and organization compared with a normal meniscus.
- Discoid meniscus in young children can sometimes present as popping or clunking that is otherwise asymptomatic to the patient and does not limit their activities. Nonoperative treatment is reasonable in this group.
- Owing to altered or absent meniscocapsular attachments and disorganized collagen makeup, discoid menisci are prone to instability or tearing, which can present similarly to tear of the normal meniscus, or in the case of an entrapped and displaced discoid tear, can result in motion limitations.
- Treatment of symptomatic discoid meniscus is composed of saucerization and rim stabilization with good outcomes. Subtotal meniscectomy should be avoided if possible.

INTRODUCTION

Discoid meniscus is the most common congenital morphologic variant of the meniscus. This most commonly occurs in the lateral meniscus and less commonly in the medial meniscus.[1] Though usually occurring unilaterally, bilateral discoid lateral menisci (DLM) have been reported in 5% to 25% of cases.[2,3] In the United States and Western Europe, the incidence of unilateral DLM has been estimated to be between 0.7% and 5%.[4–7] The true incidence of the discoid meniscus is likely underestimated due to a certain percentage remaining asymptomatic.

[a] Children's National Hospital, 111 Michigan Avenue Northwest, Washington, DC 20010, USA;
[b] The Johns Hopkins School of Medicine, 601 N Caroline St 5th Floor, Baltimore, MD 21287, USA; [c] Alberta Children's Hospital, 28 Oki TRAIL NW. Calgary, Alberta T3B 6A8, Canada; [d] Ann & Robert H. Lurie Children's Hospital of Chicago, 2515 N Clark St, Chicago, IL 60614, USA; [e] Orthopedic Center, Boston Children's Hospital, 300 Longwood Avenue, Boston, MA 02115, USA
* Corresponding author.
E-mail address: eniu@childrensnational.org

Clin Sports Med 41 (2022) 729–747
https://doi.org/10.1016/j.csm.2022.05.009
0278-5919/22/© 2022 Published by Elsevier Inc.
sportsmed.theclinics.com

EPIDEMIOLOGY

Long thought to be more prevalent in Asian populations, with reports of incidence up to 16% in Korean and Japanese patients undergoing arthroscopy,[8,9] more recent studies have delved into the racial and ethnic distributions of discoid meniscus among different populations in the United States.[10,11] Grimm and colleagues[10] looked at data from a large regional health care system database and found an overall prevalence of 4.88 per 100,000 patients. They found the highest prevalence in those of Hispanic ethnicity (6.01/100,000) and the lowest in the Black population (2.68/100,000). Those of Asian background had a prevalence of 4.38/100,000. Milewski and colleagues[11] queried the Pediatric Health Information System for patients treated with surgery for discoid meniscus in comparison to those treated surgically for a medial meniscus tear. They found that both Asian and Hispanic/Latino children had higher odds (2.41 times and 2.36 times, respectively) of undergoing surgery for discoid meniscus compared with Caucasian children. The higher prevalence of discoid meniscus in the Hispanic population was previously underappreciated and is an important diagnosis to consider in young patients of Hispanic/Latino background presenting with vague knee or leg symptoms.

ANATOMY

There is a wide spectrum of discoid meniscus anatomy. In its simplest form, a discoid meniscus is characterized by over-coverage of the tibial plateau. Other common characteristics include increased meniscal thickness, deficiency of meniscocapsular attachments, and histologic disorganization, and avascularity. Discoid meniscal thickness can be mildly increased compared with a normal meniscus or could be block-shaped and accompanied by a dysplastic appearing lateral femoral condyle (LFC) and widened lateral joint space (**Fig. 1**).

Deficient meniscocapsular attachments can lead to meniscal instability. This deficiency can both arise from the congenital lack of attachments and chronic strain on these attachments due to the abnormal meniscal anatomy leading to meniscocapsular tears and subluxation. Histologically, discoid meniscal tissue differs from the normal meniscus. Vascularity in the normal meniscus enters peripherally, leaving the central third avascular. The discoid meniscus, with its larger central component, has a larger avascular zone.[12] In addition, discoid meniscal collagen has fewer collagen fibers[13] and a disrupted appearance of the typical circular collagen network of the meniscus.[14]

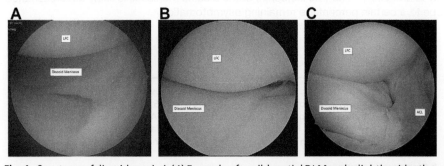

Fig. 1. Spectrum of discoid menisci. (*A*) Example of a mild partial DLM, only slightly wider than normal meniscus but with increased thickness. Note that this meniscus has a radial pattern tear. (*B*) Example of a near complete discoid meniscus with incomplete coverage of the tibial plateau and slightly increased thickness. (*C*) Example of a complete, "block-shaped" discoid lateral meniscus. ACL, anterior cruciate ligament; LFC, lateral femoral condyle.

Both the avascularity and the histologic disorganization predispose the meniscus to tearing. Tear patterns are similar to normal menisci with radial, longitudinal, horizontal cleavage, and intra-substance tears most common.

One of the enduring questions about discoid meniscus is the mechanism by which they form. An early theory[15] suggested that the normal meniscus forms via resorption of the central portion of a discoid precursor, and therefore the discoid meniscus is a normal stage of fetal meniscus development. This has since been dismissed by multiple studies[16–18] due to the rarity of discoid morphology in fetal knee specimen.[19] A recent histologic study[20] looked at surgical samples of discoid menisci in patients under 18 years of age. They observed a disorganized matrix, and cell types within the discoid tissue not found in the normal meniscus. This suggests an entirely divergent pathway of formation of the discoid; rather than a deviation during the development of the normal meniscus, the DLM could derive from a larger process of dysplastic changes in knee morphology.

CLASSIFICATION

Traditionally, DLM was classified in three primary categories by Watanabe.[21] A Watanabe Type 1 is a discoid meniscus that covers the whole lateral tibial plateau, whereas a Type 2 has overall increased width compared with a normal meniscus but incompletely covers the plateau. A Watanabe Type 3, also known as the Wrisberg variant, lacks meniscocapsular attachments posteriorly outside of the Ligament of Wrisberg and thus is unstable posteriorly. The more recently developed arthroscopic PRISM (Pediatric Research in Sports Medicine) discoid lateral meniscus classification system attempts to provide a more comprehensive description of DLM characteristics in the categories of width, height, instability, and tear pattern[22] (Fig. 2).

In the PRISM DLM classification, abnormal width is categorized as incomplete or less than 90% of the lateral tibial plateau, whereas near complete/complete is 90% or more coverage of the lateral tibial plateau. Height or "thickness" is deemed abnormal if it exceeds what is expected compared with the medial meniscal height, is thicker than appropriate for the femoral-tibial joint space, and lacks the expected central taper.

Abnormal stability is present if meniscal-capsular attachments are completely absent, or if on probing the meniscus is able to translate past the midpoint/apex of the convexity of the LFC because of insufficient meniscal-capsular attachments or a vertical tear (Fig. 3). Note that peripheral vertical tears are included in the stability rather than the tear category as their presence contributes to abnormal stability. Normal stability is the absence of these criteria. Abnormal stability is further subclassified by location. Anterior instability involves the anterior horn, with or without associated instability of the midbody. Posterior instability involves the posterior horn, with or without instability of the midbody. If both the anterior and posterior horns are involved, then the abnormal stability is classified as "anterior/posterior." Abnormal stability centered in the midbody is classified as "anterior" or "posterior," depending on which half demonstrates the predominant instability.

Finally, DLM tears are classified by presence, type, and location. These tears are classified only when located within the peripheral post-saucerization meniscus, excluding those in the central zone that would be resected during saucerization. Horizontal tears, thought to be secondary to the abnormal meniscal tissue are categorized separately from the other tear types: radial, complex, or degenerative tears. As with stability, tears are categorized as "anterior," "posterior," or "anterior/posterior" according to the predominant location of the tear. The anterior/posterior subcategory

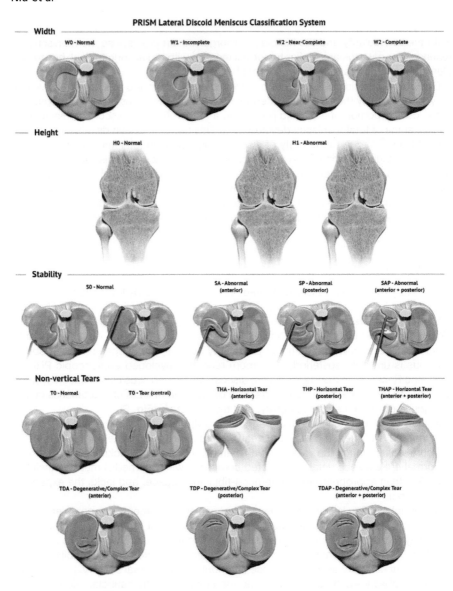

Courtesy of ©2021 Children's Orthopaedic Surgery Foundation (COSF)

Fig. 2. PRISM DLM Classification System. The five categories of width, height, instability, and tear pattern and their respective subclassifications are depicted.

is used for the anterior or posterior horn-based tears that extend past the midbody into the other horn and also for midbody radial tears.

DIAGNOSIS
Clinical Presentation

In children less than 10 years of age, discoid meniscus usually presents with a history of clunking or snapping without any history of injury. Younger patients may present with clunking in the knee, also known as "snapping knee syndrome" that is noticeable to the parent but is largely painless and does not stop the child from activity. Recurrent

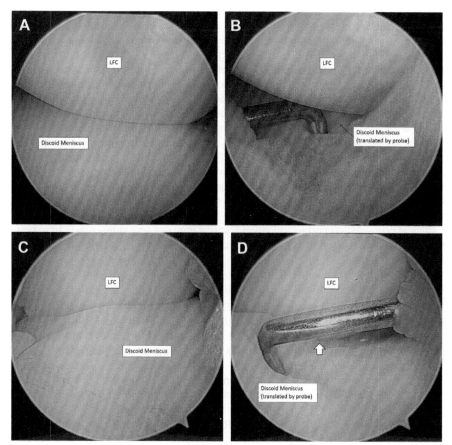

Fig. 3. Example of DLM with anterior instability. (*A*) and (*B*) show translation of the meniscus tissue using a probe from the anterolateral viewing portal. (*C*) and (*D*) show probe translation from an anteromedial (AM) viewing portal. Note that the AM viewing portal offers a superior ability to evaluate instability and tears of the anterior horn. White arrow, apex of the convexity of the LFC in the sagittal plane.

locking or symptoms of "catching" associated with a sudden fall can occur.[23] In the older child or adolescent, it may present after a minor injury or a sports injury with symptoms of a meniscal tear including joint-line pain, swelling, and locking.[24–26] Patients with an unstable or torn meniscus that is displaced may present with loss of terminal range of motion, in particular loss of terminal extension.

Clinical Examination

Keeping in mind that children are generally flexible, a gentle examination is paramount. Both knees should be examined to provide a comparison, as well as to increase patient and parent confidence by first demonstrating the examination on the unaffected knee. The patient can first be observed standing and walking, looking for asymmetry which may suggest subtle loss of terminal extension, and gauging overall alignment. Gait can be observed for antalgia or toe walking on the affected side, which can point to the loss of terminal extension and poor quad strength.

The patient can then be examined in the supine position, first observing and palpating for an effusion. The child can then be asked to actively extend and flex the knee, looking for differences in the range of motion to the contralateral side. In children and adolescents, a bulge at the anterolateral joint line in full flexion may be visualized and as the knee is extended, this may reduce, producing an audible clunk.[27] In addition, in children with symptoms of snapping or clunking, patella instability is another possible entity that should be considered and ruled out during examination. Observation of the knee during flexion and extension, looking for a J sign or abnormal patellar tracking, can rule out congenital developmental patellar subluxation or dislocation.

Special testing for meniscal signs can then be performed. Joint effusion is more likely in adolescents that have symptoms consistent with a meniscal tear, along with joint line tenderness and a positive McMurray's sign. Presence of clicking, incomplete extension, and clunking with active flexion or extension are more likely if there is meniscal instability.[28] Subtle losses to complete extension are sometimes better assessed in the prone position, looking for differences in heel height with the knees maximally extended.[29]

Clinical presentation and examination findings may not accurately predict the presence of a discoid meniscus whether intact or torn,[30] necessitating further assessment with imaging studies.

IMAGING
Radiographs

Radiographic signs (**Fig. 4**) can include wide lateral joint line, flattening or squaring of the LFC, tibial spine hypoplasia, elevation of the fibular head in relation to the tibial plateau, cupping (deepening) of the lateral tibial plateau, obliquity of the lateral tibial plateau, hypoplasia of the femoral condyle, and, in some cases, a shallow notch in the LFC.[24] These various radiographic changes suggest that there may be an encompassing process to explain the development of bony dysplasia and associated discoid meniscus.

Choi and colleagues[31] compared measurements of the lateral joint space height (LJSH), lateral tibial spine height, fibular head height (FHH), and lateral tibial plateau obliquity (LTPO) degrees in children and showed statistical differences between children with lateral discoid meniscus versus normal controls. FHH (distance between the apex of the fibular head and the lateral tibial plateau) less than 14.9 mm and LTPO

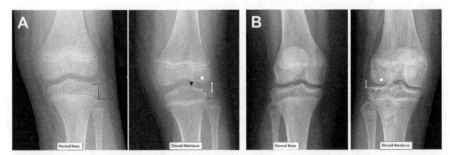

Fig. 4. Radiographic findings of DLM. (*A*) Comparison of radiographs of 8-year-old boy with normal knee versus 8-year-old boy with DLM. Note that in the case of an incompletely ossified tibial epiphysis joint space widening (*white double-headed arrow*) and tibial cupping may not be reliable findings. FHH (*red stepped line*) is significantly different between the two patients. Also seen are mild LFC squaring (*white square*), and lateral tibial spine hypoplasia (black triangle head). (*B*) Comparison of radiographs of 14-year-old girl with normal knee versus 14-year-old girl with DLM. Here, there is more pronounced joint space widening (*white double-headed arrow*), LFC squaring (*white square*), and tibial cupping (*blue curved arrow*).

greater than 17.6° were most sensitive and specific. Milewski and colleagues[32] recommended using the LJSH in weight-bearing radiographs for diagnosis in children older than age 14 as the tibial epiphysis in younger children is not completely ossified. They proposed that the diagnosis of potential discoid meniscus may be improved by using fibular height measurements across age groups (13.5 mm in discoid group vs 18.6 in control group).

Using these radiographic indices in combination can provide a predictive risk score that differs according to the patient's age.[24] Although there are significant differences in the measurements of the above parameters between discoid and non-discoid knees, radiographs should be supplemented by MRI for symptomatic patients.

Magnetic Resonance Imaging

MRI techniques should include a small field of view with thin slices, especially for younger children. Axial three-dimensional MR images have been recommended to improve diagnostic accuracy.[24]

The "bow tie" sign is the classic diagnostic sign (**Fig. 5**), showing continuity between the anterior and posterior meniscus on ≥3 consecutive sections that are 5 mm thick.[27] MRI has a high positive predictive value but low sensitivity, especially for detecting subtle peripheral detachments.[23] In older adolescents and adults, MRI was found to be 100% specific and 97.8% sensitive for diagnosis.[33]

The diagnosis of incomplete discoid meniscus is less sensitive and therefore other measurements have been recommended (**Fig. 6**). These include the ratio of lateral meniscus to tibia, that is, width of meniscal body seen on coronal view to width of lateral tibial plateau,[24] transverse meniscal diameter between the free margin and the periphery of the body on a coronal view,[34] increased width of the meniscus at the midpoint of the anterior and posterior horns on a coronal view,[27] and transverse meniscal diameter of more than 20% of the tibial width on transverse images or transverse meniscal diameter of more than 15 mm.[23] Posteromedial condylar angle and posterolateral condylar angle can be used to measure the degree of LFC hypoplasia on MRIs in adult patients. However, no pediatric patients were included in this study.[35]

MRI features of meniscal instability (**Fig. 7**), in addition to the absence of the meniscal attachments, include peri-meniscal edema, meniscal deformity, infolding and denting, abnormally large anterior or posterior horn, linear fluid at the anterior meniscal margin, and meniscal bulging.[24] Ahn and colleagues[26] classified displacement of the discoid meniscus associated with instability—none, anterocentral, posterocentral, and central.

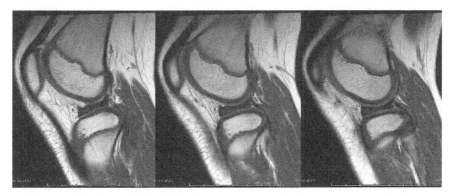

Fig. 5. MRI of the knee showing the "bow-tie" sign on three consecutive sagittal cuts.

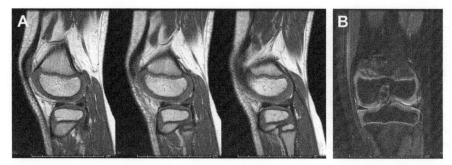

Fig. 6. MRI showing an incomplete DLM. (*A*) On sagittal views, it does not meet the criteria of the "bow-tie" sign. However, the meniscus appears thickened, particularly the posterior horn. (*B*) On coronal view, the lateral meniscus is noted to be increased in height compared with the medial meniscus.

Although the diagnosis of a discoid meniscus has become significantly more accurate with the development of MRI techniques, identification of instability or tear patterns and correlation with arthroscopic findings are areas that continue to evolve. Hampton and colleagues[30] reported 75% sensitivity and 50% specificity for MRI identification of tears within DLM. They also found that the diagnosis of a tear on MRI has a poor correlation with arthroscopic findings. Yilgor and colleagues[33] performed a similar comparison of MRI to arthroscopic findings of discoid meniscus tears and found that although MRI was highly sensitive and specific (97.8% and 100%, respectively) in determining the presence of a tear, the results were more variable when determining tear type. Sohn and colleagues[36] found that certain tear types can in fact obscure the diagnosis of a DLM. Specifically, they noted decreased ability to diagnose discoid meniscus in the presence of a large radial tear, displaced bucket handle tear, or inverted flap tear.

Given the variability of the correlation of MRI to arthroscopic findings, thorough intraoperative evaluation of the discoid meniscus for tears or instability is crucial. The PRISM DLM research group[22] developed a sequence of arthroscopic evaluation that specifically probes the anterior horn while viewing from the anteromedial portal

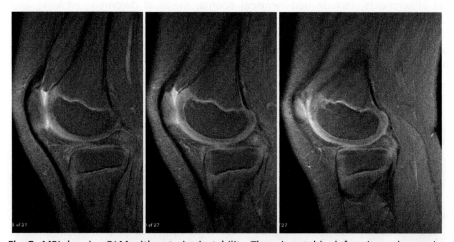

Fig. 7. MRI showing DLM with anterior instability. There is notable deformity and posterior bulging of the meniscus tissue, along with more subtle signal enhancement anterior to the meniscus.

rather than the traditional anterolateral portal (see **Fig. 3**). Systematic evaluation, in addition to a standardized classification scheme, can aid in treatment decision-making and further research in discoid saucerization and repair techniques.

TREATMENT

The natural history of the discoid meniscus, especially those with no symptoms, has not been well described in the literature. DLM have been discovered incidentally during evaluation of other injuries that have no symptoms nor any arthroscopic evidence of tearing or instability of the meniscus.[4] As such, it may be appropriate to observe asymptomatic discoid menisci.[34]

Surgery is typically recommended for the symptomatic DLM. Early surgical techniques focused on reducing mechanical symptoms through total or subtotal meniscectomy. However, modern treatment techniques seek to retain the peripheral rim of the meniscus to maintain meniscal function and reduce the iatrogenic risk of joint degeneration due to a deficient lateral meniscus.[37,38] As technology has evolved, the surgical approach has also shifted from open to arthroscopic techniques.

The procedure begins with diagnostic arthroscopy to define the discoid meniscus and any associated pathology. A 2.7-mm arthroscope and smaller instruments may be necessary for younger patients. The overall width and height of the meniscus should be assessed. The meniscus is then carefully examined for any tearing or instability. Instability may occur at any location, and careful attention must be paid to the anterior horn as the prevalence of anterior horn instability has been reported to be greater than 50% by some authors.[39] Viewing through the standard anteromedial portal has been suggested to improve the assessment of the anterior horn.[22] In a large series of 470 knees treated surgically, 63% of patients had meniscal tears, with horizontal tears being the most common.[40]

Once the pathology of the meniscus has been defined, saucerization is performed (**Fig. 8**A, B). A combination of arthroscopic biters and a motorized shaver is commonly used to excise the central portion of the meniscus and recontour the peripheral rim. Instability and displacement of the meniscus, along with the increased bulk of the discoid meniscus, may complicate saucerization, especially in smaller knees. An arthroscopic knife may be useful for saucerization along the anteromedial margin of the meniscus where the tissue may be difficult to assess or too thick for standard biters.

Optimizing the amount of resection may be a challenge, as larger meniscal remnants have been associated with higher rates of re-tearing, and over-resection may lead to insufficiency of the meniscus. Maintaining a peripheral rim of 6 to 8 mm has been suggested as a guideline by several authors and has been associated with good short- to medium-term results. Larger meniscal remnants have been associated with higher rates of re-tear[41] and a peripheral rim of less than 5 mm has also been associated with progressive degenerative changes following saucerization.[42] It is important to recognize, however, that patients being treated for discoid menisci are often younger and smaller than other meniscal surgery patients and this range is only a guideline. Other authors have suggested using the midbody of the medial meniscus as a reference point for the remaining rim.[43] Over-resection of the meniscus should also be avoided during initial saucerization as subsequent stabilization with capsule-based techniques may alter the morphology of the residual rim.

Following saucerization, peripheral meniscal tears and instability may be managed by a variety of standard meniscal repair techniques including inside-out, outside-in, and all-inside as indicated by tear pattern and location. For the treatment of anterior horn pathology, an outside-in technique may be used (see **Fig. 8**C). Again, due to the smaller

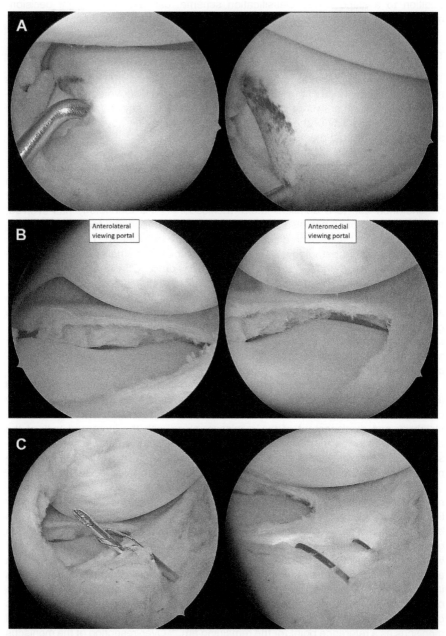

Fig. 8. Operative treatment of DLM. (*A*) The meniscus is probed for instability and tears. (*B*) After thorough arthroscopic evaluation, saucerization is completed using meniscus scissors or arthroscopic knife to initiate the process, followed by alternating biters and shaver, leaving an approximately 8 mm rim. (*C*) Outside-in capsular-based repair of anterior horn instability is performed using 0 polydioxanone suture in a vertical mattress fashion. (*D*) Horizontal cleavage tear of the posterior horn is repaired using all-inside construct. Alternatively, the inferior leaflet may be excised. (*E*) Completed saucerization and repair.

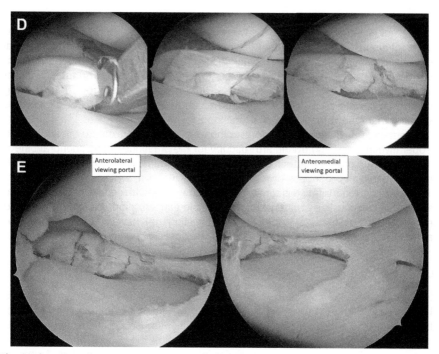

Fig. 8. (*continued*)

size of many patients undergoing surgery, caution must be used to avoid over-penetration of the posterior capsule when using capsule-based all-inside techniques.[44]

Intrasubstance degeneration and horizontal cleavage tears are often encountered during saucerization of the central meniscus. Preferential removal of the inferior or superior leaflet may be indicated based on the relative size, stability, and quality of the tissue. Partial or complete excision of one leaflet of the tear may assist in debulking a thick meniscus,[45] but may compromise the stability and size of the peripheral rim in tears extending toward the periphery. In these cases, repair of the horizontal component may be indicated (see **Fig. 8**D, E). Repair of horizontal tears with a meniscus-based all-suture technique has been described for these tears.[46]

Once saucerization and repair have been completed, the stability and function of the meniscus should be verified. Gentle probing and a dynamic examination of the knee through a range of motion may elucidate any residual instability or excess meniscal remnant. This may be addressed through additional saucerization or stabilization as indicated.

In cases with chronic degeneration of the meniscus due to abnormal morphology or instability, meniscal repair and preservation may not be possible. In such cases, unstable and degenerative tissue should be debrided back to stable margins to reduce any associated mechanical symptoms. These patients should be counseled on the risk and potential long-term complications of meniscal insufficiency. In such cases, if a young patient has lost most of the hoop stresses usually provided by the meniscus, or enough tissue has been removed, so as to constitute a "subtotal" or "total meniscectomy," lateral meniscus transplant should be considered. In the minimal evidence that exists regarding meniscus transplant in children and adolescents,[47–52] discoid meniscus that has failed prior treatment is, in fact, the most common underlying scenario. Although there is controversy regarding the optimal timing for performing meniscus transplant in these age groups, close monitoring for early degenerative changes in the lateral compartment is warranted. Our authors advocate for performing high-resolution 3-T magnet MRI as frequently as every year. The goal of the lateral meniscus transplant should be to replace the shock absorption and stabilization functions of the meniscus *before* the development of moderate chondral surface degeneration, even in the absence of symptoms. Thus, most experts agree that a young patient with grade 1 or 2 Outerbridge changes is a better candidate for a meniscus transplant than one with grade 3 or 4 changes.

The remainder of the knee and lateral compartment should be carefully evaluated on preoperative imaging and during arthroscopy for the presence of any chondral/osteochondral lesions or other pathology as up to 20% of patients may require an associated non-meniscal procedure.[41]

Postoperative rehabilitation is similar to that following typical meniscal surgery. Immediate weight-bearing is permitted following simple saucerization. Weight-bearing and range of motion restrictions following repair or stabilization may be dictated by the tear pattern, nature of the repair, and the degree/location of preoperative instability.

OUTCOMES

Literature on the outcomes of modern arthroscopic treatment of discoid meniscus is relatively sparse and is largely limited to series with small sample sizes, short-term follow-up, and little use of functional outcome measures or patient-reported outcomes. For example, Good and colleagues[39] analyzed the clinical outcomes of 23 knees in 21 patients (within a larger series of 37 knees) with more than 1 year of follow-up, with a mean follow-up time just over 3 years. The authors reported good range of motion in all patients, but knee pain in 13%, mechanical symptoms in 17%, and activity limitations in 9% at the time of most recent follow-up. Of note, although most of the patients underwent meniscal repair for instability of the posterior horn, anterior horn, or both, the authors did not differentiate outcomes based on whether or not repair had been performed. Ikeuchi[8] reviewed the clinical results in 23 knees which had undergone meniscectomy with mean follow-up of 4.3 years, reporting 78% good or excellent results, and 22% fair. Interestingly, the authors found better results in those with total meniscectomy than those with partial meniscectomy. Atay and colleagues[53] reported on 34 knees in 34 patients who underwent arthroscopic partial meniscectomy with a mean follow-up of 5.6 years, citing 39% excellent results, 46% good results, and 15% fair results. However, a significant percentage showed flattening of the femoral condyle on radiographic review. Vandermeer and colleagues[54] investigated the outcomes of 25 knees in 22 patients with the lateral discoid meniscus, most of them underwent partial lateral meniscectomy, or "saucerization." Only 55% had good or excellent results at a mean of 4.5 years postoperatively, and more than one-third of patients could not resume a normal postoperative activity level. Aicroth and colleagues[3] reported on 48 knees that underwent open total meniscectomy, 6 knees that underwent arthroscopic partial lateral meniscectomy, and 8 knees that underwent no treatment, given a stable posterior horn and the absence of tears. Because 84% of their patients had a good or excellent result, they recommended total meniscectomy for any patients with posterior instability and cited the development of arthritic changes in post-meniscectomy pediatric knee as a "matter for conjecture."

Most recently, Logan and colleagues[40] reviewed 470 cases in 401 patients with the discoid meniscus. Amomg them 18% were initially managed non-operatively and more than one-third of the patients subsequently required surgery at a median of 7.9 months post-diagnosis. Of the 419 patients who underwent surgery at any point,

17% required reoperation, mostly for meniscal re-tear, and another 16% reported ongoing pain or mechanical symptoms at final follow-up. Although 54% underwent saucerization alone and 46% saucerization and repair/stabilization, comparative analysis of the cohorts with and without repair was not explored.

Most studies with longer term follow-up greater than 10 years have focused on the outcomes of subtotal or total meniscectomy. These are instructive through their demonstration of relatively high rates of progression of degenerative changes and poor outcomes, overall. For example, Washington and colleagues[6] reviewed the outcomes of 18 patients treated with one or more meniscectomy surgeries over the period of 1955 to 1983 at the Hospital for Special Surgery, with a mean follow-up of 17 years. Although 13 knees had good or excellent outcomes using the Ikeuchi scale,[8] one-third of the patients had only fair outcomes, with common complaints of intermittent symptoms and mechanical symptoms. However, no degenerative changes were seen on the knees (50%) that underwent long-term radiographic review.

Habata and colleagues[55] investigated the radiographic and lower extremity alignment implications of "total resection" of lateral discoid meniscus in 37 knees in 32 patients at a mean of 14.5 years postoperatively. The authors reported moderate or severe joint space narrowing in 11% of knees, with worse rates of degenerative changes and a more lateralized mechanical axis in those patients who underwent resection at older ages. In another series of Japanese patients with a mean follow-up of 16 years, Okazaki and colleagues[56] similarly showed more severe degenerative changes, as well as poorer IKDC (International Knee Documentation Committee) scores, in the patients who had undergone discoid treatment at older ages. However, both studies' results may be less applicable to pediatric orthopedic surgeons considering age-based approaches to discoid meniscus. The subpopulations found to have poorer outcomes were treated with arthroscopy well into adulthood, whereas younger patients tended to have minimal degenerative findings and overall good outcomes if treated in childhood. In contrast, Raber and colleagues[57] reported on 20-year follow-up on a series of 17 knees in 14 children (mean age: 9 years, range 3–14 years) in Switzerland, all of them had undergone total meniscectomy. Long-term radiographic follow-up revealed osteoarthritic changes in 59% of knees, with an identical percentage showing clinical symptoms consistent with osteoarthrosis.

Overall, outcomes of surgical treatment of discoid meniscus are good, and may be better than attempted non-operative treatment, which has been associated with conversion to surgery in over one-third of cases.[40] However, despite increasing awareness of meniscal instability patterns in knees with discoid meniscus, particularly anterior horn instability, few studies have focused on the outcomes of saucerization with repair, which can be considered the modern gold standard of care in a substantial percentage of cases. Owing to known abnormalities in the integrity and quality of discoid meniscus tissue, re-tear and reoperation are not uncommon regardless of technique. However, due to concerning rates of degenerative changes observed in longer term studies, efforts toward meniscal preservation should be favored over subtotal and total meniscectomy. Longer term comparative studies investigating the results of repair are sorely needed to better understand which cases may benefit from varying degrees of stabilization, and which may be better suited for nihilistic approaches.

ASSOCIATED CONDITIONS
Bilateral Discoid

Bilateral DLM are uncommon (5%–20% of those with symptomatic discoid); however, reported prevalence varies and is likely underestimated, with a study by Ahn and colleagues[58] of 33 Asian males with unilateral symptomatic discoid, finding that nearly all (32) had MRI confirmed discoid on the asymptomatic contralateral knee. They also found that the DLM were similar in morphology between the symptomatic and asymptomatic sides. Patel and colleagues[2] studied bilateral DLM—16 patients symptomatic bilaterally and 60 patients symptomatic on one side only. They found that those with bilateral symptoms requiring treatment were younger (10.4 vs 12.5 years of age), and more often presented with complete or Wrisberg-type DLM. The possibility of contralateral side DLM that may eventually need treatment should be discussed, especially with younger patients who have specific types of discoid morphology.

Osteochondritis Dissecans

Osteochondritis dissecans (OCD) of the LFC in association with DLM has been well documented. Takigami and colleagues[59] studied 133 patients with symptomatic complete DLM and found that 14.5% of the affected knees had a concurrent lateral OCD and discoid. They found that predictive factors were males, younger patients (5–11 years), as well as those with a central shift based on the MRI classification of DLM tears by Ahn and colleagues.[26]

The pathway by which either pathology occurs independently is not well understood; even less so how they occur in conjunction with each other. However, it would follow that the altered joint forces of the lateral compartment as a result of a DLM, and especially in the setting of a torn discoid, would contribute to the formation of OCD. Some authors have studied anatomic factors including the type of discoid and alterations in the shape of the LFC to begin to elucidate this relationship. Deie and colleagues[60] studied 38 knees with lateral femoral OCD. They found that 19 occurred with complete discoid, 15 incomplete DLM, and 4 occurred in conjunction with a normal meniscus. They found that complete discoid, both with and without tear, more commonly occurred with OCD in zone 4 (more central area, Cahill and Berg classification) of the LFC, and incomplete discoid occurred more commonly with a zone 5 (more peripheral and lateral) OCD. Kamei and colleagues[61] evaluated the shape of the LFC in patients with concomitant OCD and DLM compared with those with DLM only. They found that those with concomitant findings had a higher LFC prominence ratio, or a more squared-off appearance of the LFC compared with the medial femoral condyle. They suggest that those patients with DLM who form OCD may have experienced more excessive stress across the LFC, leading to both this difference in shape and development of the OCD.

OCD following surgical treatment of DLM, particularly partial or subtotal meniscectomy, is also well established and an important factor to consider in long-term follow-up of these patients. Hashimoto and colleagues[62] studied patients who underwent arthroscopic surgery for DLM, with mean follow-up over 4 years. They found that 7.8% developed postoperative OCD, with younger age (below 10 years of age at the time of surgery) and subtotal meniscectomy as predictors for OCD.

Discoid Medial Meniscus

Discoid medial meniscus (DMM) is far rarer than DLM. Although true incidence is likely underestimated, studies looking at registries of knees undergoing surgery for the meniscus estimate the incidence of medial discoid to be between 0.06% and 0.3%.[1,63–65] The presentation, physical examination findings, and treatment of DMM are similar to DLM. Some authors[66] advocate a lower threshold for surgical intervention in cases of DMM due to the natural decreased mobility of the medial compared with lateral meniscus, potentially increasing the stress across the meniscus and predisposing it to tears. Outcome data are mainly limited to smaller case series,[1,63,66,67] but overall support improved outcomes with rim preserving saucerization and rim stabilization over subtotal meniscectomy. Further studies with larger series are needed to evaluate the long-term outcomes of DMM.

SUMMARY

Discoid meniscus is a spectrum of disorders with accordingly diverse clinical presentations. There are various physical examination and radiographic findings that are suggestive of a discoid meniscus, which can be confirmed by MRI. Treatment of symptomatic patients, especially those with loss of terminal motion due to a displaced unstable or torn discoid, is surgical. Although MRI can be useful to identify tearing and instability, it is not always consistent in identifying tear types and may not always perfectly guide treatment. Careful evaluation and reevaluation during surgery are necessary to ensure proper preservation of the rim and stabilization of the meniscus. Outcome of discoid treatment is superior in cases of saucerization with and without repair over subtotal or total meniscectomy. Long-term outcomes of untreated tears or subtotal and total meniscectomy include progression of degenerative changes and arthritis of the knee. Further directions in research should focus on patient-reported outcomes data with longer term follow-up results of rim preservation with and without repair of discoid.

CLINICS CARE POINTS

- Discoid meniscus is a spectrum of abnormality but generally possess the key features of wider and thicker meniscal tissue with altered collagen makeup and organization compared with a normal meniscus.

- Discoid meniscus in young children can sometimes present as popping or clunking that is otherwise asymptomatic to the patient and does not limit their activities. Nonoperative treatment is reasonable in this group.

- Owing to altered or absent meniscocapsular attachments and disorganized collagen makeup, discoid menisci are prone to instability or tearing, which can present similarly to tear of the normal meniscus, or in the case of an entrapped and displaced discoid tear, can result in motion limitations.

- Treatment of symptomatic discoid meniscus is composed of saucerization and rim stabilization with good outcomes. Subtotal meniscectomy should be avoided if possible.

DISCLOSURE

The authors have nothing to disclose.

REFERENCES

1. Tachibana Y, Yamazaki Y, Ninomiya S. Discoid medial meniscus. Arthroscopy 2003;19(7):E12–8.
2. Patel NM, Cody SR, Ganley TJ. Symptomatic bilateral discoid menisci in children: a comparison with unilaterally symptomatic patients. J Pediatr Orthop 2012; 32(1):5–8.
3. Aichroth PM, Patel DV, Marx CL. Congenital discoid lateral meniscus in children. A follow-up study and evolution of management. J Bone Joint Surg Br 1991;73(6): 932–6.

4. Dickhaut SC, DeLee JC. The discoid lateral-meniscus syndrome. J Bone Joint Surg Am 1982;64(7):1068–73.
5. Neuschwander DC, Drez D Jr, Finney TP. Lateral meniscal variant with absence of the posterior coronary ligament. J Bone Joint Surg Am 1992;74:1186–90.
6. Washington ER 3rd, Root L, Liener UC. Discoid lateral meniscus in children. Long-term follow-up after excision. J Bone Joint Surg Am 1995;77(9):1357–61.
7. Jordan MR. Lateral Meniscal Variants: Evaluation and Treatment. J Am Acad Orthop Surg 1996;4(4):191–200.
8. Ikeuchi H. Arthroscopic treatment of the discoid lateral meniscus. Technique and long-term results. Clin Orthop Relat Res 1982;167:19–28.
9. Seong SC, Park MJ. Analysis of the discoid meniscus in Koreans. Orthopedics 1992;15(1):61–5.
10. Grimm NL, Pace JL, Levy BJ, et al. Demographics and Epidemiology of Discoid Menisci of the Knee: Analysis of a Large Regional Insurance Database. Orthop J Sports Med 2020;8(9). 2325967120950669.
11. Milewski MD, Coene RP, McFarlane KH, et al. Nationwide Ethnic/Racial Differences in Surgical Treatment of Discoid Meniscus in Children: A PHIS Database Study. J Pediatr Orthop 2021;41(8):490–5.
12. Arnoczky SP, Warren RF. Microvasculature of the human meniscus. Am J Sports Med 1982;10(2):90–5.
13. Atay OA, Pekmezci M, Doral MN, et al. Discoid meniscus: an ultrastructural study with transmission electron microscopy. Am J Sports Med 2007;35(3):475–8.
14. Papadopoulos A, Kirkos JM, Kapetanos GA. Histomorphologic study of discoid meniscus. Arthroscopy 2009;25(3):262–8.
15. Smillie IS. The congenital discoid meniscus. J Bone Joint Surg Br 1948;30B(4):671–82.
16. Kaplan EB. Discoid lateral meniscus of the knee joint; nature, mechanism, and operative treatment. J Bone Joint Surg Am 1957;39-A(1):77–87.
17. Clark CR, Ogden JA. Development of the menisci of the human knee joint. Morphological changes and their potential role in childhood meniscal injury. J Bone Joint Surg Am 1983;65(4):538–47.
18. Le Minor JM. Comparative morphology of the lateral meniscus of the knee in primates. J Anat 1990;170:161–71.
19. Turati M, Anghilieri FM, Accadbled F, et al. Discoid meniscus in human fetuses: A systematic review. Knee 2021;30:205–13.
20. Tudisco C, Botti F, Bisicchia S. Histological Study of Discoid Lateral Meniscus in Children and Adolescents: Morphogenetic Considerations. Joints 2021;7(4):155–8.
21. Watanabe M, Takeda S, Ikeuchi H. Atlas of arthroscopy. 2nd edition. New York: Springer-Verlag; 1969.
22. Lee RJ, Nepple JJ, Schmale GA, Niu EL, Beck JJ, Milewski MD, Finlayson CJ, Joughin VE, Stinson ZS, Pace JL, PRISM Meniscus Research Interest Group, Heyworth BE. Reliability of a New Arthroscopic Discoid Lateral Meniscus Classification System: A Multicenter Video Analysis. Am J Sports Med: in press.
23. Morrissey RT, Weinstein SL. Sports Medicine in the Growing child. Lovell and Winter's pediatric Orthopaedics. 6th edition. RT Morrissey and SL Weinstein; 2006. p. 1393–4.
24. Tyler PA, Jain V, Ashraf T, et al. Update on imaging of the discoid meniscus. Skeletal Radiol 2021. https://doi.org/10.1007/s00256-021-03910-9.
25. Yamaguchi N, Chosa E, Tajima T, et al. Symptomatic discoid lateral meniscus shows a relationship between types and tear patterns, and between causes of

clinical symptom onset and the age distribution. Knee Surg Sports Traumatol Arthrosc 2021. https://doi.org/10.1007/s00167-021-06635-3.

26. Ahn JH, Lee YS, Ha HC, et al. A novel magnetic resonance imaging classification of discoid lateral meniscus based on peripheral attachment. Am J Sports Med 2009;37(8):1564–9.

27. Siow HM, Ganley TJ. Discoid lateral meniscus. Pediatric orthopaedic surgery: operative techniques. MS Kocher and MB Millis Elsevier; 2011. p. 376.

28. Jin B, Zhen J, Wei X, et al. Evaluation of the Peripheral Rim Instability of the Discoid Meniscus in Children by Using Weight-Bearing Magnetic Resonance Imaging. J Comput Assist Tomogr 2021;45(2):263–8.

29. Beck JJ, Niu EL, Cruz AI Jr, et al. Physical Exam for Sports Medicine Knee Injuries in Pediatric Patients. JPOSNA 2021;3(4). Available at: https://www.jposna.org/ojs/index.php/jposna/article/view/369.

30. Hampton M, Hancock G, Christou A, et al. Clinical presentation, MRI and clinical outcome scores do not accurately predict an important meniscal tear in a symptomatic discoid meniscus. Knee Surg Sports Traumatol Arthrosc 2021;29(9): 3133–8.

31. Choi SH, Ahn JH, Kim KI, et al. Do the radiographic findings of symptomatic discoid lateral meniscus in children differ from normal control subjects? Knee Surg Sports Traumatol Arthrosc 2015;23(4):1128–34.

32. Milewski MD, Krochak R, Duarte AJ, et al. Do Age and Weightbearing Radiographs Affect Lateral Joint Space and Fibular Height Measurements in Patients With Discoid Lateral Meniscus? Orthop J Sports Med 2018;6(3). 2325967118760534.

33. Yilgor C, Atay OA, Ergen B, et al. Comparison of magnetic resonance imaging findings with arthroscopic findings in discoid meniscus. Knee Surg Sports Traumatol Arthrosc 2014;22(2):268–73.

34. Sohn DW, Bin SI, Kim JM, et al. Discoid lateral meniscus can be overlooked by magnetic resonance imaging in patients with meniscal tears. Knee Surg Sports Traumatol Arthrosc 2018;26(8):2317–23.

35. Kocher MS, Logan CA, Kramer DE. Discoid Lateral Meniscus in Children: Diagnosis, Management, and Outcomes. J Am Acad Orthop Surg 2017;25(11): 736–43.

36. Xu Z, Chen D, Shi D, et al. Evaluation of posterior lateral femoral condylar hypoplasia using axial MRI images in patients with complete discoid meniscus. Knee Surg Sports Traumatol Arthrosc 2016;24(3):909–14.

37. Ahn JH, Kim KI, Wang JH, et al. Long-term results of arthroscopic reshaping for symptomatic discoid lateral meniscus in children. Arthroscopy 2015;31(5): 867–73.

38. Smuin DM, Swenson RD, Dhawan A. Saucerization Versus Complete Resection of a Symptomatic Discoid Lateral Meniscus at Short- and Long-term Follow-up: A Systematic Review. Arthroscopy 2017;33(9):1733–42.

39. Good CR, Green DW, Griffith MH, et al. Arthroscopic treatment of symptomatic discoid meniscus in children: classification, technique, and results. Arthroscopy 2007;23(2):157–63.

40. Logan CA, Tepolt FA, Kocher SD, et al. Symptomatic Discoid Meniscus in Children and Adolescents: A Review of 470 Cases. J Pediatr Orthop 2021;41(8): 496–501.

41. Hayashi LK, Yamaga H, Ida K, et al. Arthroscopic meniscectomy for discoid lateral meniscus in children. J Bone Joint Surg Am 1988;70(10):1495–500.

42. Yamasaki S, Hashimoto Y, Takigami J, et al. Risk Factors Associated With Knee Joint Degeneration After Arthroscopic Reshaping for Juvenile Discoid Lateral Meniscus. Am J Sports Med 2017;45(3):570–7.

43. Kim SH, Ahn J, Kim TW, et al. Midbody of the medial meniscus as a reference of preservation in partial meniscectomy for complete discoid lateral meniscus. Knee Surg Sports Traumatol Arthrosc 2019;27(8):2558–67.

44. Shea KG, Dingel AB, Styhl A, et al. The Position of the Popliteal Artery and Peroneal Nerve Relative to the Menisci in Children: A Cadaveric Study. Orthop J Sports Med 2019;7(6). 2325967119842843.

45. Tsujii A, Matsuo T, Kinugasa K, et al. Arthroscopic minimum saucerization and inferior-leaf meniscectomy for a horizontal tear of a complete discoid lateral meniscus: Report of two cases. Int J Surg Case Rep 2018;53:372–6.

46. Pace JL, Luczak SB, Kanski G, et al. Discoid Lateral Meniscus Saucerization and Treatment of Intrasubstance Degeneration Through an Accessory Medial Portal Using a Small Arthroscope. Arthrosc Tech 2021;10(9):e2165–71.

47. Kocher MS, Tepolt FA, Vavken P. Meniscus transplantation in skeletally immature patients. J Pediatr Orthop B 2016;25(4):343–8.

48. Tuca M, Luderowski E, Rodeo S. Meniscal transplant in children. Curr Opin Pediatr 2016;28(1):47–54.

49. Zaffagnini S, Espinosa M, Neri MP, et al. Treatment of Meniscal Deficiency with Meniscal Allograft Transplantation and Femoral Osteotomy in a Patient with History of Lateral Discoid Meniscus: 15-Year Follow-up Case Report. JBJS Case Connect 2020;10(1):e0079.

50. Smith RA, Vandenberg CD, Pace JL. Management of Long-Term Complications in the Setting of Lateral Meniscal Deficiency After Saucerization of a Discoid Lateral Meniscus in an Adolescent Patient: A Case Report and Review of the Literature. JBJS Case Connect 2018;8(4):e102.

51. Middleton S, Asplin L, Stevenson C, et al. Meniscal allograft transplantation in the paediatric population: early referral is justified. Knee Surg Sports Traumatol Arthrosc 2019;27(6):1908–13.

52. Riboh JC, Tilton AK, Cvetanovich GL, et al. Meniscal Allograft Transplantation in the Adolescent Population. Arthroscopy 2016;32(6):1133–40.e1.

53. Atay OA, Doral MN, Leblebicioğlu G, et al. Management of discoid lateral meniscus tears: observations in 34 knees. Arthroscopy 2003;19(4):346–52.

54. Vandermeer RD, Cunningham FK. Arthroscopic treatment of the discoid lateral meniscus: results of long-term follow-up. Arthroscopy 1989;5(2):101–9.

55. Habata T, Uematsu K, Kasanami R, et al. Long-term clinical and radiographic follow-up of total resection for discoid lateral meniscus. Arthroscopy 2006;22(12):1339–43.

56. Okazaki K, Miura H, Matsuda S, et al. Arthroscopic resection of the discoid lateral meniscus: long-term follow-up for 16 years. Arthroscopy 2006;22(9):967–71.

57. Räber DA, Friederich NF, Hefti F. Discoid lateral meniscus in children. Long-term follow-up after total meniscectomy. J Bone Joint Surg Am 1998;80(11):1579–86.

58. Ahn JH, Lee SH, Yoo JC, et al. Bilateral discoid lateral meniscus in knees: evaluation of the contralateral knee in patients with symptomatic discoid lateral meniscus. Arthroscopy 2010;26(10):1348–56.

59. Takigami J, Hashimoto Y, Tomihara T, et al. Predictive factors for osteochondritis dissecans of the lateral femoral condyle concurrent with a discoid lateral meniscus. Knee Surg Sports Traumatol Arthrosc 2018;26(3):799–805.

60. Deie M, Ochi M, Sumen Y, et al. Relationship between osteochondritis dissecans of the lateral femoral condyle and lateral menisci types. J Pediatr Orthop 2006; 26(1):79–82.

61. Kamei G, Adachi N, Deie M, et al. Characteristic shape of the lateral femoral condyle in patients with osteochondritis dissecans accompanied by a discoid lateral meniscus. J Orthop Sci 2012;17(2):124–8.

62. Hashimoto Y, Nishino K, Reid JB 3rd, et al. Factors Related to Postoperative Osteochondritis Dissecans of the Lateral Femoral Condyle After Meniscal Surgery in Juvenile Patients With a Discoid Lateral Meniscus. J Pediatr Orthop 2020;40(9): e853–9.

63. Dickason JM, Del Pizzo W, Blazina ME, et al. A series of ten discoid medial menisci. Clin Orthop Relat Res 1982;168:75–9.

64. Marchetti ME, Jones DC, Fischer DA, et al. Bilateral discoid medial menisci of the knee. Am J Orthop (Belle Mead Nj) 2007;36(6):317–21.

65. Lukas K, Livock H, Kontio K, et al. Bilateral Discoid Medial Menisci: A Case Report and Review of the Literature. J Am Acad Orthop Surg Glob Res Rev 2020;4(8). e20.00069.

66. Song IS, Kim JB, Lee JK, et al. Discoid Medial Meniscus Tear, with a Literature Review of Treatments. Knee Surg Relat Res 2017;29(3):237–42.

67. Pinar H, Akseki D, Karaoglan O, et al. Bilateral discoid medial menisci. Arthroscopy 2000;16:96–101.

Meniscus Repair in Pediatric Athletes

Brendan Shi, MD[a], Zachary Stinson, MD[b], Marie Lyne Nault, MD[c], Jennifer Brey, MD[d], Jennifer Beck, MD[e],*

KEYWORDS

- Pediatric • Meniscus • Meniscus repair • Meniscectomy • Rehabilitation
- Platelet-rich plasma

KEY POINTS

- Stable and peripheral tears may heal with nonoperative management. However, meniscus tears that cause persistent pain and discomfort, mechanical symptoms, or instability are indicated for surgical treatment.
- Pediatric patients with meniscus tears have a higher success rate after meniscus repair than the adult population and do poorly after meniscectomy.
- When performing all-inside or inside-out repairs for posterior meniscus tears in pediatric patients, it is important to understand the relationship between repair site and neurovascular structures.

INTRODUCTION AND BACKGROUND

As understanding of the biological and functional importance of the meniscus has increased over the past century, treatment of meniscus tears has evolved. Early investigators describe the presence of pain and joint dysfunction from meniscus injury; however, the meniscus was thought of as a vestigial, embryologic remnant shaped as a "semilunar cartilage."[1,2] Thus, early treatment of meniscus tears often consisted of total meniscectomy with little consideration for retention or repair. Longer term follow-up of total meniscectomy patients showed poor results. Increasing joint reactive forces led to early osteoarthritis and poor overall outcomes.[3] As recognition and acceptance of these results widened, the treatment of meniscus tears has appropriately shifted. In pediatric patients with acute, traumatic meniscus tears, treatment focuses on maintenance of meniscus function, preferentially through repair or partial meniscectomy if unsalvagable.[4–8]

[a] UCLA Department of Orthopaedic Surgery; [b] Nemours Children's Health; [c] Pediatric Orthopaedic Surgery, University of Montreal; [d] Department of Orthopaedic Surgery, University of Louisville; [e] Orthopaedic Institute for Children/UCLA Department of Orthopaedic Surgery, 403 W Adams Blvd, Los Angeles, CA 90007, USA
* Corresponding author.
E-mail address: jjbeck@mednet.ucla.edu

Clin Sports Med 41 (2022) 749–767
https://doi.org/10.1016/j.csm.2022.05.010
0278-5919/22/© 2022 Elsevier Inc. All rights reserved.

Youth sports participation has increased dramatically over the past 50 years, and the rate of meniscus injury has increased proportionally.[9] Along with anterior cruciate ligament (ACL) tears, meniscus tears have been shown to be the most common pediatric sports injuries requiring surgery.[10] Data from 2020 report the rate of meniscus tears in adolescent athletes as 0.51 per 10,000 athlete exposures.[2] Improvements in MRI quality have made diagnosis of meniscus tears more accurate, especially in younger, smaller patients. Improved imaging techniques have also improved surgical planning,[11] and proliferation of new arthroscopic techniques and tools has expanded the options for meniscus repair in smaller knees with more complex tear patterns. Finally, the rate of meniscus repair has increased, with better outcomes reported in pediatric than adult populations.[2,3,9]

Many of the principles of pediatric meniscus management are derived from the broader adult meniscus literature, but there are a few key differences between skeletally immature and mature patients. First, as the meniscus is fully vascularized at birth and does not achieve the adult pattern of peripheral 10% to 30% vascularization until 10 years of age[12,13] (**Fig. 1**), the pediatric population should have improved healing potential than their adult counterparts. This combined with possible higher levels of resident stem cells, and a more robust inflammatory response may explain the association between younger age and higher meniscus repair success rates.[13,14] Second, a host of long-term studies have demonstrated poor clinical outcomes associated with meniscectomy in the pediatric population.[9,15] The preservation of meniscal tissue is critical in younger patients to prevent the accumulation of increased knee contact stress, subsequent arthritis, and limitations in range of motion.[15,16]

PATIENT EVALUATION
History

A pediatric patient with a meniscus tear will often relate a history of an acute onset of knee pain. Common mechanisms include twisting injury, varus or valgus contact injuries, or landing incorrectly. Unlike adults, patients may have a rapid effusion due to increased vascularity of the pediatric meniscus. Patients who have acute loss of range of motion or large effusions may present earlier due to difficulty with ambulation

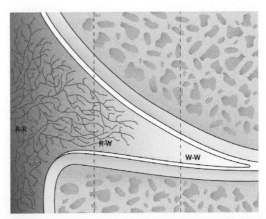

Fig. 1. Vascularity of fully mature meniscus. R-R, red-red; R-W, red-white; W-W, white-white zones. (*From* Vinagre G, Cruz F, Alkhelaifi K, D'Hooghe P. Isolated meniscus injuries in skeletally immature children and adolescents: state of the art. J ISAKOS. 2021 May 21:jisakos-2020-000496. https://doi.org/10.1136/jisakos-2020-000496. Epub ahead of print. PMID: 34021035.)

and activities of daily living and are more likely to have displaced meniscus tears. Pain and effusions may quickly improve with nonoperative treatment (rest, ice, anti-inflammatories, brace wear) causing delayed presentation of nondisplaced tears. However, continued pain, especially with cutting, pivoting, or deep squatting activities, is common findings in more chronic tears. Patients with a history of painless mechanical symptoms or inability to achieve full range of motion in the knee should also be evaluated for a congenital discoid meniscus.[17]

Physical Examination

Physical examination should begin with examination manuevers that comfort and relax the patient as guarded examinations can make diagnosis of meniscus injuries very difficult. If possible, examination of lower extremity alignment and gait should occur first. An acutely injured patient may be dependent on crutches, have an antalgic gait with shortened stance on the injured leg, or lack full extension at heel strike. A child with an unstable, discoid meniscus may walk with a circumduction gait to "pop" the knee into extension during swing phase.

Sitting and supine examination of the patient can occur on an examination table or a parents lap to facilitate comfort. Often, watching the patient get onto the table or into a sitting position can uncover important physical findings such as strength, range of motion limitations, or positional apprehension. Loss of normal patella contour and fullness of the infrapatellar soft spots on visual inspection are suggestive of an effusion.

Knee examinations should include the range of motion testing. Placing one finger over the joint line during the range of motion can often detect mechanical symptoms. Limitations in both passive and active ranging may indicate an incarcerated bucket-handle meniscus tear, displaced meniscus tear, or congenital discoid meniscus. Patients with acute injuries will often lose active range of motion while retaining full passive motion. Thorough palpation of the knee including distal femoral physis, proximal tibial physis, and tibial tubercle apophysis should be completed, with pain along the joint line being a sensitive marker for meniscus pathology.[18]

Meniscus-specific tests include the McMurray test, Apley grind, and Thessaly testing. The McMurray test is performed with the patient supine. The examination begins with the hip and knee flexed to 90°. The foot is either internally or externally rotated to evaluate for the lateral and medial meniscus, respectively. The knee is then slowly extended. The McMurray examination maneuver tests for tears of the posterior and body segments of the meniscus. Apley grind testing is performed by having the patient lay supine on the examination table. The knee is flexed to 90° and the foot is compressed and rotated internally and externally. Thessaly testing is performed by having the patient stand with the hips in slight flexion. The injured leg is then flexed to 30 to 45° and the patient's pelvis is rotated. Pain or reproduction of symptoms is considered a positive test. Positive findings with any of these tests should initiate further workup for meniscus pathology. McMurray's test has a sensitivity of 61% and a specificity of 84%. Joint line tenderness and Thessaly testing have a sensitivity and specificity of around 80% each.[18]

During examination, patients should be assessed for concomitant injuries such as ligament tears, osteochondritis dissecans (OCD), or tibial spine fractures. Active strength testing of the hip flexors, quadriceps, and hamstrings should be completed last to reduce guarding and may help rule out muscle strains and target areas for rehabilitation if nonoperative treatment is pursued.

Supine examination of any pediatric patient with knee pain or limp should include examination of the hips and ankles as well. Loss of motion or recreation of knee pain with hip range of motion may indicate hip pathology such as a slipped capital femoral epiphysis, septic joint, or Legg-Calve-Perthes. Referred pain from an ankle injury should also be considered.

Imaging

Radiographs

Imaging for evaluation of knee injuries begins with plain radiographs to rule out fractures, dislocations, osteochondral lesions, or physeal injuries. Four views of the knee, including weight bearing anterior-posterior (AP), lateral, tunnel, and merchant or sunrise views are recommended. Evidence of osteoarthritis may support the diagnosis of chronic meniscus injury. Standing lower extremity alignment radiographs can evaluate for mechanical axis deviations. Correction of these deviations should be considered in complex or recurrent tears.

MRI

MRI has become the gold standard for radiographic diagnosis of meniscus tears. The sensitivity and specificity of MRI diagnosis of meniscus tears are high 89% and 88%, respectively, for medial meniscus tears and 78% and 95%, respectively, for lateral meniscus tears.[19] MRI is also useful for diagnosis of concomitant conditions such as OCD, ACL tears, or discoid meniscus.[2]

MRI scans are also useful for surgical planning. MRIs can reveal the tear location, pattern, and displacement, as well as presence of a bucket-handle variant or root tear.[5,20,21] Bucket-handle meniscus tears often are diagnosed by the presence of the "double-posterior cruciate ligament (PCL)" sign (**Fig. 2**).

As noted by Francavilla and colleagues, the increased vascularity of the pediatric meniscus can often be misdiagnosed as an intra-substance tear of the posterior horns of the menisci[13] (**Fig. 3**). Great care needs to be taken to correlate the patient's presentation, physical examination findings, and age with the meniscus appearance on MRI.[22]

NONOPERATIVE MANAGEMENT

Initial management of pediatric meniscus tears is determined by tear size, location, and displacement, as well as symptom chronicity and associated injuries. There is

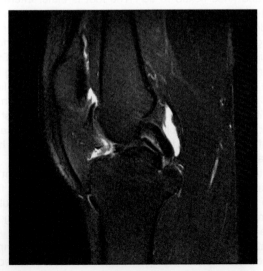

Fig. 2. MRI depicting "double-PCL" sign seen in bucket-handle medial meniscus tears.

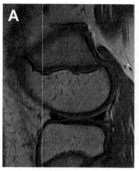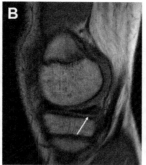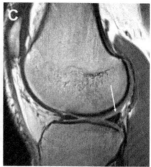

Fig. 3. MRI depicting (A) normal meniscus morphology, (B) vascular channel in patient without meniscus tear, and (C) true lateral meniscus tear.

limited understanding regarding the natural history of pediatric and adolescent meniscus tears, and careful consideration should be given to the use of nonoperative management in the appropriate clinical context. Patients with a suspected meniscus tear based on palpation alone with an absence of knee effusion or mechanical symptoms, unrestricted knee motion and a stable knee examination may not need advanced imaging or surgery. Nonoperative management is appropriate for patients with small, isolated, peripheral, nondisplaced tears. According to adult literature, stable meniscus tears (less than 3 mm of displacement), longitudinal meniscus tears less than 10 mm in length, and partial meniscus tears can also successfully heal with nonoperative management.[1,23] Younger age and tears involving the medial meniscus are risk factors for failure of nonoperative treatment in patients who had stable meniscus tears left alone at the time of ACL reconstruction.[24]

The nonoperative approach includes weight-bearing restrictions, bracing, ice, and anti-inflammatory medications. A prolonged course of activity modification (avoiding impact activities, cutting, or pivoting activities) should be used until symptoms have completely resolved. The use of a brace may be considered in the early course of a nonoperative approach and can assist in promoting activity restriction. This can include a straight knee immobilizer and/or a hinged type brace depending on symptom severity and patient comfort. As symptoms resolve, knee bracing or immobilization should be discontinued in favor of regaining strength and motion. There is no evidence of prevention of further meniscus injury with bracing as a patient returns back to activities. Also, a course of structured outpatient physical therapy may be used to focus on maintaining knee range of motion, neuromuscular control, and symptom relief. Following symptom resolution, strength and functional movements can be initiated to assist in return to sports and activities. Although physical therapy has proven success in managing degenerative meniscus tears in adults with osteoarthritis,[25] there are no studies that specifically evaluate the use of physical therapy for meniscus tears in pediatric patients.

SURGICAL TREATMENT INDICATIONS

Although meniscus tears with minimal symptoms may be observed and managed, nonoperatively, acute, large, displaced tears and subacute or chronic tears that cause persistent pain and discomfort, mechanical symptoms, or knee instability should be addressed surgically. Knee locking, or acute deficits in range of motion, suggests the presence of a displaced meniscus tear and is an indication for surgery.

As in the adult population, certain tear morphologies are more amenable to repair. Simple tears have a higher rate of repair success than complex tears,[26] and peripheral repairs have a higher success rate than more central tears.[27] Similar to findings from the adult literature, the ideal candidates for repair are peripheral, vertical, longitudinal tears in the lateral meniscus.[26,28] However, studies focusing on pediatric patients have found that meniscus repairs extending into the red-white zone can also achieve high healing rates.[14,28]

Owing to their distinct biologic characteristics and potential long-term sequella, meniscus injuries in pediatric patients require a different surgical approach than meniscus injuries in the adult population by focusing on meniscus retention as much as resolution of patients' symptoms. An attempt at repair should be the gold standard for all meniscus tears undergoing surgical intervention in a pediatric population. In cases of complex tears deemed irreparable at time of surgery, as much of the meniscus should be preserved as possible, as even a 10% decrease in contact area can increase contact stresses by 65%.[29]

SURGICAL TECHNIQUES

Meniscus preservation is particularly important in the pediatric population given the potential long-lasting effects of altered meniscus mechanics. An effective repair that leads to healing may require several surgical techniques with the three most commonly used meniscus suturing techniques being inside-out, all-inside, and outside-in.

With the development of new implants that are increasingly efficient, recent studies have suggested that the results of all-inside techniques may be comparable to the traditional gold standard inside-out technique.[30] However, although a systematic review by Fillingham and colleagues found no difference with respect to failure rate, functional outcomes, or complication rates between the two techniques,[31] Westermann and colleagues reported a 16% failure rate for all-inside meniscus repairs compared with 10% for inside-out.[32] Additional high quality and adequately powered studies are still needed to determine the optimal repair technique. Regardless of the technique used, there are important technical principles to follow to optimize the chance of success.

After the patient has been placed supine on the operating table and anesthetized, a full knee examination should be performed to assess stability and range of motion before establishing arthroscopic portals. In patients over 3 years of age, a traditional 4.0 mm arthroscope can be used for visualization, but a smaller arthroscope should be considered for younger patients. After establishing portals, it is a key to perform a thorough debridement of the anterior fat pad and plicas to ease the passage of instruments into the knee. Appropriately sized arthroscopic shavers and biters should be requested in smaller knees to avoid iatrogenic chondral damage. In the case of tight medial compartment hindering visualization, a medial collateral ligament release or piecrusting can be performed to protect the articular cartilage from potential iatrogenic trauma by sharp arthroscopic instruments.

After the tear has been fully evaluated in terms of location, size, displacement, and morphology, it should be prepared with a rasp or shaver before any repair is performed to stimulate a biologic healing response. Any irreparable meniscus portions should be resected, taking care to retain as much meniscus as possible.

Inside-Out Technique

The inside-out technique is the traditional gold standard of meniscus repair. It allows for consistent suture placement, securing the sutures over the capsule, and is preferentially used to treat tears in the posterior horn and body of the meniscus. In addition, it remains the preferred technique for the repair of displaced bucket-handle tears or tears with unstable reduction (**Fig. 4**). Drawbacks include the need for additional incisions and risk of injury to posterolateral and posteromedial structures. As the assistant plays an important role in the procedure, it is ideal to be assisted by someone familiar with the technique.

Technique pearls:

1. Mark relevant surgical anatomy (ie, peroneal or saphenous nerve) before repair to avoid iatrogenic injury during suture placement.
2. Start with a traction suture placed within the leading edge of the tear, commonly the body of the meniscus, to reduce the meniscus and prevent further displacement. This suture may be used throughout the remainder of the case to keep the unstable meniscus reduced (see **Fig. 4**C).
3. Make a posterolateral or posteromedial incision depending on the location of the affected meniscus. The previously placed traction suture is a good indicator of where the incision should be (**Fig. 5**B).
4. Use dedicated cannulas to pass needles with a size 2.0 suture in both the superior and inferior borders of the meniscus. Distance between sutures should be 3 to 5 mm. Vertical suture patterns are used most frequently, but the optimal configuration depends on the tear pattern and tissue deformation is present (see **Fig. 4**F).
5. Use an instrument such as a small spatula in the counter incision to protect neurovascular structures from exiting needles (see **Fig. 5**C).
6. Visualize the meniscus during tension to avoid overtightening of the sutures.
7. Once the repair is completed, knee range of motion can be performed with visualization of the repair arthroscopically to ensure no displacement occurs.

All-Inside Technique

The all-inside technique has grown in popularity due to ease of use and lack of needing an accessory incision. In a recent systematic review of inside-out versus all-inside

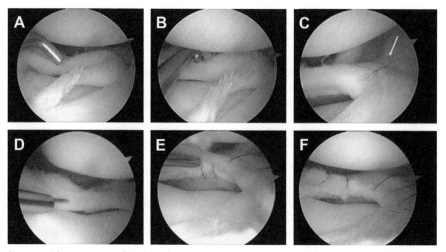

Fig. 4. Inside-out repair. (*A, B*) Probe demonstrating bucket-handle tear. (*C*) Traction suture used to reduce tear. (*D*) Suture passer above and below meniscus. (*E, F*) Deployment of sutures perpendicular to tear.

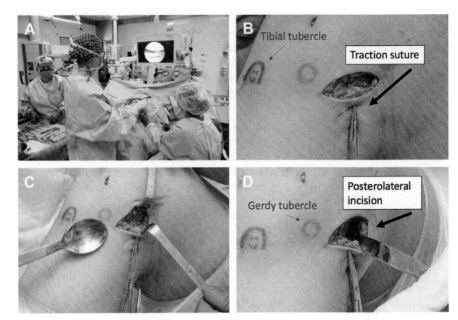

Fig. 5. Skin incision placement for inside-out repairs.

meniscus repairs, no difference was found with respect to healing or functional outcomes.[30] However, a limited number of studies have suggested that the all-inside technique requires lower operative time.[30] Given the increasing number of proprietary systems on the market, it is a key for orthopedic surgeons using this technique to familiarize themselves with the chosen implant system. Size of instrumentation should be noted and can limit its application in smaller knees.

The most popular all-inside repair technique is based on capsular fixation. The classic tear that is repaired by this technique is a vertical tear in the posterior horn. Recently published studies cite the anatomic location of the neurovascular bundle in relationship to all-inside repair techniques of the posterior horn[33–35] and should be reviewed as part of preoperative planning (**Fig. 6**).

Technique pearls:
1. Consider making pre-holes with an 18G needle to prevent the tip of the implant from slipping over the meniscus.
2. When entering the knee joint, keep the tip of the implant needle in view to avoid damaging the cartilage.
3. Needle tip direction should avoid the neurovascular bundle location. New implants allow curving of the device to improve access while avoiding dangerous areas.
4. Flex the knee for posterior horn fixation to move the neurovascular bundle away from the capsule.
5. Ensure the implant has passed through the capsule before deployment. Depth of needle penetration can be altered based on patient size and anatomy. Unsuccessful implant deployment can lead to the failure of meniscus healing or intra-articular displacement.

The second all-inside repair technique is one that does not rely on fixation to the capsule but represents a standard suture technique with arthroscopic knots (**Fig. 7**).

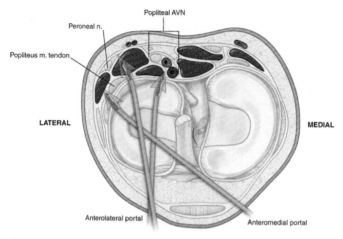

Fig. 6. Location of neurovascular structures at risk during knee arthroscopy. (*From* Yen YM, Fabricant PD, Richmond CG, et al. Proximity of the neurovascular structures during all-inside lateral meniscal repair in children: a cadaveric study. *J Exp Orthop*. 2018;5(1):50. Published 2018 Dec 18. https://doi.org/10.1186/s40634-018-0166-0)

This technique is useful for radial tears, where capsular fixation is often impossible, or horizontal tears when the goal is to compress the two leaflets.

Outside-In Technique

The outside-in suture technique is ideal for repairing tears in the anterior horn of the menisci. Similar to all-inside and inside-out techniques, the outside-in technique has been shown to have high success rates. It uses small incisions and does not leave behind intra-articular anchors or hardware. Finally, as it is typically used for anterior tears, it is associated with lower rates of neurovascular injuries.

Technique pearls:
1. Mark relevant surgical anatomy (ie, peroneal or saphenous nerve) before repair to avoid iatrogenic injury during suture placement.
2. Moving the camera to the medial portal may allow improved visualization of anterior horn lateral meniscus tears and increase working space.
3. Larger gauge monofilament sutures should be used to facilitation ease of passage through spinal needles.
4. When advancing the spinal needle under the anterior edge of the meniscus, take care to avoid iatrogenic tibial plateau chondral damage.
5. Once the repair is complete, make a small incision between the external sutures, dissect deep to the anterior joint capsule, and tie the sutures with proper tension over the capsule.

Root Repair

Indication and techniques for meniscus root repair have increased recently due to the increased recognition of meniscus root tears as a cause of long-term instability and poor outcomes. These tears are often reported in the presence of other intra-articular injuries in children and adolescents.[5,20] Utilization of posteromedial or posterolateral portals and a 70° arthroscope may ease repair. If being performed concomitantly with an ACL reconstruction, it is vital to avoid tibial tunnel convergence.

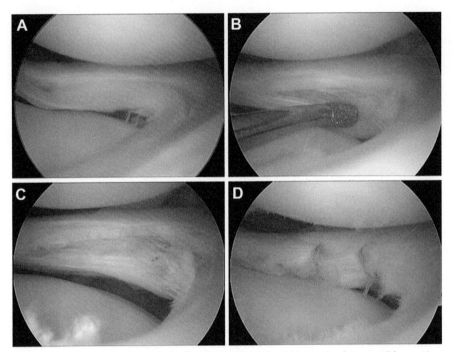

Fig. 7. All-inside repair. (*A*) Longitudinal tear. (*B, C*) Debridement of irreparable portions exposing horizontal tear. (*D*) Simple interrupted sutures to reduce horizontal tear.

For example, in a lateral meniscus root repair, place the tunnel lateral to the intended exit point for the ACL.

Technique pearls:
1. Enhance visualization using an accessory portal or mini-notch plasty.
2. Use luggage tag sutures to improve the strength of repair. Multiple types of meniscal forceps or suture passers are available and knee size should be considered when determining preferred equipment.
3. Use a tibial tunneling guide for ACL reconstruction to make one or two tunnels to the root anchor site, pending preferred technique.
4. Insert a suture passer into the tunnel(s) to bring the sutures down to the anteromedial border of the tibia and avoid convergence with other tunnels.

Principles of Meniscectomy

Despite the surgeon's best efforts, sometimes it is impossible to repair a meniscus tear. Three situations that may necessitate partial meniscectomy include re-tears with degenerative changes, chronically displaced bucket handles that are irreducible or chronically deformed, and partially or completely detached parrot beak tears. In these situations, the goal of the meniscectomy is to resect the least amount of tissue necessary to end up with a stable meniscus.

Technique pearls:
1. Determine the extent of the tear by serially assessing the mobility of the remaining meniscus with a probe.

2. Use biters and other manual instruments to delicately resect damaged or unstable tissue. Use shavers to remove debris and clean up frayed edges. Take care when resecting near the popliteal hiatus as meniscus tissue can be more narrow at this location.
3. Trim the contour of the remaining meniscus to prevent further tears.
4. Protect as much peripheral meniscus and capsular attachments as possible.
5. Document the location of the lesion and the percent of resected versus retained meniscus for future follow-up.

POSTOPERATIVE MANAGEMENT

The goal of postoperative management is to strike the appropriate balance between protecting the recently manipulated or repaired tissue while minimizing the effects of immobilization and deconditioning. Patients who undergo partial meniscectomies may begin weight bearing and range of motion as tolerated immediately postoperatively.[36] However, the literature on postoperative management of meniscus repairs is more varied. Although the general consensus is to protect the repaired meniscus with partial weight bearing and restricted range of motion for 4 to 6 weeks, specific weight bearing regimen and timing of weight bearing or range of motion advancement remains surgeon-dependent with little consensus.

In the meniscus repair literature, reported postoperative weight-bearing restrictions range from complete non-weight bearing for 6 to 12 weeks,[37–39] to partial weight bearing for 4 to 6 weeks,[28,40,41] and to immediate weight bearing.[42,43] Range of motion limitations are similarly varied, ranging from locked extension for 4 weeks[40] to unrestricted range of motion.[44,45] Postoperative regimen remains so highly surgeon specific that it is often disparate at a single institution within the same study.[12]

Biomechanical studies have shown that specific regions of the meniscus are at risk with different movements. The posterior aspects of both lateral and medial menisci are compressed most with deep flexion,[46] although the medial meniscal root is stressed most significantly with internal femoral rotation.[47] In longitudinal meniscus tear patterns, some studies suggest that physiologic loading may aid in healing by causing compression at the repair site.[48]

Proponents of an accelerated rehabilitation protocol[42,43] have shown promising outcomes in small sample sizes, finding no difference in healing rate as assessed by second-look arthroscopy, functional outcome scores, and postoperative MRI. In patients undergoing concurrent ACL reconstruction at the time of meniscus repair, there was no increased risk of clinical failure when following an accelerated rehabilitation program.[38]

Despite these preliminary findings, however, there remains a lack of strong evidence focusing on the effect of early weight bearing and motion on different meniscus tear morphologies. Furthermore, the impact of weight bearing combined with twisting or pivoting movements has not yet been assessed. With such heterogeneity, it is reasonable to adopt an individualized postoperative rehabilitation regimen. Posterior or complex tears may benefit from more restrictive protocols,[46] whereas simple longitudinal lateral meniscus tears may be able to progress more rapidly. Throughout the postoperative period, it is imperative for the clinician and patient to remain vigilant for new pain, swelling, or mechanical symptoms and modify their regimen as needed.

TREATMENT COMPLICATIONS

While rare, the most serious short-term risks associated with meniscus repair include neurovascular damage, infection, and deep venous thrombosis (DVT). The reported rate of DVT within the first 90 days after knee arthroscopy is 0.25%, and this number is likely even lower in the pediatric population.[49]

The highest risk of neurovascular damage is seen in inside-out or all-inside repair of the posterior horn of the lateral meniscus (PHLM).[30] Recent studies have defined anatomic relationships between the PHLM and key neurovascular structures including the peroneal nerve, saphenous nerve, and popliteal neurovascular bundle in the pediatric population. During pediatric PHLM repair, the average distance between the all-inside device and the peroneal nerve and popliteal artery is as low as 3.2 mm and 1.9 mm, respectively[33] (see **Fig. 6**). These distances are larger in men[50] and increase with age/skeletal maturity[34] and patient size.[50] The popliteal tendon may be used as a lateral reference point to establish a safe zone for PHLM repairs (**Fig. 8**).[35]

A neurovascular examination should always follow meniscus repairs. If abnormalities are found, ultrasound, MRI, or angio-computed tomography may be performed. If a vascular injury is identified, a revision surgery must be quickly planned in collaboration with the vascular surgeon.

Compared with inside-out repairs, all-inside meniscus repairs have a lower rate of posterior neurovascular structure injury or irritation. However, they have been associated with hardware irritation and chondral damage,[30] likely due to implant malposition, breakage, or migration.

In the case of a complete or near-complete meniscectomy, given the young age of the patient, the knee must be closely monitored for the appearance of degenerative changes in the compartment. Assessment of limb alignment should be performed for consideration of guided growth or osteotomy to off-load the affected compartment. A follow-up with weight-bearing radiographs of both lower limbs can be done every year to evaluate the joint space. In the case of radiographic joint height decrease and advanced imaging showing chondral degradation, discussion should be held with the patient and family and shared decision-making used to evaluate the indication for a meniscal transplant. Currently, the presence of knee symptoms (pain, swelling, and so forth) is required as an indication for meniscal transplant in addition to radiographic findings.

TREATMENT OUTCOMES

Long-term studies have now established that partial meniscectomy in the pediatric population is associated with early onset arthritis and pain. Abdon and colleagues showed that at an average of 16.8 years post-op, 36% of meniscectomy patients had decreased knee range of motion, 45% suffered grade 1 instability, and 89% of knees demonstrated joint space narrowing.[15] An 80% of meniscectomy patients have been found to have radiographic signs of early osteoarthritis at 5.5 years after surgery. Clinical outcomes are similarly poor,[51] with less than 50% of patients demonstrating excellent or good results at long-term follow-up.

On the other hand, meniscus repair in pediatric patients has been shown to produce good results,[27,52] with greater than 80% of simple meniscus tears achieving clinical success after repair (no pain, mechanical signs or symptoms, or subsequent surgeries). The key factors that have been shown to influence likelihood of clinical success after meniscus repair include age, presence of concomitant ACL reconstruction, and location and morphology of the tear itself. Higher rates of clinical success have been noted in the adolescent population with open physes compared with those with closed physes.[14] With regard to morphology and location of tear, medial meniscus tears heal at a lower rate than lateral tears,[26,27] possibly due to the higher biomechanical loads imparted on the medial meniscus.[53] Complex tears have far lower rates of healing when compared with simple or bucket-handle

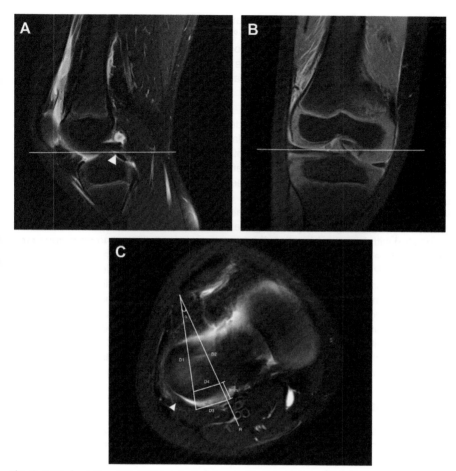

Fig. 8. MRI depicting the distance between popliteal tendon and posterior neurovascular bundle.

tears,[26,27] with a reported 13% success rate in isolated complex meniscus repairs. Complex meniscus tears repaired in conjunction with ACL reconstruction enjoy higher clinical success rates than those repaired in isolation (57% vs 13%).[26] Unlike in the adult literature, however, the benefit of concomitant ACL reconstruction has not been shown to extend to simple or bucket-handle tears.[26]

As the pediatric meniscus achieves similar vascularity to its adult counterpart by age 10, the association between zone of injury and healing potential is similar to findings from the adult population. Tears occurring less than 3 mm from the rim have a higher chance of healing than those with rim width of 3 to 6 mm.[27] Despite this, there are benefits to attempting repair in the red-white or even white-white zone in the pediatric population. Vanderhave and colleagues reported successful 2 year clinical outcomes in 31 out of 33 red-white zone repairs and all 9 white-white zone tears,[14] suggesting that the adolescent knee may obtain good clinical outcomes even when tears extend into the avascular zone.

Most of the current outcomes data are limited to clinical assessment and lack patient reported outcomes and adequate advanced imaging to determine meniscus healing. Miao and colleagues reported that the accuracy of clinical assessment is only around 73% compared with 85% to 91% for standard MRI.[54] Other studies have found that MR arthrogram is superior to conventional MRI for detecting recurrent tears.[55,56] Further studies using objective measures of healing are needed to better characterize the timing and degree of healing after meniscus repair.

Biologic Augmentation

Although studies on adult patients have demonstrated encouraging results regarding biologic augmentation (ie, platelet-rich plasma [PRP], stem cells, bone marrow aspirate) of meniscus repairs,[30,57] the effect of biologic additions remains unknown in pediatric meniscus repairs. The protective effect of concomitant ACL reconstruction on meniscus repair integrity in adults has been attributed to the increased bleeding and growth factor delivery within the joint, supporting a possible benefit of biologic augmentation in isolated meniscus repairs. A 2018 randomized controlled trial on adults demonstrated that augmenting meniscus repair with intra-operative PRP was associated with improved functional outcomes and meniscal healing rates compared with saline injection.[58] Similar benefits were found with a bone marrow venting procedure (BMVP), with 100% of patients in the BMVP augmentation group demonstrating meniscus healing at second-look arthroscopy at 35 weeks postoperatively compared with 76% in the control group.[57] Finally, PRP injections demonstrated a protective effect in patients who had an isolated meniscus repair.[59] This effect was not seen in patients who had concomitant ACL reconstruction, suggesting that the bone tunnel drilling in ACL reconstruction provides sufficient bleeding and growth factors. Despite the promising results in adult literature, further studies are needed to determine the utility of biologic adjuvants in pediatric meniscus surgery.

SUMMARY AND FUTURE DIRECTIONS

Meniscus tears are one of the most common pediatric sports injuries. Although the diagnosis of a meniscus tear can often be made based on patient history and physical examination findings alone, radiographs and MRI should be obtained for all surgical candidates to confirm the diagnosis, assess for concomitant pathologies such as discoid meniscus, and aid in surgical planning. Patients with meniscus tears causing persistent pain, loss of range of motion, instability, or mechanical symptoms are candidates for surgery.

In all but the most complex tears, meniscus repair should be attempted before any consideration of partial meniscectomy. Younger patients can expect a high rate of clinical success after meniscus repair. On the other hand, partial meniscectomy has been associated with poor long-term results. Posterior or meniscus body tears can be repaired with either inside-out or all-inside approaches, whereas anterior tears are best addressed with an outside-in approach. Predictors of a successful repair include young age, lateral meniscus involvement, simple tear morphology, peripheral tears, and concomitant ACL reconstruction.

There remain significant knowledge gaps and opportunities for further research. Current outcomes data are largely limited to functional scores and clinical assessment only. Studies using higher sensitivity imaging modalities such as MR arthrograms would be useful to correlate clinical outcomes with radiologic outcomes and better characterize both the timing and quality of postoperative meniscus healing. Recent studies have demonstrated the benefit of delivering local biologic augmentation (PRP or BMVP) to the site of meniscus repair, but further studies with objective postoperative outcome measures are needed to confirm these findings.

Finally, there is a paucity of data focusing on the appropriate postoperative rehabilitation protocol after meniscus repair. The appropriate regimen likely depends on both the location and morphology of the meniscus tear, but given the lack of detailed biomechanical data on the topic, there is almost no consensus in the literature regarding specific weight bearing or range of motion protocols. Objective data on meniscal healing will also help inform postoperative rehabilitation protocols and the appropriate timing of weight bearing and range of motion liberalization.

CLINICS CARE POINTS

- Meniscus tears are increasingly common in the pediatric population and typically present as knee pain, loss of range of motion, and swelling after a non-contact twisting injury.

- Nonoperative management with bracing and physical therapy is reasonable in stable, non-displaced, small peripheral tears in the red-red zone of the meniscus.

- Surgical indications include large, unstable tears, loss of range of motion, and persistent symptoms despite nonoperative management.

- In surgical candidates, meniscus repair should be attempted given the high rate of successful repair and the poor reported long-term outcomes after meniscectomies.

- All-inside and inside-out meniscus repair techniques are appropriate for posterior or meniscal body tears; care must be taken to avoid posterior neurovascular structures.

- Complex tears or chronically displaced bucket-handle tears that cannot be repaired may require a partial meniscectomy.

- Biologic augmentation in the form of bone marrow venting procedure or platelet-rich plasma may improve postoperative meniscus healing, but studies are currently lacking on its efficacy.

DISCLOSURE

The authors have nothing to disclose.

REFERENCES

1. Chambers H, Chambers R. The natural history of meniscus tears. J Pediatr Orthop 2019;39(Issue 6, Supplement 1 Suppl 1):S53–5. Available at: http://ovidsp.ovid.com/ovidweb.cgi?T=JS&NEWS=n&CSC=Y&PAGE=fulltext&D=ovft&AN=01241398-201907001-00014.

2. Gee SM, Tennent DJ, Cameron KL, et al. The burden of meniscus injury in young and physically active populations. Clin Sports Med 2020;39(1):13–27.

3. Lee WQ, Gan JZ, Lie DTT. Save the meniscus – clinical outcomes of meniscectomy versus meniscal repair. J Orthop Surg (Hong Kong) 2019;27(2). 2309499019849813. Available at: https://journals.sagepub.com/doi/full/10.1177/2309499019849813.

4. Lee TQ. Current biomechanical concepts for rotator cuff repair. Clin Orthop Surg 2013;5(2):89–97.

5. Faucett SC, Geisler BP, Chahla J, et al. Meniscus root repair vs meniscectomy or nonoperative management to prevent knee osteoarthritis after medial meniscus root tears: Clinical and economic effectiveness. Am J Sports Med 2019;47(3): 762–9. Available at: https://journals.sagepub.com/doi/full/10.1177/0363546518755754.

6. Feeley B, Lau B. Biomechanics and clinical outcomes of partial meniscectomy. J Am Acad Orthop Surg 2018;26(24):853–63. Available at: https://www.ncbi.nlm.nih.gov/pubmed/30247309.

7. Feeley BT, Liu S, Garner AM, et al. The cost-effectiveness of meniscal repair versus partial meniscectomy: A model-based projection for the united states. The knee 2016;23(4):674–80. Available at: https://www.clinicalkey.es/playcontent/1-s2.0-S0968016016300035.

8. Lau BC, Conway D, Mulvihill J, et al. Biomechanical consequences of meniscal tear, partial meniscectomy, and meniscal repair in the knee. JBJS Rev 2018; 6(4):e3. Available at: https://www.ncbi.nlm.nih.gov/pubmed/29613868.

9. Mosich GM, Lieu V, Ebramzadeh E, et al. Operative treatment of isolated meniscus injuries in adolescent patients: A meta-analysis and review. Sports health 2018;10(4):311–6. Available at: https://journals.sagepub.com/doi/full/10.1177/1941738118768201.

10. Yang B, Liotta E, Paschos N. Outcomes of meniscus repair in children and adolescents. Curr Rev Musculoskelet Med 2019;12(2):233–8. Available at: https://www.ncbi.nlm.nih.gov/pubmed/31123921.

11. Nguyen JC, De Smet AA, Graf BK, et al. MR imaging–based diagnosis and classification of meniscal tears. Radiographics 2014;34(4):981–99. Available at: https://www.ncbi.nlm.nih.gov/pubmed/25019436.

12. Kramer DE, Micheli LJ. Meniscal tears and discoid meniscus in children: Diagnosis and treatment. J Am Acad Orthop Surg 2009;17(11):698–707. Available at: http://www.jaaos.org/content/17/11/698.abstract.

13. Francavilla M, Restrepo R, Zamora K, et al. Meniscal pathology in children: Differences and similarities with the adult meniscus. Pediatr Radiol 2014;44(8):910–25. Available at: https://www.ncbi.nlm.nih.gov/pubmed/25060615.

14. Vanderhave K, Moravek J, Sekiya J, et al. Meniscus tears in the young athlete: Results of arthroscopic repair. J Pediatr Orthop 2011;31(5):496–500. Available at: http://ovidsp.ovid.com/ovidweb.cgi?T=JS&NEWS=n&CSC=Y&PAGE=fulltext&D=ovft&AN=01241398-201107000-00004.

15. Abdon P, Turner MS, Pettersson H, et al. A long-term follow-up study of total meniscectomy in children. Clin orthopaedics Relat Res 1990;(257):166–70. Available at: https://www.ncbi.nlm.nih.gov/pubmed/2379357.

16. Marc Manzione Peter D, Pizzutillo Alan B, Peoples Paul A. Schweizer. Meniscectomy in children: A long-term follow-up study. Am J Sports Med 1983;11(3): 111–5. Available at: http://ajs.sagepub.com/content/11/3/111.abstract.

17. Bhan K. Meniscal tears: Current understanding, diagnosis, and management. Curēus (Palo Alto, CA) 2020;12(6):e8590. Available at: https://search.proquest.com/docview/2429379394.

18. Smith BE, Selfe J, Thacker D, et al. Incidence and prevalence of patellofemoral pain: A systematic review and meta-analysis. PLoS One 2018;13(1):e0190892. Available at: https://www.ncbi.nlm.nih.gov/pubmed/29324820.

19. Phelan N, Rowland P, Galvin R, et al. A systematic review and meta-analysis of the diagnostic accuracy of MRI for suspected ACL and meniscal tears of the knee. Knee Surg Sports Traumatol Arthrosc 2016;24(5):1525–39. Available at: https://www.ncbi.nlm.nih.gov/pubmed/26614425.

20. Wilson PL, Wyatt CW, Romero J, et al. Incidence, presentation, and treatment of pediatric and adolescent meniscal root injuries. Orthop J Sports Med 2018;6(11). 2325967118803888. Available at: https://journals.sagepub.com/doi/full/10.1177/2325967118803888.

21. Kennedy MI, Strauss M, LaPrade RF. Injury of the meniscus root. Clin Sports Med 2020;39(1):57–68.

22. Takeda Y, Ikata T, Yoshida S, et al. MRI high-signal intensity in the menisci of asymptomatic children. J Bone Joint Surg Br 1998;80(3):463–7. Available at: https://www.ncbi.nlm.nih.gov/pubmed/9619937.

23. Weiss C, Lundberg M, Hamberg P, et al. Non-operative treatment of meniscal tears. J Bone Joint Surg Am 1989;71(6):811–22. Available at: http://ovidsp.ovid.com/ovidweb.cgi?T=JS&NEWS=n&CSC=Y&PAGE=fulltext&D=ovft&AN=00004623-198971060-00003.

24. Duchman KR, Westermann RW, Spindler KP, et al. The fate of meniscus tears left in situ at the time of anterior cruciate ligament reconstruction. Am J Sports Med 2015;43(11):2688–95. Available at: https://journals.sagepub.com/doi/full/10.1177/0363546515604622.

25. Katz JN, Brophy RH, Chaisson CE, et al. Surgery versus physical therapy for a meniscal tear and osteoarthritis. N Engl J Med 2013;368(18):1675–84.

26. Krych AJ, Pitts RT, Dajani KA, et al. Surgical repair of meniscal tears with concomitant anterior cruciate ligament reconstruction in patients 18 years and younger. Am J Sports Med 2010;38(5):976–82. Available at: https://journals.sagepub.com/doi/full/10.1177/0363546509354055.

27. Krych AJ, McIntosh AL, Voll AE, et al. Arthroscopic repair of isolated meniscal tears in patients 18 years and younger. Am J Sports Med 2008;36(7):1283–9. Available at: http://ajs.sagepub.com/content/36/7/1283.abstract.

28. Noyes FR, Chen RC, Barber-Westin SD, et al. Greater than 10-year results of red-white longitudinal meniscal repairs in patients 20 years of age or younger. Am J Sports Med 2011;39(5):1008–17. Available at: https://journals.sagepub.com/doi/full/10.1177/0363546510392014.

29. Baratz ME, Fu FH, Mengato R. Meniscal tears: The effect of meniscectomy and of repair on intraarticular contact areas and stress in the human knee. Am J Sports Med 1986;14(4):270–5. Available at: https://journals.sagepub.com/doi/full/10.1177/036354658601400405.

30. Grant JA, Wilde J, Miller BS, et al. Comparison of inside-out and all-inside techniques for the repair of isolated meniscal tears. Am J Sports Med 2012;40(2):459–68. Available at: https://journals.sagepub.com/doi/full/10.1177/0363546511411701.

31. Fillingham YA, Riboh JC, Erickson BJ, et al. Inside-out versus all-inside repair of isolated meniscal tears: An updated systematic review. Am J Sports Med 2017;45(1):234–42. Available at: https://journals.sagepub.com/doi/full/10.1177/0363546516632504.

32. Westermann RW, Duchman KR, Amendola A, et al. All-inside versus inside-out meniscal repair with concurrent anterior cruciate ligament reconstruction: A meta-regression analysis. Am J Sports Med 2017;45(3):719–24. Available at: https://journals.sagepub.com/doi/full/10.1177/0363546516642220.

33. Yen Y, Fabricant P, Richmond C, et al. Proximity of the neurovascular structures during all-inside lateral meniscal repair in children: A cadaveric study. J Exp Ortop 2018;5(1):1–5.

34. Shea KG, Dingel AB, Styhl A, et al. The position of the popliteal artery and peroneal nerve relative to the menisci in children: A cadaveric study. Orthop J Sports Med 2019;7(6). 2325967119842843. Available at: https://journals.sagepub.com/doi/full/10.1177/2325967119842843.

35. Beck JJ, Shifflett K, Greig D, et al. Defining a safe zone for all-inside lateral meniscal repairs in pediatric patients: A magnetic resonance imaging study. Arthroscopy 2019;35(1):166–70.

36. Koch M, Memmel C, Zeman F, et al. Early functional rehabilitation after meniscus surgery: Are currently used orthopedic rehabilitation standards up to date? Rehabil Res Pract 2020;2020:3989535–8.

37. Haklar U, Kocaoglu B, Nalbantoglu U, et al. Arthroscopic repair of radial lateral meniscus [corrected] tear by double horizontal sutures with inside-outside technique. The knee 2008;15(5):355–9. Available at: https://www.ncbi.nlm.nih.gov/pubmed/18684627.

38. Barber FA. Accelerated rehabilitation for meniscus repairs. Arthroscopy 1994; 10(2):206–10.

39. Donald Shelbourne K, Patel DV, Adsit WS, et al. Rehabilitation after meniscal repair. Clin Sports Med 1996;15(3):595–612.

40. Bloome DM, Blevins FT, Paletta GA, et al. Meniscal repair in very young children. Arthroscopy 2000;16(5):545–9.

41. Logan M, Watts M, Owen J, et al. Meniscal repair in the elite athlete. Am J Sports Med 2009;37(6):1131–4. Available at: https://journals.sagepub.com/doi/full/10.1177/0363546508330138.

42. Mariani PP, Santori N, Adriani E, et al. Accelerated rehabilitation after arthroscopic meniscal repair: A clinical and magnetic resonance imaging evaluation. Arthroscopy 1996;12(6):680–6.

43. Lind M, Nielsen T, Faunø P, et al. Free rehabilitation is safe after isolated meniscus repair. Am J Sports Med 2013;41(12):2753–8. Available at: https://journals.sagepub.com/doi/full/10.1177/0363546513505079.

44. Barber FA, Click SD. Meniscus repair rehabilitation with concurrent anterior cruciate reconstruction. Arthroscopy 1997;13(4):433–7.

45. Oâ€™Shea JJ, Donald Shelbourne K. Repair of locked bucket-handle meniscal tears in knees with chronic anterior cruciate ligament deficiency. Am J Sports Med 2003;31(2):216–20. Available at: http://ajs.sagepub.com/content/31/2/216.abstract.

46. Vedi V, Williams A, Tennant SJ, et al. Meniscal movement. an in-vivo study using dynamic MRI. J Bone Joint Surg Br 1999;81(1):37. Available at: https://www.ncbi.nlm.nih.gov/pubmed/10067999.

47. Stärke C, Kopf S, Roland L, et al. Tensile forces on repaired medial meniscal root tears. Arthroscopy 2013;29(2):205–12. Available at: https://www.clinicalkey.es/playcontent/1-s2.0-S0749806312017069.

48. McCulloch P, Jones H, Hamilton K, et al. Does simulated walking cause gapping of meniscal repairs? J Exp Ortop 2016;3(1):1–10. Available at: https://www.ncbi.nlm.nih.gov/pubmed/26979177.

49. Maletis G, Inacio M, Reynolds S, et al. Incidence of symptomatic venous thromboembolism after elective knee arthroscopy. J Bone Joint Surg Am 2012;94(8):714–20. Available at: http://ovidsp.ovid.com/ovidweb.cgi?T=JS&NEWS=n&CSC=Y&PAGE=fulltext&D=ovft&AN=00004623-201204180-00006.

50. Schachne JM, Heath MR, Yen Y, et al. The safe distance to the popliteal neurovascular bundle in pediatric knee arthroscopic surgery: An age-based magnetic resonance imaging anatomic study. Orthop J Sports Med 2019;7(7). 2325967119855027. Available at: https://journals.sagepub.com/doi/full/10.1177/2325967119855027.

51. Mcdermott ID, Amis AA. The consequences of meniscectomy. J Bone Joint Surg Br 2006;88(12):1549–56. Available at: https://www.ncbi.nlm.nih.gov/pubmed/17159163.

52. Shieh A, Bastrom T, Roocroft J, et al. Meniscus tear patterns in relation to skeletal immaturity. Am J Sports Med 2013;41(12):2779–83. Available at: https://journals.sagepub.com/doi/full/10.1177/0363546513504286.

53. Becker R, Becker R, Wirz D, et al. Measurement of meniscofemoral contact pressure after repair of bucket-handle tears with biodegradable implants. Arch Orthop Trauma Surg 2005;125(4):254–60. Available at: https://www.ncbi.nlm.nih.gov/pubmed/15365717.

54. Miao Y, Yu J, Ao Y, et al. Diagnostic values of 3 methods for evaluating meniscal healing status after meniscal repair. Am J Sports Med 2011;39(4):735–42. Available at: https://journals.sagepub.com/doi/full/10.1177/0363546510388930.

55. Yamasaki S, Hashimoto Y, Nishida Y, et al. Assessment of meniscal healing status by magnetic resonance imaging T2 mapping after meniscal repair. Am J Sports Med 2020;48(4):853–60. Available at: https://journals.sagepub.com/doi/full/10.1177/0363546520904680.

56. Kececi B, Kaya Bicer E, Arkun R, et al. The value of magnetic resonance arthrography in the evaluation of repaired menisci. Eur J Orthop Surg Traumatol 2015;25(1):173–9. Available at: https://www.ncbi.nlm.nih.gov/pubmed/24719084.

57. Kaminski R, Kulinski K, Kozar-Kaminska K, et al. Repair augmentation of unstable, complete vertical meniscal tears with bone marrow venting procedure: A prospective, randomized, double-blind, parallel-group, placebo-Controlled Study. Arthroscopy 2019;35(5):1500–8.e1.

58. Kaminski R, Kulinski K, Kozar-Kaminska K, et al. A prospective, randomized, double-blind, parallel-group, placebo-controlled study evaluating meniscal healing, clinical outcomes, and safety in patients undergoing meniscal repair of unstable, complete vertical meniscal tears (bucket handle) augmented with platelet-rich plasma. Biomed Research International 2018;2018:9315815–9.

59. Everhart JS, Cavendish PA, Eikenberry A, et al. Platelet-rich plasma reduces failure risk for isolated meniscal repairs but provides no benefit for meniscal repairs with anterior cruciate ligament reconstruction. Am J Sports Med 2019;47(8):1789–96. Available at: https://journals.sagepub.com/doi/full/10.1177/0363546519852616.

Sex and Gender Differences in Pediatric Knee Injuries

Bianca R. Edison, MD, MS[a,*], Nirav Pandya, MD[b], Neeraj M. Patel, MD, MPH, MBS[c], Cordelia W. Carter, MD[d]

KEYWORDS

• Knee injuries • Gender • Disparities

KEY POINTS

- With the implementation of Title IX, athletic participation has increased for both sexes with a closing gap in participation disparities.
- Differences in anatomy, hormone production, biomechanics, strength profiles, neuromuscular patterns, and sex hormones can contribute to differences in knee injury rates and patterns in male and female athletes.
- Understanding the relationships between intrinsic and extrinsic factors for sports-related injuries of the knee will inform policy and strategic initiatives to prevent these injuries in male and female athletes alike.

In assessing disability and outcomes related to health, differences may fall under effects of sex and/or gender. Sex refers to the genotype of one's chromosomal makeup present in cells. Gender refers to one's phenotypical identity that encompasses cultural, behavioral, environmental and psychosocial factors. Biological differences between males and females alone cannot fully explain worldwide differences in health outcomes throughout history, thus the importance of analyzing the existence and effects of gender disparities. Gender includes complex relationships between people and can reflect the distribution of power and intricate social processes within those relationships.[1] Gender operates as an important but modifiable determinant of health on interpersonal, institutional and societal levels[2] and intersects with other causes of inequities and marginalization. This article aims at addressing disparities that have been found for pediatric knee injuries along sex and gender categories. In reporting

a Orthopaedics, Children's Hospital Los Angeles, University Southern California, Los Angeles, CA, USA; b Department of Pediatric Orthopaedics, University of California San Francisco Benioff Children's Hospitals, 747 52nd Street, Oakland, CA 94609, USA; c Division of Orthopaedic Surgery, Ann & Robert H. Lurie Children's Hospital of Chicago, 225 E Chicago Ave, Box 69, Chicago, IL 60611, USA; d Department of Orthopedic Surgery, NYU-Langone Medical Center, 301 East 17th Street, New York, NY 1000, USA
* Corresponding author. Children's Hospital Los Angeles, Children's Orthopaedic Center, 4650 Sunset Boulevard, Mailstop #69, Los Angeles, CA 90027.
E-mail address: bedison@chla.usc.edu

Clin Sports Med 41 (2022) 769–787
https://doi.org/10.1016/j.csm.2022.06.002
0278-5919/22/© 2022 Elsevier Inc. All rights reserved.

sportsmed.theclinics.com

on these differences, the aim is not to ascribe superiority to one group over another but to offer evidence-based information to sports medicine clinicians to deliver more nuanced and personalized care or help inform policy and advocacy.

Title IX, a federal civil rights law passed as part of the Education Amendments of 1972, protects people from discrimination based on sex in education programs or activities that receive Federal financial assistance.[3] However, it took another 16 years with the passage of the 1988 Civil Rights Restoration Act to reinforce compliance with Title IX. Both the number of sports played in schools and female participants have risen since 1972. The number of girls playing high school sports since the passage of Title IX has increased more than 1000%, and women playing varsity sports rose more than 600%.[3] This rise in female participation also paralleled an increase in youth male athlete participation as well. The current ratio stands at 2 female for every 3 male athletes.[3]

YOUTH SPORTS AND INJURY

A 2011 survey found approximately 27 million youth from 6 to 17 years participate in team sports in the United States,[4] and the National Council of Youth Sports survey reported that 60 million children aged 6 to 18 years participate in organized sports.[5] The percentage of young persons participating in sports continued to grow through 2019, although a disparity in participation rates between males and females persisted. According to the 2017 Youth Risk Behavior Survey, 60% of boys and 49% of girls in high school reported participating in at least one sport in the previous year.[6] In that same year, the National Youth Sports Strategy committee reported that 58% of youth ages 6 to 17 years participated in team sports or took a sports lesson in the prior 12 months; however, participation rates were distinctly lower for females and for traditionally underserved populations including racial and ethnic minorities, youth with disabilities, youth who identify as LGBTQ+ and those from lower income households.[7] According to Aspen Project Play, in 2019, 43.5% of males and 34.8% of females ages 13 to 17 years played a sport regularly.[8]

Sport and recreation participation serves as a leading cause of injury in youth 11 to 18 years of age.[9] One study reported an injury rate of 2.29 per 1000 athlete exposures across nine major sports over the 2018 to 2019 season,[10] but that data does not include injuries from all youth participation or injuries incurred outside of the high school setting. Another data source, the National SAFE KIDS Campaign, estimates that more than 3.5 million children are injured annually playing sports or participating in recreational activities,[11] and some estimate of all sports injuries, approximately 45% to 54% are due to overuse.[12] Literature has cited discrepancies in injury patterns and incidence rates between adolescent male and female athletes; some research has shown evidence that female athletes sustain more overuse injuries as compared with male cohorts[13] with differences attributed to flexibility discrepancies, physiologic, anatomic factors, as well as sports and background characteristics.

Knee injuries, common in interscholastic sports, account for 15.2% of all sport-related injuries.[14] Nearly 54% of young adolescents experience knee pain on a yearly basis.[15] A retrospective study found the most frequent location of overuse injuries in pediatric patients involved the lower extremity and more than half of those injuries occurred in the knee.[16] These injuries carry both short and long-term health deficits. Individuals with youth sport-related knee injuries report more symptoms such as pain and range of motion deficits, demonstrate suboptimal balance, and are found to have higher risk of obesity 3 to 10 years post-injury than peers without knee injury.[17] Additional studies show that despite full medical clearance, adolescent athletes with a previous knee injury experience decreased knee-specific and general health-related quality of life than their peers who do not endure a knee injury.[18] These detrimental effects also extend into socio-emotional learning and psychological functioning, which can negatively impact interpersonal relationships and school functioning.[18,19] Amidst sweeping injury rates, the youth sports culture also faces a grim epidemic: burnout. According to the Sports and Fitness Industry Association, 37.9% of children played team sports on a regular basis in 2013, which decreased from 44.5% in 2008[20] (**Fig. 1**). Burnout is defined as a response to chronic stress when a previously enjoyable activity no longer exists as such.[21,22] Understanding the differences that exist with injury patterns, location, risk factors, as well as short and long-term effects can help sports medicine clinicians address ways to evaluate, manage and prevent such injuries.

PATELLOFEMORAL PAIN SYNDROME

Patellofemoral pain syndrome (PFPS) exists as the most frequently diagnosed condition in adolescents and adults with symptomatic knee complaints.[23] PFPS, characterized by discomfort around or behind the patella, occurs when an unnecessary load onto the patellofemoral joint occurs, such as high impact running, jumping or lower impact, such as ascending or descending stairs, or squatting. Some research proposes an equal incidence in this condition in athletes while others report a higher incidence of PFPS in female athletes.[5,23–25] A prospective study of 810 youth basketball

KIDS ARE LEAVING SPORTS
SIGNIFICANT DECLINE IN PARTICIPATION AMONG 6-12 YEAR OLDS

	BASKETBALL	SOCCER	TRACK & FIELD	BASEBALL	FOOTBALL	SOFTBALL
2008	5.7 M	5.6 M	847 K	5.3 M	1.8 M	1.3 M
2013	5.5 M	5.0 M	731 K	4.5 M	1.3 M	862 K
	-3.9%	-10.7%	-13.7%	-14.4%	-28.6%	-31.3%

2.6M fewer kids playing these sports alone in past 5 years.

...AND ARE LESS PHYSICALLY ACTIVE THROUGH SPORTS

2008 ---------------- 9M ACTIVE KIDS

-8.8%

2013 ---------------- 8.2M ACTIVE KIDS

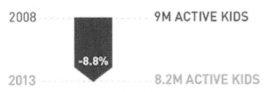

Fig. 1. Around 37.9% of children played team sports on a regular basis in 2013, which decreased from 44.5% in 2008. (*Courtesy of* Aspen Institute's Project Play Initiative.)

players found PFPS to be significantly more common in females than in males (7.3% as opposed to 1.2%, P<.05).[25] The pathophysiology of PFPS remains multifaceted and is connected to several nonmodifiable and modifiable risk factors.

Sex-related disparities in the incidence of PFPS have been connected to anatomic differences in males and females that contribute to improper tracking of the patella in relation to the patellofemoral contact area of the knee joint. Females have been found to have wider pelvises, which can translate to a larger Q angle, the acute angle formed by the quadriceps muscle and patellar tendon.[26] A larger Q angle in females has been associated with greater dynamic lateral shift during quadriceps muscle contraction[27] (**Fig. 2**); however, more recent studies have challenged this notion and propose that the Q angle may not affect one's risk of developing PFPS as originally thought. One study found a negative correlation between one's Q angle and peak knee abduction moments ($P = .005$).[28] When comparing females with PFPS to controls, other researchers found no difference between the affected subjects' and controls' Q angle, nor was there any significant difference between the symptomatic versus asymptomatic knees in those with PFPS.[29]

Additional research has proposed altered lower extremity and proximal kinematics lead to increased risk of developing PFPS. Meyer and colleagues found adolescent females who demonstrated greater than 15 Nm of knee abduction during landing had increased risk of developing PFPS.[30] Significant dynamic knee loading during a task that involves higher impact on the knee joint can contribute to patellofemoral pain syndrome. Adolescent females have been found to demonstrate increased malalignment and more dynamic knee valgus during a drop jump as compared with age-matched males.[31] Hip strength deficits can also increase risk for PFPS in females. When measuring hip isometric strength in female athletes, the imbalance of hip adductor/abductor isometric strength ratio was found to be 23% higher in the PFPS group as compared with the control group ($P = .1$),[32] leading to improper

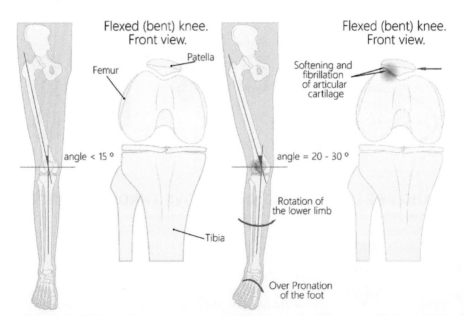

Fig. 2. Biomechanics in asymptomatic knee (*Left*) and in patellofemoral syndrome (*Right*). (Source: Aksanaku/Shutterstock.com.)

patellofemoral loading. Supporting the notion disparities in the incidence and risk for PFPS in females as compared with males stem more from impaired neuromuscular control, Foss and colleagues found no difference in BMI, BMI z-score or body fat percentage between adolescent female athletes with PFPS and those without.[33] In males, landing with decreased knee flexion and increased hip external rotation can increase risk of developing PFPS. In female athletes, landing with less hip abduction and increased knee internal rotation can increase the risk of PFPS.[34] Taking these nuanced differences into account when developing targeted intervention or preventative programs for groups of athletes can be integral.

Variables related to training load and environment have also been examined when assessing risk of PFPS. Some studies underscore overuse of the patellofemoral joint and overloading as a major risk factor for PFPS as opposed to anatomic differences,[29] particularly during adolescent growth spurts. Disparities in coaching and sport training can also affect one's risk. Early specialization in a single sport during this time can also increase a young female athlete's risk of developing PFPS 1.5x greater than age-matched controls ($P = .038$).[35] All factors need to be considered, and training and conditioning programs may need to be modified for a particular athlete group based on their gender to reduce the risk of such an overuse-type injury.

OSTEOCHONDRITIS DISSECANS

Osteochondritis dissecans (OCD), a condition characterized by the separation of subchondral bone from the articular surface of a joint, most commonly affects the knee (followed by the elbow and talus), usually involves the medial femoral condyle, and is bilateral in 30% to 40% of pediatric patients (**Fig. 3**).[36] The exact causes or pathophysiological reasons of OCD is not fully elucidated and remains at the center of debate, although it is increasingly understood to be a repetitive overuse injury that results in compromised vascularity of the osteoarticular surface.[37,38] Sex differences in the incidence of OCD have been reported, with males being disproportionately affected. In one cross-sectional study of pediatric patients in the United States from 2007 to 2011, the male:female ratio for OCD was 3.1:1 and only 1 out of 41 female patients had bilateral disease. The male:female ratio remained similar when comparing younger (6–11 years) and older (12–19 years) groups. The older male patients had the greatest incidence of disease (18.1 per 100,000) as compared with the younger female patients (2.3 per 100,000).[39]

Some argue sex disparities may be influenced by participation in competitive sports, as the mean age of OCD appears to be decreasing over the years, and there is growing prevalence among female cohorts. Other theories to support this trend include an increased risk in those athletes playing in multiple leagues simultaneously, early sport specialization, those with increased intensive training and longer hours of training.[39] Knowing risk factors can help athletes, parents, and coaches adjust training schedules to avoid the development of OCD of the knee as a result of overuse. Increasing awareness of signs and symptoms of OCD—persistent and worsening activity-related knee pain, swelling and mechanical symptoms such as catching or locking - may promote early identification and treatment of this injury. Although the risk of OCD is higher in males, no sex differences have been described in terms of treatment algorithms or long-term outcomes.

ANTERIOR CRUCIATE LIGAMENT INJURIES

Injuries of the anterior cruciate ligament (ACL) have received much of the attention in research and prevention efforts for young athletes. An estimated 250,000 ACL injuries

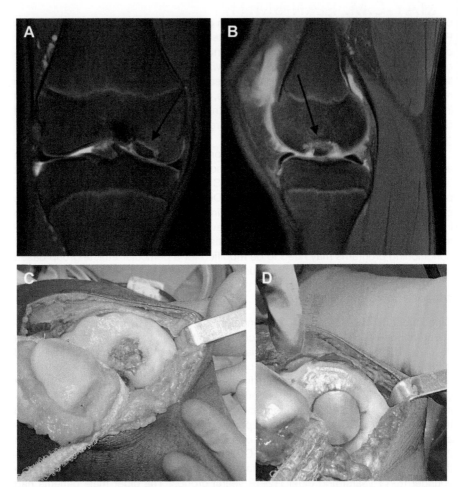

Fig. 3. Figures 3A and 3B are coronal and sagittal T2-weighted MRI cuts demonstrating a large, unstable and fragmented OCD lesion of the medial femoral condyle in an 18-year-old male. Figure 3C demonstrates the appearance of the condyle at the time of surgical treatment. 3D is the final appearance following placement of an osteochondral allograft.

occur yearly in the United States, more than 50% of which are sustained by youth aged 15 to 25 years.[40] At a cost of $17,000-$25,000 per injury,[41] surgical and rehabilitative expenses amount to an astounding $6,250,000,000 per year. Furthermore, this injury can increase a young athlete's risk of long-term sequelae such as osteoarthritis by as much as 80%,[42,43] potentially increasing the burden on the health care system. The ACL, one of the major stabilizing intracapsular ligaments in the knee, functions to prevent anterior displacement of the tibia and is essential for maintaining stability and control in cutting and pivoting movement patterns (**Fig. 4**).[44] However, this stabilizing ligament can tear in 70 milliseconds,[45] and despite reconstruction options, some athletes may not regain their preinjury performance level following surgical treatment.[46] In young athletes, and in female athletes in particular, injuries to the anterior cruciate ligament (ACL) create the most total time lost from sport and recreational physical activity.[47,48]

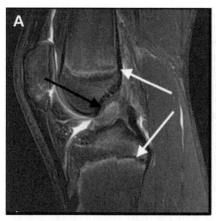 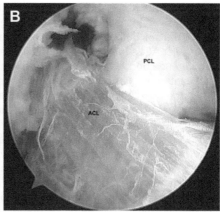

Fig. 4. Fig. 4A is a sagittal T2-weighted MRI image of the knee of an 11-year-old female, demonstrating a torn ACL (*black arrow*) and incompletely closed physes (*white arrows*). Fig. 4B is an intraoperative arthroscopic view of a completed ACL reconstruction using autograft iliotibial band and a physeal-sparing technique.

Adolescent females have been reported to have 2 to 10× risk of ACL injury as compared with their male counterparts.[49,50] Further research has shown that being female, a college athlete, and participating in soccer or rugby are independent risk factors for a first-time noncontact ACL injury.[51] In high school athletes, injuries to the ACL are found at higher rates in females as compared with male counterparts (4.6% vs 2.5%), with high school girls' basketball sustaining the highest rate (6%), followed by girls' soccer (5%), girls' volleyball (5%) and girls' gymnastics (5%).[52] Another study found female athletes having greater than 2 times the risk of ACL injury as compared with male counterparts at both high school (IRR 2.30) and collegiate (IRR 2.49) levels.[53] This stands in contrast to professional-level gender-comparable sports that see similar injury rates between sexes.[54] Interestingly, in contradistinction to the well-documented increased vulnerability of adolescent females to ACL injury when compared with their male peers, recent research has revealed that among pediatric athletes aged less than 12 years, males have almost double the risk of ACL injury as their female counterparts.[55,56] Given this shift in ACL injury prevalence to females during the pubescent years, one must take into account sex-based differences along not only anatomic, hormonal and biomechanical factors, but also age-related factors when making recommendations for sport participation and training.

There are a variety of anatomic differences between males and females that have been theorized to predispose a young athlete to ACL injury. Some differences are based in the knee and others are based more proximally in the hip; some sex-based differences are more general, such as body shape. The ACL size and orientation can be influenced by the femoral notch shape and width. Irrespective of one's sex, researchers have theorized that smaller femoral notches have increased risk of ACL injury. However, it remains unclear if a smaller ACL is weaker and more prone to tear. Controlling for height, the size of an ACL in female athletes has been found to be smaller as compared with males.[45] However, conflicting evidence exists for intercondylar notch anatomy and notch-width-index (NWI) differences between males and females. One study evaluated 100 high school basketball players via MRI and found no correlation between ACL size and notch size, thus suggesting one cannot predict ACL size from intercondylar notch size.[57] In another prospective study of Division I athletes, individuals with intercondylar notch stenosis have increased risk of ACL injury. However, there was no statistically significant difference found when comparing the NWI, the sex of the athlete, and the incidence of ACL tear.[58] In summary, females have smaller ACLs than males, although there is not a clear relationship between this size difference and ACL injury risk. Additionally, individuals – male or female – with a stenotic intercondylar notch are more prone to ACL tear.

When the posterior tibial slope (PTS)—the angle formed between a line perpendicular to the mid-diaphysis of the tibia and the tibial plateau's posterior inclination – is increased, the tibia becomes more anterior relative to the femur. During quadriceps contraction, this may result in higher forces through the ACL, thus increasing a risk of tear.[59,60] In one recent study, females who sustained ACL injuries were found to have higher PTS angles than did males with ACL injuries.[61] In another study, females with ACL tears were found on MRI to have a mean PTS angle of 10.9° as compared with 8.2° in the sex-matched control group. Males with ACL tear were not found to have any significant difference as compared with the male control group.[62] Thus, anatomic variations including decreased notch width and increased posterior tibial slope contribute to an increased risk of ACL tear, although the role that sex plays in mediating this risk is yet to be fully determined.

Similar to patellofemoral syndrome, it has been suggested that the increased quadriceps angle (Q angle) observed in females may contribute to an enhanced vulnerability to ACL injury. The Q angle has been found to be up to 4.9° greater in females as compared with males[63]; however, research has not found a direct correlation between Q-angle and ACL injury. In a study comparing both male and female athletes with a history of ACL tear to matched controls without ACL injury, although females had larger Q-angles, no association with ACL tear was identified. Other predictors found to increase risk of ACL injury included anterior pelvic tilt and navicular drop, though those did not vary significantly when comparing sexes.[64]

Biomechanical and neuromuscular control differences involving muscle activation patterns, landing characteristics and core stability in the setting of ACL injury have been extensively studied, and differences between males and females have been identified (**Table 1**). After the onset of puberty and the start of peak growth velocity, decreased core stability can stem from increased overall body mass, increased tibia and femur length, and increased height of center of mass.[65] Some argue that ACL injury risk is heightened when these rapid changes to the musculoskeletal system occur in the setting of decreased muscular strength. Namely, as young adolescents experience increases in height and mass, knee abduction loads increase and place higher load forces on the ACL.[66] It is during rapid growth and peak height velocity that muscles and tendons lengthen, but muscle strength and hypertrophy may not occur at the same rate, and differences between males and females in the development of skeletal muscle strength have been well-documented. On average, girls reach their peak height velocity at 12 years and boys at 14 years.[67]

Other biomechanical studies have found that adolescent females demonstrate decreased knee flexion, increased quadriceps activity and decreased hamstring activity during tests of neuromuscular control, referred to as a "quadriceps dominant" strategy.[45] Males are generally found to first activate the hamstrings instead of the quadriceps; the hamstrings have multiple attachment points and can pull the tibia more posteriorly, thus providing more stability to the ACL.[68] Female athletes have also been found to take significantly longer time to recruit maximum hamstring torque during isokinetic testing when compared with males.[45] Differences in muscle firing patterns during electromyogram (EMG) testing have been described between males and females: one net effect of these differences is greater dynamic anterior tibial

Table 1
Summarizes the anatomic and biomechanical/neuromuscular factors hypothesized to contribute to risk of ACL injury

Proposed Anatomic and Biomechanical/Neuromuscular Risk Factors for ACL Injury in Young Female and Male Athletes.

Anatomic	Association with ACL Injury?	Sex Difference?
Higher Q-angle	Weak	Yes, higher in females
Decreased notch width	Yes	Does not seem to be sex dependent
Increased posterior slope	Yes	Some support for sex difference
Smaller ACL size	Weak	Yes, smaller in females
Neuromuscular		
Increased lateral trunk displacement	Yes	Yes, increased in females
Increased truncal motion/decreased core stability	Yes	Yes, increased trunk motion in females
Decreased hip-and knee-flexion angles	Yes	Yes, decreased in females
Increased hip adduction and internal rotation moments	Yes	Yes, increased in females
Increased knee abduction moment	Yes	Yes, increased in females
Increased dynamic knee valgus	Yes	Yes, increased in females
Increased Quadriceps: Hamstring activity ratio	Yes	Yes, "quad-dominant" pattern in females
Limb asymmetry	Yes	Yes, higher in females

translation in females which places more strain on the ACL.[69] Across multiple studies, females have been consistently found to have greater peak knee abduction angles as compared with their male counterparts,[70,71] and ACL injury risk may stem from a lack of reflex muscle activation in response to valgus knee movement.

Trunk dominance, the inability to maintain control of the trunk during three-dimensional movements, also increases risk of ACL injury. In one recent prospective study, lateral displacement of the trunk was the greatest risk factor for ACL injury in females but was not found in male athletes.[72] After the onset of puberty, females typically undergo a shift in weight distribution to their trunk, which changes their center of mass further from the ground. Without proper training to strengthen the supportive muscles to accommodate this change in center of gravity, excessive lateral trunk lean can occur and thus increase ACL injury risk by putting greater strain on the ACL.[73]

The concept of leg dominance, or favoring one side resulting in asymmetry of strength and control, has also been found to contribute to sex-based differences in ACL injuries. Females tend to use one leg more dominantly whereas males tend to have more symmetric leg strength. One recent study used vertical jump testing to assess lower limb neuromuscular asymmetry in young basketball and volleyball players. These authors found significantly greater asymmetry between dominant and nondominant legs in the female athletes than in the males. Additionally, a higher percentage of female athletes (31.6% vs 24.4%) had a limb asymmetry index (ASI) greater than 15%, a known risk factor for injury.[74]

Asymmetry leads to unequal weight distribution between feet upon landing, which results in a shift of the body's center of mass away from the foundation of support.[75]

One recent study reported significant side-to-side differences in hamstring-to-quadriceps peak torque ratios in females.[76] Other researchers found significant differences in dynamic knee valgus angles when comparing dominant and nondominant legs in female high school athletes.[77] In younger athletes, females were found to demonstrate more asymmetrical single-limb preference in landing with peak vertical ground reaction force, which was further accentuated after a fatiguing exercise.[78] Anatomic and neuromuscular risk factors for ACL injury are summarized in **Table 1**.

The ACL, like other ligaments in the body, has hormone receptors for estrogen, testosterone and relaxin.[79,80] Given the differences in circulating levels of these hormones between young male and female athletes, it has been hypothesized that sex-based discrepancies in ACL injury rates may be attributable to the effects of sex hormones on the mechanical properties of the ACL. In contrast to males, females have increased generalized joint laxity after the onset of puberty.[81] In female athletes, increased general joint laxity has been associated with increased ACL injury risk. ACL laxity has been found to increase at peak levels of estrogen and progesterone.[82] Although some research has shown ACL tear to occur more frequently during the ovulatory phase of the menstrual cycle,[83] other research demonstrates ACL injuries in females to cluster near the 1st or 2nd day of the menstrual cycle.[84] Interestingly, one recent cross-sectional study reported significant differences in motor unit recruitment between vastus medialis and vastus medialis oblique muscles in the ovulatory and midluteal phases of a female's menstrual cycle.[85]

Sex hormones may affect neuromuscular maturation, growth and control. Before puberty, girls and boys maintain a similar body composition. During puberty, due to differences in endocrine and hormonal factors, males and females diverge regarding the development of lean muscle mass, fat mass, bone mass, and leg length.[86] After the age of 12 to 14 years, muscle mass tends to plateau in females, yet increases at an accelerated rate in males. Some attribute that continued muscle mass climb to rises in testosterone.[87] During puberty, males undergo a large testosterone surge, affecting muscle mass and strength. This strength can facilitate better maintenance of one's center of gravity and reduce trunk lean during athletic maneuvers. Females only experience a small testosterone surge during puberty, thus resulting in smaller increases in muscle mass and strength from hormone stimulation alone.[75]

Training and sport participation trends cannot be ignored when assessing differences in risk and incidence of ACL injury between youth females and males. Some researchers have reported similar or slightly larger proportion of ACL injuries in prepubescent boys as compared with age-matched female peers.[56,73] Participation in organized sports, particularly without focused conditioning/training, remains a factor for ACL injury. There is a higher propensity for male youth to play contact organized sports at a higher rate than females.[88] However, young female athletes have a higher ACL injury rate when compared with male counterparts after the age of 12. Although the effects of pubertal growth and differences in neuromuscular control and strength contribute to these effects, we then see a shift that older adolescent males from ages 17 to 19 exhibit higher incidence of ACL injury when compared with age-matched female athletes.[56] Again, later attainment of puberty for males could be a factor, but the attrition rate of female athlete participation at these ages may also contribute.[89,90] Males in this age range have also been found to play team sports at a greater rate as compared with females compared with individual sports. One study revealed despite steady growth in female sports participation, with females comprising approximately 42% of high school athletes and 43% of collegiate athletes, females only make up 24% of those who report playing sports on any given day, 12% of those playing sports in public parks, and 26% of those registered for intramural sports.[91] In young adult cohorts, the risk again shifts toward females; in young adult athletes, when matching sport, females experience higher rates of ACL injury as compared with males, both at high level competition level and on a recreational level.[92] Clearly, a variety of factors contribute to an individual young athlete's risk of ACL injury, some of which are intrinsic (eg, tibial slope, physiologic-developmental level, chronologic age and sex) and some of which are extrinsic, such as sport participation pattern and neuromuscular functioning. Importantly, many of the sex-based differences that are best understood to contribute to a young female athlete's heightened ACL injury risk are extrinsic factors (unrelated to sex) associated with neuromuscular firing patterns that may be corrected through focused training and injury prevention programs.

INJURY PREVENTION

To address injury rates, improve movement control, and assume a more proactive approach, several injury-prevention programs have been developed, mostly centering around ACL injury prevention. As previously discussed, altered or reduced motor control during sports can create biomechanical deficits that underlie injury risk. In 2008, the International Olympic Committee put forth a statement regarding injury prevention programs, detailing those effective and well-designed programs should include strength and power exercises, neuromuscular training, plyometric and agility exercises as well as proper warm-up.[54] Additionally, programs should train and emphasize correct cutting and landing techniques, to include landing softly, articulating through the entire foot, engaging knee and hip flexion, and avoiding dynamic valgus of the knee.[54] Neuromuscular training programs have been found to be significantly effective in athletes in ACL risk reduction, particularly for female athletes, resulting in up to 67% risk reduction[93] through biomechanical optimization and focusing on posterior chain strength development.[66] In a systematic review, three neuromuscular training programs were found to be effective in reducing injury risk: (1) Sportsmetrics, (2) Knee Injury Prevention Program (KIPP), and (3) Prevent Injury and Enhance Performance (PEP) program.[94] In addition to plyometric training, robust resistance training is also imperative for youth athletes regarding strength and control adaptations.[95] However, despite the importance of resistance training programs, girls and women participate at much lower levels than boys and men. Frequency also becomes important to maintain proper muscle/body memory. A meta-analysis found that programs with higher neuromuscular training sessions (at least 2 or more per week, exceeding 30 minutes per session) provided higher preventative effects and benefit for high school female athletes.[96] Awareness also poses a barrier to proper involvement. In a study of female collegiate athletes, although the vast majority (85%) knew that females were at higher risk of ACL injury, only 33% were familiar with the concept of ACL injury-prevention programs, and a staggering 15% had only participated in such programs.[97]

GENDER DISPARITIES AFFECTING INJURY

It is clear that sex-based disparities exist regarding risk and incidence of knee injuries for young athletes. However, solely focusing on biological or physiologic traits without considering wider societal influences that impact gender behaviors and norms likely limits sports medicine practitioners from fully addressing these issues. One recent study of worldwide trends reported that annual ACL injury rates have decreased among boys and men whereas they are stagnant for girls and women.[98] This suggests that a more nuanced approach to assess the complex interplay between biology, physiology, and social influences is needed to inform best practices for intervention and prevention.

One may argue that from the outset, females face a biased environment that limits their opportunities to safely participate in sports by failing to provide accessible training for both injury prevention and performance optimization. Fox and colleagues argue that women in sport have been ostracized historically; only since 1972 have women been able to compete in the Boston marathon as before that point, event organizers feared that the female physiology could not handle the physical demand.[99] Although progress has been made in terms of female participation in sports over the ensuing half-century, perhaps less focus has been placed on ensuring that female athletes receive adequate training and preparation to be able to participate safely. In fact, environmental and sociocultural stereotypes still exist that can place female athletes at a stark disadvantage. Gender inequities in terms of access to adequate training facilities and sports nutrition were exposed during the 2021 NCAA basketball tournament, with glaring differences in the quality of the weight rooms and meals provided for male and female athletes reported in the lay press.[100] A recent external report further detailed massive, systematic gender disparities for NCAA basketball programs.[101] Without equitable access to the myriad components of sport participation – training facilities, coaching expertise, sports nutrition – females may be at a higher risk of knee injury because of their unique (and inferior) experience, rather than their unique biology. Furthermore, framing female athletes as suboptimal and unable to withstand rigorous training and propagating the outdated message that a female's biologic makeup dooms her to injury from the start likely widen the gender gap in sports participation, as some female athletes may avoid sports out of fear that their bodies will set them up for injury.

Both intrinsic and extrinsic factors need to be acknowledged and addressed to properly address inequities in injuries to further benefit all athletes. Biological and social factors influence each other in ways that while not explicitly or empirically measurable, are plausible.[102] Such factors as training rooms, coaching, environment of play, all need to be considered and examined to ensure they are optimal for groups of athletes to enhance performance and minimize risk of injury.[103]

Although a detailed review of the literature regarding transgender athletes is outside the scope of this article, it is important to note that gender differences in sports participation and sports-related knee injuries are not limited to girls/women and boys/men but include a spectrum of athletes including those who are nonbinary or transgender. Transgender athletes are a particularly vulnerable population, with lower reported levels of physical activity and sport participation than cis-gendered individuals. Barriers to sports participation are manifold, and include: inadequate changing facilities/locker rooms, personal body dissatisfaction, fear of not being accepted by teammates, prior negative sporting experiences, and backlash from other athletes and parents.[104] As a result, little is known about the risk of sports-related musculoskeletal injuries for transgender athletes, and this is an area of active research.

FUTURE DIRECTIONS

Research looking at the intersectionality of biological differences between sexes while assessing the impact of societal and social disparities from gender categories in youth athlete populations is imperative. Furthermore, gender cannot be a binary category. Sports medicine health professionals and the field need to remain knowledgeable regarding those athletes who are nonbinary or who have transitioned from one gender category to another as those nuanced details need to be considered when caring for an individual athlete or recommending a particular rehab or training regimen. Research in this area is lacking and offers opportunity to enrich our field.

SUMMARY

Athletic participation has increased for both sexes with a closing gap in participation disparities. Differences in anatomy, hormone production, biomechanics, strength and neuromuscular training can contribute to differences in knee injury rates and patterns in males and females. However, the intersection of social influences with biological factors needs to be taken into account. Understanding the relationships between intrinsic and extrinsic factors will better help inform intervention, strategic initiatives, and policy. With the advancement of information regarding youth sports and injury patterns, there are still large opportunities to advance the field with further research.

CLINICS CARE POINTS

- Adolescent females have been found to have 2-10x risk of ACL injury as compared to their male counterparts. In high school athletes, injuries to the ACL are found at higher rates in females as compared to male counterparts (4.6% versus 2.5%), with high school girls' basketball sustaining the highest rate (6%), followed by girls' soccer (5%), girls' volleyball (5%) and girls' gymnastics (5%).

- Differences exist in biomechanical and neuromuscular control in youth males and females in the setting of ACL injury risk, including activation patterns, landing, and stability.

- Early specialization in a single sport during adolescence can increase a young female athlete's risk of developing patellofemoral pain syndrome 1.5x greater than age-matched controls.

- Solely focusing on biological or physiological trait differences between youth male and female athletes without considering wider sociological influences that impact gender behaviors and norms limit sports medicine practitioners and stakeholders from fully addressing these issues.

DISCLOSURE

The authors have nothing to disclose.

REFERENCES

1. Manandhar M, Hawkes S, Buse K, et al. Gender, health and the 2030 agenda for sustainable development. Bull World Health Organ 2018;96(9):644.
2. Marmot M. Social determinants of health inequalities. Lancet 2005;365(9464): 1099–104.
3. Ladd Amy L. The sports bra, the ACL, and Title IX—the game in play. Clin Orthop Relat Res 2014;472(6):1681–4.
4. Jacobs, Cameron. "Sporting Goods Manufacturers Association Research/ Sports Marketing Surveys." 1 May 2011. U.S. Trends in Team Sports Report. 1 October 2021. Available at: http://www.sfia.org/reports/280_2011-U.S-Trends-in-Team-Sports-Report. Accessed October 1, 2021.
5. Stracciolini A, Casciano R, Friedman HL, et al. A closer look at overuse injuries in the pediatric athlete. Clin J Sport Med 2015;25(1):30–5.
6. Available at: https://www.cdc.gov/healthyyouth/data/yrbs/data.htm. Accessed October 1, 2021.
7. Available at: https://health.gov/sites/default/files/2019-10/National_Youth_Sports_Strategy.pdf. Accessed October 1, 2021.

8. Available at: https://www.aspenprojectplay.org/state-of-play-2020/ages-13-17. Accessed October 15, 2021.

9. Whittaker JL, Toomey CM, Nettel-Aguirre A, et al. Health-related Outcomes after a Youth Sport-related Knee Injury. Med Sci Sports Exerc 2019;51(2):255–63.

10. Comstock, Dawn R. and Lauren Pierpoint. "High School RIO." 1 12 2019. National High School Sports-Related Injury Surveillance Study: 2018-2019 School Year. 10 10 2021. Available at: https://coloradosph.cuanschutz.edu/docs/librariesprovider204/default-document-library/2018-19.pdf?sfvrsn=d26400b9_2. Accessed October 10, 2021.

11. Ferguson RW. "Safe Kids Worldwide Analysis of CPSC NEISS data." 1 August 2013. 10 10 2021. Available at: https://www.safekids.org/sites/default/files/documents/ResearchReports/game_changers_-_stats_stories_and_what_communites_are_doing_to_protect_young_athletes.pdf. Accessed October 10, 2021.

12. Valovich McLeod TC, Decoster LC, Loud KJ, et al. 46. "National Athletic Trainers' Association position statement: prevention of pediatric overuse injuries. J Athl Train 2011;46(2):206–20.

13. Powell JW, Barber-Foss KD. Sex-related injury patterns among selected high school sports. Am J Sports Med 2000;28(3):385–91.

14. Ingram JG, Fields SK, Yard EE, et al. Epidemiology of knee injuries among boys and girls in US high school athletics. Am J Sports Med 2008;36(6):1116–22.

15. Louw QA, Manilall J, Grimmer KA. Epidemiology of knee injuries among adolescents: a systematic review. Br J Sports Med 2008;42(1):2–10.

16. Valasek AE, Young JA, Huang L, et al. Age and Sex Differences in Overuse Injuries Presenting to Pediatric Sports Medicine Clinics. Clin Pediatr 2019;58(7):770–7.

17. Whittaker JL, Woodhouse LJ, Nettel-Aguirre A, et al. Osteoarthritis and ca. "Outcomes associated with early post-traumatic osteoarthritis and other negative health consequences 3–10 years following knee joint injury in youth sport. Osteoarthritis Cartilage 2015;23(7):1122–9.

18. Lam KC, Markbreiter JG. The impact of knee injury history on health-related quality of life in adolescent athletes. J Sport Rehabil 2019;28(2):115–9.

19. Varni JW, Burwinkle TM, Seid M. The PedsQL™ as a pediatric patient-reported outcome: Reliability and validity of the PedsQL™ Measurement Model in 25,000 children. Expert Rev Pharmacoeconomics Outcomes Res 2005;5(6):705–19.

20. Aspen-Institute. "Aspen Institute Project Play." 27 January 2015. Sport for all play for life: A playbook to get every kid in the game. 2021. Available at: https://www.aspenprojectplay.org/sport-for-all-play-for-life. Accessed October 10, 2021.

21. Smith RE. Toward a cognitive-affective model of athletic burnout. J Sport Exerc Psychol 1986;8(1):36–50.

22. DiFiori JP, Benjamin HJ, Brenner JS, et al. Overuse injuries and burnout in youth sports: a position statement from the American Medical Society for Sports Medicine. Br J Sports Med 2014;48(4):287–8.

23. Boling M, Padua D, Marshall S, et al. Gender differences in the incidence and prevalence of patellofemoral pain syndrome. Scand J Med Sci Sports 2010;20(5):725–30.

24. Stracciolini A, Casciano R, Levey Friedman H, et al. Pediatric sports injuries: a comparison of males versus females. Am J Sports Med 2014;42(4):965–72.

25. Foss KD, Myer GD, Magnussen RA, et al. Diagnostic differences for anterior knee pain between sexes in adolescent basketball players. J Athl Enhanc 2014;3(1):1814.

26. Horton MG, Hall TL. Quadriceps femoris muscle angle: normal values and relationships with gender and selected skeletal measures. Phys Ther 1989;69(11): 897–901.

27. Lankhorst NE, Bierma-Zeinstra SM, van Middelkoop M. Factors associated with patellofemoral pain syndrome: a systematic review. Br J Sports Med 2013;47(4): 193–206.

28. Park SK, Stefanyshyn DJ. Greater Q angle may not be a risk factor of patellofemoral pain syndrome. Clin Biomech 2011;26(4):392–6.

29. Thomee R, Renström P, Karlsson J, et al. Patellofemoral pain syndrome in young women: I. A clinical analysis of alignment, pain parameters, common symptoms and functional activity level. Scand J Med Sci Sports 1995;5(4):237–44.

30. Myer GD, Ford KR, Di Stasi SL, et al. High knee abduction moments are common risk factors for patellofemoral pain (PFP) and anterior cruciate ligament (ACL) injury in girls: is PFP itself a predictor for subsequent ACL injury? Br J Sports Med 2015;49(2):118–22.

31. Schmitz RJ, Shultz SJ, Nguyen AD. Dynamic valgus alignment and functional strength in males and females during maturation. J Athl Train 2009;44(1):26–32.

32. Magalhães E, Silva APM, Sacramento SN, et al. Isometric strength ratios of the hip musculature in females with patellofemoral pain: a comparison to pain-free controls. J Strength Cond Res 2013;27(8):2165–70.

33. Foss KDB, Hornsby M, Edwards NM, et al. Is body composition associated with an increased risk of developing anterior knee pain in adolescent female athletes? Phys Sportsmed 2012;40(1):13–9.

34. Boling MC, Nguyen AD, Padua DA, et al. Gender-specific risk factor profiles for patellofemoral pain. Clin J Sport Med 2021;31(1):49–56.

35. Hall R, Foss KB, Hewett TE, et al. Sport specialization's association with an increased risk of developing anterior knee pain in adolescent female athletes. J Sport Rehabil 2015;24(1):31–5.

36. Williams JS Jr, Bush-Joseph CA, Bach BR Jr. Osteochondritis dissecans of the knee. Am J knee Surg 1998;11(4):221–32.

37. Cahill BR. Osteochondritis dissecans of the knee: treatment of juvenile and adult forms. J Am Acad Orthop Surg 1995;3(4):237–47.

38. Glancy GL. Juvenile osteochondritis dissecans. Am J knee Surg 1999;12(2): 120–4.

39. Kessler JI, Nikizad H, Shea KG, et al. The demographics and epidemiology of osteochondritis dissecans of the knee in children and adolescents. Am J Sports Med 2014;42(2):320–6.

40. Griffin LY, Albohm MJ, Arendt EA, et al. Understanding and preventing noncontact anterior cruciate ligament injuries: a review of the Hunt Valley II meeting, January 2005. Am J Sports Med 2006;34(9):1512–32.

41. Myer GD, Ford KR, Hewett TE. Rationale and clinical techniques for anterior cruciate ligament injury prevention among female athletes. J Athl Train 2004; 39(4):352.

42. Kessler MA, Behrend H, Henz S, et al. Function, osteoarthritis and activity after ACL-rupture: 11 years follow-up results of conservative versus reconstructive treatment. Knee Surg Sports Traumatol Arthrosc 2008;16(5):442–8.

43. Lohmander LS, Englund PM, Dahl LL, et al. The long-term consequence of anterior cruciate ligament and meniscus injuries: osteoarthritis. Am J Sports Med 2007;35(10):1756–69.

44. Dugan SA. Sports-related knee injuries in female athletes: what gives? Am J Phys Med Rehabil 2005;84(2):122–30.

45. Ireland ML. The female ACL: why is it more prone to injury? Orthop Clin 2002; 33(4):637–51.

46. Ardern CL, Taylor NF, Feller JA, et al. Fifty-five per cent return to competitive sport following anterior cruciate ligament reconstruction surgery: an updated systematic review and meta-analysis including aspects of physical functioning and contextual factors. Br J Sports Med 2014;48(21):1543–52.

47. Loes MD, Dahlstedt LJ, Thomée R. A 7-year study on risks and costs of knee injuries in male and female youth participants in 12 sports. Scand J Med Sci Sports 2000;10(2):90–7.

48. Alentorn-Geli E, Myer GD, Silvers HJ, et al. Prevention of non-contact anterior cruciate ligament injuries in soccer players. Part 1: Mechanisms of injury and underlying risk factors. Knee Surg Sports Traumatol Arthrosc 2009;17(7): 705–29.

49. Malone TR. 2, 36-39. "Relationship of gender in anterior cruciate ligament injuries of NCAA divison I basketball players. J South Orthop Assoc 1992;2:36–9.

50. Hewett TE, Lindenfeld TN, Riccobene JV, et al. The effect of neuromuscular training on the incidence of knee injury in female athletes. Am J Sports Med 1999;27(6):699–706.

51. Beynnon BD, Vacek PM, Newell MK, et al. The effects of level of competition, sport, and sex on the incidence of first-time noncontact anterior cruciate ligament injury. Am J Sports Med 2014;42(8):1806–12.

52. LaBella CR, Hennrikus W, Hewett TE. Anterior cruciate ligament injuries: diagnosis, treatment, and prevention. Pediatrics 2014;133(5):e1437–50.

53. Stanley LE, Kerr ZY, Dompier TP, et al. Sex differences in the incidence of anterior cruciate ligament, medial collateral ligament, and meniscal injuries in collegiate and high school sports: 2009-2010 through 2013-2014. Am J Sports Med 2016;44(6):1565–72.

54. Renstrom P, Ljungqvist A, Arendt E, et al. Non-contact ACL injuries in female athletes: an International Olympic Committee current concepts statement. Br J Sports Med 2008;42(6):394–412.

55. Koch PP, Fucentese SF, Blatter SC. Complications after epiphyseal reconstruction of the anterior cruciate ligament in prepubescent children. Knee Surg Sports Traumatol Arthrosc 2016;24(9):2736–40.

56. Bloom DA, Wolfert AJ, Michalowitz A, et al. ACL Injuries Aren't Just for Girls: The Role of Age in Predicting Pediatric ACL Injury. Sports health 2020;12(6):559–63.

57. Anderson AF, Dome DC, Gautam S, et al. Correlation of anthropometric measurements, strength, anterior cruciate ligament size, and intercondylar notch characteristics to sex differences in anterior cruciate ligament tear rates. Am J Sports Med 2001;29(1):58–66.

58. Souryal TO, Moore HA, Evans JP. Bilaterality in anterior cruciate ligament injuries: associated intercondylar notch stenosis. Am J Sports Med 1988;16(5): 449–54.

59. Sutton KM, Bullock JM. Anterior cruciate ligament rupture: differences between males and females. J Am Acad Orthop Surg 2013;21(1):41–50.

60. Giffin JR, Vogrin TM, Zantop T, et al. Effects of increasing tibial slope on the biomechanics of the knee. Am J Sports Med 2004;32(2):376–82.

61. Hohmann E, Bryant A, Reaburn P, et al. Is there a correlation between posterior tibial slope and non-contact anterior cruciate ligament injuries? Knee Surg Sports Traumatol Arthrosc 2011;19(1):109–14.

62. Terauchi M, Hatayama K, Yanagisawa S, et al. Sagittal alignment of the knee and its relationship to noncontact anterior cruciate ligament injuries. Am J Sports Med 2011;39(5):1090–4.

63. Conley S, Rosenberg A, Crowninshield R. The female knee: anatomic variations. J Am Acad Orthop Surg 2007;15:S31–6.

64. Hertel J, Dorfman JH, Braham RA. Lower extremity malalignments and anterior cruciate ligament injury history. J Sports Sci Med 2004;3(4):220–5.

65. Myer GD, Brent JL, Ford KR, et al. A pilot study to determine the effect of trunk and hip focused neuromuscular training on hip and knee isokinetic strength. Br J Sports Med 2008;42(7):614–9.

66. Quatman-Yates CC, Myer GD, Ford KR, et al. A longitudinal evaluation of maturational effects on lower extremity strength in female adolescent athletes. Pediatr Phys Ther 2013;25(3):271.

67. Krabak BJ, Snitily B, Milani CJ. Running injuries during adolescence and childhood. Phys Med Rehabil Clin 2016;27:179–202.

68. Huston LJ, Wojtys EM. Neuromuscular performance characteristics in elite female athletes. Am J Sports Med 1996;24(4):427–36.

69. Chappell JD, Creighton RA, Giuliani C, et al. Kinematics and electromyography of landing preparation in vertical stop-jump: risks for noncontact anterior cruciate ligament injury. Am J Sports Med 2007;35(2):235–41.

70. Earl JE, Monteiro SK, Snyder KR. Differences in lower extremity kinematics between a bilateral drop-vertical jump and a single-leg step-down. J Orthop Sports Phys Ther 2007;37(5):245–52.

71. Kernozek TW, Torry MR, van Hoof H, et al. Gender differences in frontal and sagittal plane biomechanics during drop landings. Med Sci Sports Exerc 2005;37(6):1003–12.

72. Zazulak BT, Hewett TE, Reeves NP, et al. Deficits in neuromuscular control of the trunk predict knee injury risk: prospective biomechanical-epidemiologic study. Am J Sports Med 2007;35(7):1123–30.

73. Stracciolini A, Stein CJ, Zurakowski D, et al. Anterior cruciate ligament injuries in pediatric athletes presenting to sports medicine clinic: a comparison of males and females through growth and development. Sports Health 2015;7(2):130–6.

74. Fort-Vanmeerhaeghe A, Gual G, Romero-Rodriguez D, et al. Lower Limb Neuromuscular Asymmetry in Volleyball and Basketball Players. J Hum Kinet 2016;50: 135–43.

75. Dharamsi A, LaBella C. Prevention of ACL injuries in adolescent female athletes. Contemp Pediatr 2013;30(7):12–9.

76. Hewett TE, Stroupe AL, Nance TA, et al. Plyometric training in female athletes: decreased impact forces and increased hamstring torques. Am J Sports Med 1996;24(6):765–73.

77. Ford KR, Myer GD, Hewett TE. Valgus knee motion during landing in high school female and male basketball players. Med Sci Sports Exerc 2003;35(10): 1745–50.

78. Briem K, Jónsdóttir KV, Árnason Á, et al. Effects of sex and fatigue on biomechanical measures during the drop-jump task in children. Orthop J Sports Med 2017;5(1). 2325967116679640.

79. Faryniarz DA, Bhargava M, Lajam C, et al. Quantitation of estrogen receptors and relaxin binding in human anterior cruciate ligament fibroblasts. In Vitro Cell Dev Biol Anim 2006;42(7):176–81.

80. Lovering RM, Romani WA. Effect of testosterone on the female anterior cruciate ligament. Am J Physiol Regul Integr Comp Physiol 2005;289(1):R15–22.

81. Falciglia F, Guzzanti V, Di Ciommo V, et al. Physiological knee laxity during pubertal growth. Bull NYU Hosp Jt Dis 2009;67:325.

82. Heitz NA, Eisenman PA, Beck CL, et al. Hormonal changes throughout the menstrual cycle and increased anterior cruciate ligament laxity in females. J Athl Train 1999;34(2):144.

83. Wojtys EM, Huston LJ, Lindenfeld TN, et al. Association between the menstrual cycle and anterior cruciate ligament injuries in female athletes. Am J Sports Med 1998;26(5):614–9.

84. Hewett TE, Zazulak BT, Myer GD. Effects of the menstrual cycle on anterior cruciate ligament injury risk: a systematic review. Am J Sports Med 2007;35(4):659–68.

85. Tenan MS, Peng YL, Hackney AC, et al. Menstrual cycle mediates vastus medialis and vastus medialis oblique muscle activity. Med Sci Sports Exerc 2013;45(11):2151–7.

86. Wells JC. Sexual dimorphism of body composition. Best Pract Res Clin Endocrinol Metab 2007;21(3):415–30.

87. Loomba-Albrecht LA, Styne DM. Effect of puberty on body composition. Curr Opin Endocrinol Diabetes Obes 2009;16(1):10–5.

88. Veliz P, Shakib S. Gender, academics, and interscholastic sports participation at the school level: A gender-specific analysis of the relationship between interscholastic sports participation and AP enrollment. Sociological focus 2014;47(2):101–20.

89. Senne JA. Examination of gender equity and female participation in sport. Sport J 2016;19:1–9.

90. Guthold R, Stevens GA, Riley LM, et al. Worldwide trends in insufficient physical activity from 2001 to 2016: a pooled analysis of 358 population-based surveys with 1· 9 million participants. Lancet Glob Health 2018;6(10):e1077.

91. Deaner RO, Geary DC, Puts DA, et al. A sex difference in the predisposition for physical competition: males play sports much more than females even in the contemporary US. PloS one 2012;7(11):e49168.

92. Montalvo AM, Schneider DK, Yut L, et al. What's my risk of sustaining an ACL injury while playing sports?" A systematic review with meta-analysis. Br J Sports Med 2019;53:1003–12.

93. Myer GD, Sugimoto D, Thomas S, et al. The influence of age on the effectiveness of neuromuscular training to reduce anterior cruciate ligament injury in female athletes: a meta-analysis. , 41. "The influence of age on the effectiveness of neuromuscular training to reduce anterior cruciate ligament injury in female athletes: a meta-analysis. Am J Sports Med 2013;41(1):203–15.

94. Noyes FR, Barber-Westin SD. Neuromuscular retraining intervention programs: Do they reduce noncontact anterior cruciate ligament injury rates in adolescent female athletes? Arthroscopy 2014;30(2):245–55.

95. Lesinski M, Prieske O, Granacher U. Effects and dose–response relationships of resistance training on physical performance in youth athletes: a systematic review and meta-analysis. Br J Sports Med 2016;50(13):781–95.

96. Sugimoto D, Myer GD, Foss KDB, et al. Dosage effects of neuromuscular training intervention to reduce anterior cruciate ligament injuries in female athletes: meta-and sub-group analyses. Sports Med 2014;44(4):551–62.

97. Tanaka MJ, Jones LC, Forman JM. Awareness of anterior cruciate ligament injury-preventive training programs among female collegiate athletes. J Athl Train 2020;55(4):359–64.

98. Sanders TL, Maradit Kremers H, Bryan AJ, et al. Incidence of anterior cruciate ligament tears and reconstruction: a 21-year population-based study. Am J Sports Med 2016;44(6):1502–7.

99. Fox A, Bonacci J, Hoffmann S, et al. Anterior cruciate ligament injuries in Australian football: should women and girls be playing? You're asking the wrong question. BMJ open Sport Exerc Med 2020;6(1):e000778.

100. Available at: https://onherturf.nbcsports.com/2021/03/25/ncaa-womens-mens-basketball-weight-rooms-discrepancies/. Accessed Octobe 20, 2021.

101. Fischels, Josie. NPR. 3 August 2021. 17 10 2021. Available at: https://www.npr.org/2021/08/03/1024481199/report-ncaa-undervalues-womens-basketball-prioritizes-mens-teams. Accessed October 17, 2021.

102. Springer KW, Stellman JM, Jordan-Young RM. Beyond a catalogue of differences: a theoretical frame and good practice guidelines for researching sex/gender in human health. Social Sci Med 2012;74(11):1817–24.

103. Parsons JL, Coen SE, Bekker S. Anterior cruciate ligament injury: towards a gendered environmental approach. Br J Sports Med 2021;55(2021):984–90.

104. Dubon ME, Abbott K, Carl RL. Care of the Transgender Athlete. Curr Sports Med Rep December 2018;17(12):410–8.

The Impact of Race, Insurance, and Socioeconomic Factors on Pediatric Knee Injuries

Neeraj M. Patel, MD, MPH, MBS[a],*, Bianca R. Edison, MD, MS[b],
Cordelia W. Carter, MD[c], Nirav K. Pandya, MD[d]

KEYWORDS

- Pediatric sports • Knee injury • Disparities • Anterior cruciate ligament • Meniscus
- Osteochondritis dissecans • Tibial spine • Tibial eminence

KEY POINTS

- Race and insurance status affect the timing of anterior cruciate ligament (ACL) reconstruction, concomitant intra-articular pathology, and postoperative outcomes in children and adolescents.
- Insurance status affects the timing of meniscal surgery as well as the feasibility of repair.
- Access to care is a major contributor to disparities in the care of pediatric knee injuries.
- Further research is necessary to clearly identify the etiology of these disparities so that action can be taken to remedy them.

INTRODUCTION

While the landscape of American health care continues to evolve, disparities persist along the lines of race, ethnicity, socioeconomic status (SES), and other factors.[1–4] Some of the most frequently discussed inequalities relate to infant mortality, pulmonary disease, and general access to care.[5–7] Similar disparities have been studied in orthopedic surgery and sports medicine.[8–12] The purpose of the current review is to discuss the ways in which race, insurance, and socioeconomic factors impact the risk, evaluation, management, and outcomes of knee injuries in children and adolescents. An improved understanding of these issues may allow for the development of

No authors have any relevant financial conflicts of interest.
[a] Ann & Robert H. Lurie Children's Hospital of Chicago, 225 East Chicago Avenue, Box 69, Chicago, IL 60611, USA; [b] Children's Hospital Los Angeles, 4650 Sunset Blvd, Los Angeles, CA 90027, USA; [c] New York University Langone Orthopedic Hospital, 301 E 17th St, New York, NY 10010, USA; [d] University of California San Francisco Benioff Children's Hospital, 747 52nd St, Oakland, CA 94609, USA
* Corresponding author.
E-mail address: neepatel@luriechildrens.org

strategies to limit the negative ramifications of disparities on young athletes with knee injuries.

Anterior Cruciate Ligament Injury

Anterior cruciate ligament rupture is a relatively common injury with an incidence that continues to increase in the pediatric population. Dodwell and colleagues reported that the rate of ACL reconstruction in New York increased from 17.6/100,000 to 50.9/100,000 over a span of 20 years. Reconstruction was six times more common in patients with commercial health insurance compared with those with Medicaid.[13] Other studies have noted similar increases in annual incidence within the pediatric population.[14,15] Prompt, effective treatment is important in children and adolescents, as delayed intervention or recurrent knee instability may result in more frequent meniscal injury and poorer outcomes.[16–18] At least 2 meta-analyses demonstrate the negative impact of delayed surgery or nonoperative treatment in young patients. Ramski and colleagues reported that children treated without surgery had over 12 times the chance of a medial meniscus injury, more pathologic laxity, and inability to return to previous levels of athletic participation.[19] A larger, more recent meta-analysis by James and colleagues found that reconstruction later than 12 weeks after injury resulted in 4.3 times higher odds of any concomitant meniscus tear and 3.2 times higher odds of an irreparable meniscus tear. Nonoperative treatment was associated with high rates of residual instability and meniscus injury and low rates of return to sports.[20]

While the rising incidence of pediatric ACL injuries and the consequences of delayed treatment is well recognized, research on the impact of various demographic factors on management and outcomes continues to grow. Several studies have investigated the effect of insurance and SES on children and adolescents with ACL tears. Pierce and colleagues contacted the offices of 42 surgeons on 2 separate occasions with a fictitious scenario of a 14-year-old man with an acute ACL rupture, first with Medicaid, then with private insurance. Ninety percent offered the privately insured patient an appointment within 2 weeks, compared with 14% for the patient with Medicaid.[21]

Clinical studies reflect similar problems with access to care. A retrospective analysis of 121 children and adolescents revealed that those with public insurance had 12.4 and 7.8 times higher odds of waiting greater than 3 and 6 months for surgery, respectively. These patients also had 2.5 times higher odds of a significant meniscus tear than those with private insurance. Surgical delay beyond 6 months was also associated with worse patient-reported outcomes.[22] Similarly, Williams and colleagues reported that patients with commercial insurance had a mean time of 56 days between injury and initial presentation compared with 136 days for those with public insurance. Publicly insured patients with a meniscus tear were more likely to require debridement rather than repair and more likely to have significant chondral injuries.[23] Bram and colleagues also found a longer delay between injury and surgery for children with Medicaid, as well as less postoperative physical therapy visits and lower rate of clearance for sports.[24] At least one study found a higher rate of postoperative stiffness in patients with public insurance (22%) than with private insurance (9%).[25]

While insurance is often considered a marker of SES in the aforementioned articles, others have attempted to evaluate it in different ways. In addition to insurance status, Newman and colleagues studied the impact of median household income based on the home ZIP code. The authors found that those with median income in the 75th percentile or higher had a significantly shorter wait between injury and surgery compared with those below the 75th percentile.[26] Another retrospective study found that median household income was significantly correlated with time between injury and magnetic resonance imaging (MRI), injury and surgery, and initial orthopedic evaluation and surgery.[25]

The impact of race and ethnicity on pediatric ACL injury is studied less frequently than insurance and SES. The study by Bram and colleagues is one of the few that analyzed these factors. Even when controlling for insurance status and other factors, Black and Hispanic patients experienced greater delays to surgery and were more likely to have an irreparable meniscus tear. These children averaged fewer postoperative physical therapy sessions, had greater residual strength deficits, and were less likely to meet return to sport criteria.[24] The systematic review by Ziedas and colleagues, while not limited to children and adolescents, found that a minority of the 22 included studies specifically analyzed race or ethnicity. In addition to citing the results of Bram and colleagues, the authors also noted that Hispanic patients were more likely to have injuries to the lateral meniscus or both menisci.[27,28]

Some of the aforementioned studies have found higher ACL reinjury rates in white and privately insured patients. This is in contrast to the delayed treatment and more severe meniscal pathology seen in publicly insured patients and those from racial and ethnic minority communities. For example, Bram and colleagues studied 915 children and adolescents and found that those with private insurance had 1.3 times higher odds of postoperative graft failure compared with those with Medicaid.[24] The meta-analysis by Ziedas and colleagues included adult patients but found a higher risk of revision ACL reconstruction, contralateral ACL reconstruction, and non-ACL knee surgery in white patients.[27] Dodwell and colleagues noted a higher incidence of primary ACL reconstruction in those with private insurance.[13] These results are similar to those of a study reporting a higher rate of stress fractures in white and privately insured children in New York.[29] The specific reasons for these findings are unclear, but may be related to the type and intensity of sports participation. It is possible that those with more resources and access to multi-seasonal, extra-scholastic club sports may have more athletic exposures that risk reinjury.[30,31] Further research is needed to better understand the causative factors driving such trends.

As disparities exist at every step in the care of pediatric ACL injuries, additional study is needed to elucidate the manners in which these issues arise throughout the care process: from initial evaluation at the time of injury to the final stages of return to play and beyond. Once these mechanisms are better understood, direct action is necessary to improve care. A team-based approach that examines each step of the process will allow for improved outcomes for patients and families, preventing the cascade of negative consequences of an unstable, degenerative knee.

Meniscus Injury

The meniscus serves as a load transmitter, shock absorber, and stabilizer for the knee.[32] Impaired meniscal function may result in a higher risk of degenerative changes, ultimately leading to premature osteoarthritis.[33–35] For example, loss of 20% of the meniscus results in a 350% increase in contact forces through the articular cartilage.[36] Such changes are especially worrisome in children and adolescents, whose knees may face greater demands than those of adults and require maintained function over a longer period of time. For these reasons, the treatment paradigm in young patients has shifted from resection to repair whenever possible.[37] Prompt, effective treatment of meniscus injuries may, therefore, have a substantial impact on future knee function in children and adolescents.

Several studies have investigated the impact of insurance status on the treatment of meniscus injuries. Johnson and colleagues analyzed 237 patients aged 22 years or younger. The authors found significantly longer times for referral, orthopedic evaluation, and surgery for publicly insured and uninsured patients.[38] Similarly, Olson and Pandya studied 49 patients younger than 18 years and found that those with public insurance waited for an average of 230 days longer for surgery than those with private insurance. These patients also experienced longer delays in initial presentation and advanced imaging.[39] Another retrospective study of 52 patients with a bucket-handle meniscus tear similarly found increased delays in the initial presentation, advanced imaging, and surgery for patients with Medicaid or Charity Care. Of note, this study included adults as well as adolescents. The authors noted that 87% of tears treated within 6 weeks of injury were repairable compared with 19% treated after 6 weeks, but only 20% of underinsured patients underwent surgery within 6 weeks of injury.[40]

Finally, a nationwide investigation of meniscal allograft transplantation (MAT) in the pediatric population found that patients undergoing MAT had twice the odds of having private insurance compared with those undergoing simple, primary meniscus procedures such as repair or meniscectomy.[41] On the other hand, as previously noted, those with government insurance are more likely to sustain irreparable tears and possibly a higher risk of subsequent meniscal insufficiency.[23,24,40] Therefore, there exists the possibility that publicly insured patients are more likely to experience postmeniscectomy syndrome, but less likely to undergo MAT for such sequelae. Further research is required to determine long-term outcomes of pediatric patients with meniscus injuries, especially along the lines of insurance status and other demographic factors. The impact of race and ethnicity, for example, has not been studied in this context.

Other Knee Injuries

An understanding of the influence of demographic factors on other pediatric knee injuries continues to evolve. Osteochondritis dissecans (OCD) is a focal pathology of the subchondral bone most commonly seen in children and adolescents that may affect the articular cartilage. Ineffective treatment can result in osteoarthritis and poor outcomes.[42–44] Kessler and colleagues analyzed the epidemiology of juvenile OCD in a managed care health system with more than 1 million patients. Compared with white children, the incidence of OCD was higher in black patients, who made up only 8.6% of the overall population but 27.6% of those with an OCD lesion.[45] The reasons for this finding are unclear. Another study found that black children are less likely to successfully heal an OCD lesion in the knee. In this retrospective analysis of 204 lesions, non-healing OCD was found in 25% of black patients compared with 9.4% of white patients.[46] Previous studies have sought to describe predictors of OCD healing, but these have not included race, ethnicity, SES, or other such demographic factors. For example, Wall and colleagues found that larger lesions and those with swelling or mechanical symptoms are less likely to heal with nonoperative treatment, but did not include any demographic factors beyond age and sex in the analysis.[47] A similar study did report on race, but all subjects were white, raising questions regarding the generalizability of the results to a broader population.[48] The impact of race, SES, and other demographic factors on the evaluation and treatment of OCD require further investigation.

Fracture of the tibial spine, or tibial eminence, is another knee pathology that is mostly unique to children and adolescents. Prompt, effective treatment aims to restore knee motion, stability, and kinematics. This avulsion of the ACL is relatively rare, with an incidence of 3 per 100,000 children.[49] The rarity of the injury and potential difficulty identifying small fracture fragments on x-ray may result in missed diagnosis and delayed management. A study of pediatric knee injuries in a national malpractice claims database found that tibial spine fractures were the most commonly missed injury.[50] These issues may be compounded by demographic factors, as with ACL and meniscus injuries, but there is little data on such trends. A recent multicenter study of 434 children and adolescents with a tibial spine fracture reported that those with public insurance were 5.3 times more likely to obtain MRI greater than 3 weeks after injury. Similarly, those that underwent surgery 3 or more weeks after injury were 2.5 times more likely to have government insurance. These patients were also more likely to be immobilized postoperatively in a cast rather than a hinged brace.[51] The long-term impact of such disparities remains unclear and merits further research.

Access to Care

The etiology of the aforementioned disparities is multifactorial and likely related to a number of historical, political, social, and economic factors. Fundamental to efficient, effective care is access to quality health care. A number of studies suggest that this can be a major impediment to timely diagnosis and treatment. Skaggs and colleagues called 50 orthopedic practices in California with hypothetical scenarios of a 10 year old with an acute fracture, first with Medicaid and then with private insurance. Only 1/50 offices offered an appointment within 7 days for Medicaid compared with all 50 for the child with commercial insurance.[52] The authors then expanded their study to a national sample of 250 orthopedic practices and arrived at similar results.[53] In their study of 168 pediatric sports medicine patients that required knee MRI, Beck and colleagues found that children with government insurance had longer delays between injury and MRI (34 vs 67 days) and initial clinic visit and MRI (11 vs 40 days) compared with those with private insurance. There was no difference in the rate of positive findings on imaging or need for surgery.[54]

Other research has similarly found disparities in access to care along the lines of insurance status in broader orthopedic contexts. For example, while musculoskeletal urgent care centers have proliferated in recent years, a recent study reported that only 13% of such facilities in Connecticut accepted all patients regardless of insurance type and 66% did not accept any form of Medicaid. Furthermore, these centers were located in areas with median household incomes greater than the state median.[55] While centers like this could serve as an effective "front line" for children with acute knee injuries, the aforementioned trends may disproportionately affect the large proportion of pediatric patients with public insurance. Similar trends were found in access to outpatient orthopedic care in North Carolina and across the United States.[56,57] Another important first line in the evaluation and triage of acute sports injuries is the athletic trainer. However, such staff is not available in all schools. A study of 14 urban and suburban high schools in Michigan noted that 84.4% of white athletes had access to an athletic trainer at school compared with 40.6% of black athletes.[58] In California, only 13% of schools use a full-time, certified athletic trainer, and the majority either had no trainer at all or used unqualified health personnel in this role. When using the percentage of students eligible for reduced-price lunch as a marker of SES, about 66% of students in schools without an athletic trainer met this criterion compared with 50% of students in schools with a trainer.[59] Such results underscore the substantial disparities in access to first-line professionals such as athletic trainers that may subsequently impact timely, effective evaluation and management of acute sports injuries.

Other Barriers to Care

Trust in the health care system and cultural differences in seeking care may also affect the evaluation and treatment of pediatric patients with acute injuries. In one study, black adults were 37% less likely to trust their physicians than white adults, and were more likely to be concerned about personal privacy and the potential for harmful experimentation in hospitals.[60] Another survey of low-income residents in southern Florida found that the perception of racism accounted for residual differences in health care trust between black and white patients.[61] While some of these findings may be rooted in American medical history that includes unethical and discriminatory practices such as the Tuskegee experiment, at least one study suggests that this specific historic event alone may not explain differences in current mistrust in the health care system.[62] Rather, this may be related to broader experiences with structural and personal racism both in the past and present. For example, a study of college athletic medical staff found that participants believed black athletes experience less pain than white athletes. Specifically, this assumption was made primarily when participants assumed black athletes had a lower SES than their white counterparts.[63] Similarly, black patients with a long bone fracture were 66% less likely than white patients to receive analgesics in the emergency department despite similar reports of pain.[64] Another study found that Medicaid insurance and Hispanic ethnicity were associated with lower usage of regional anesthesia for arthroscopic surgery in pediatric patients.[65] Such findings point to current, disparate practices that may impact trust in the health care system as well as patient satisfaction and outcomes.

SUMMARY

As has been described in various other medical fields, disparities persist in pediatric sports medicine along the lines of race, ethnicity, insurance status, and other demographic factors. When considered in the context of knee injuries in children and adolescents, these inequalities affect evaluation, treatment, and outcomes. The long-term effects can be far-reaching, including sports and physical activity participation, comorbid chronic disease, and socio-emotional health. Further research is needed to more concretely identify the etiology of these disparities so that effective, equitable care is provided for all children.

CLINICS CARE POINTS

- Race and insurance status are associated with the timing of ACL reconstruction, concomitant intra-articular injuries, and outcomes in the pediatric population.
- Insurance status is associated with the timing of meniscus surgery and the feasibility of repair.

REFERENCES

1. Chen J, Vargas-Bustamante A, Mortensen K. Ortega AN. Racial and ethnic disparities in health care access and utilization under the affordable care act. Med Care 2016;54(2):140–6.
2. Bailey ZD, Krieger N, Agénor M, et al. Structural racism and health inequities in the USA: evidence and interventions. Lancet 2017;389(10077):1453–63.
3. Dickman SL, Himmelstein DU, Woolhandler S. Inequality and the health-care system in the USA. Lancet 2017;389(10077):1431–41.
4. Buchmueller TC, Levinson ZM, Levy HG, et al. Effect of the affordable care act on racial and ethnic disparities in health insurance coverage. Am J Public Health 2016;106(8):1416–21.

5. Matthews TJ, MacDorman MF. Infant mortality statistics from the 2010 period linked birth/infant death data set. Natl Vital Stat Rep 2013;62(8):1–26.
6. Eisner MD, Blanc PD, Omachi TA, et al. Socioeconomic status, race and COPD health outcomes. J Epidemiol Community Health 2011;65(1):26–34.
7. Flores G. Technical report–racial and ethnic disparities in the health and health care of children. Pediatrics 2010;125(4):e979–1020.
8. Dy CJ, Lyman S, Do HT, et al. Socioeconomic factors are associated with frequency of repeat emergency department visits for pediatric closed fractures. J Pediatr Orthop 2014;34(5):548–51.
9. Kim CY, Wiznia DH, Hsiang WR, et al. The Effect of Insurance Type on Patient Access to Knee Arthroplasty and Revision under the Affordable Care Act. J Arthroplasty 2015;30(9):1498–501.
10. Medford-Davis LN, Lin F, Greenstein A, et al. "I broke my ankle": access to orthopedic follow-up care by insurance status. Acad Emerg Med 2017;24(1):98–105.
11. Nuño M, Drazin DG, Acosta FL Jr. Differences in treatments and outcomes for idiopathic scoliosis patients treated in the United States from 1998 to 2007: impact of socioeconomic variables and ethnicity. Spine J 2013;13(2):116–23.
12. Sterling RS. Gender and race/ethnicity differences in hip fracture incidence, morbidity, mortality, and function. Clin Orthop Relat Res 2011;469(7):1913–8.
13. Dodwell ER, Lamont LE, Green DW, et al. 20 years of pediatric anterior cruciate ligament reconstruction in New York State. Am J Sports Med 2014;42(3):675–80.
14. Beck NA, Lawrence JTR, Nordin JD, et al. ACL tears in school-aged children and adolescents Over 20 Years. Pediatrics 2017;139(3):e20161877.
15. Tepolt FA, Feldman L, Kocher MS. Trends in Pediatric ACL Reconstruction From the PHIS Database. J Pediatr Orthop 2018;38(9):e490–4.
16. Funahashi KM, Moksnes H, Maletis GB, et al. Anterior cruciate ligament injuries in adolescents with open physis: effect of recurrent injury and surgical delay on meniscal and cartilage injuries. Am J Sports Med 2014;42(5):1068–73.
17. Kolin DA, Dawkins B, Park J, et al. ACL Reconstruction Delay in Pediatric and Adolescent Patients Is Associated with a Progressive Increased Risk of Medial Meniscal Tears. J Bone Joint Surg Am 2021;103(15):1368–73.
18. Dumont GD, Hogue GD, Padalecki JR, et al. Meniscal and chondral injuries associated with pediatric anterior cruciate ligament tears: relationship of treatment time and patient-specific factors. Am J Sports Med 2012;40(9):2128–33.
19. Ramski DE, Kanj WW, Franklin CC, et al. Anterior cruciate ligament tears in children and adolescents: a meta-analysis of nonoperative versus operative treatment. Am J Sports Med 2014;42(11):2769–76.
20. James EW, Dawkins BJ, Schachne JM, et al. Early operative versus delayed operative versus nonoperative treatment of pediatric and adolescent anterior cruciate ligament injuries: a systematic review and meta-analysis. Am J Sports Med 2021;49(14):4008–17.
21. Pierce TR, Mehlman CT, Tamai J, et al. Access to care for the adolescent anterior cruciate ligament patient with Medicaid versus private insurance. J Pediatr Orthop 2012;32(3):245–8.
22. Zoller SD, Toy KA, Wang P, et al. Temporal relation of meniscal tear incidence, severity, and outcome scores in adolescents undergoing anterior cruciate ligament reconstruction. Knee Surg Sports Traumatol Arthrosc 2017;25(1):215–21.
23. Williams AA, Mancini NS, Solomito MJ, et al. Chondral injuries and irreparable meniscal tears among adolescents with anterior cruciate ligament or meniscal tears are more common in patients with public insurance. Am J Sports Med 2017;45(9):2111–5.

24. Bram JT, Talathi NS, Patel NM, et al. Affect the care of pediatric anterior cruciate ligament injuries? Clin J Sport Med 2020;30(6):e201–6.
25. Patel AR, Sarkisova N, Smith R, et al. Socioeconomic status impacts outcomes following pediatric anterior cruciate ligament reconstruction. Medicine (Baltimore) 2019;98(17):e15361.
26. Newman JT, Carry PM, Terhune EB, et al. Delay to reconstruction of the adolescent anterior cruciate ligament: the socioeconomic impact on treatment. Orthop J Sports Med 2014;2(8). 2325967114548176.
27. Ziedas A, Abed V, Swantek A, et al. Social determinants of health influence access to care and outcomes in patients undergoing anterior cruciate ligament reconstruction: a systematic review. Arthroscopy 2021;38(2):583–94.
28. Navarro RA, Inacio MC, Maletis GB. Does racial variation influence preoperative characteristics and intraoperative findings in patients undergoing anterior cruciate ligament reconstruction? Am J Sports Med 2015;43(12):2959–65.
29. Patel NM, Mai DH, Ramme AJ, et al. Is the incidence of paediatric stress fractures on the rise? Trends in New York State from 2000 to 2015. J Pediatr Orthop B 2020; 29(5):499–504.
30. Hyde ET, Omura JD, Fulton JE, et al. Disparities in Youth Sports Participation in the U.S., 2017-2018. Am J Prev Med 2020;59(5):e207–10.
31. Kanters MA, Bocarro JN, Edwards MB, et al. School sport participation under two school sport policies: comparisons by race/ethnicity, gender, and socioeconomic status. Ann Behav Med 2013;45(Suppl 1):S113–21.
32. Bellisari G, Samora W, Klingele K. Meniscus tears in children. Sports Med Arthrosc Rev 2011;19(1):50–5.
33. Englund M, Roos EM, Lohmander LS. Impact of type of meniscal tear on radiographic and symptomatic knee osteoarthritis: a sixteen-year followup of meniscectomy with matched controls. Arthritis Rheum 2003;48(8):2178–87.
34. McDermott ID, Amis AA. The consequences of meniscectomy. J Bone Joint Surg Br 2006;88(12):1549–56.
35. Roos H, Laurén M, Adalberth T, et al. Knee osteoarthritis after meniscectomy: prevalence of radiographic changes after twenty-one years, compared with matched controls. Arthritis Rheum 1998;41(4):687–93.
36. Rao AJ, Erickson BJ, Cvetanovich GL, et al. The meniscus-deficient knee: biomechanics, evaluation, and treatment options. Orthop J Sports Med 2015;3(10). 2325967115611386.
37. Pekari TB, Wang KC, Cotter EJ, et al. Contemporary surgical trends in the management of symptomatic meniscal tears among United States Military Servicemembers from 2010 to 2015. J Knee Surg 2019;32(2):196–204.
38. Johnson TR, Nguyen A, Shah K, et al. Impact of insurance status on time to evaluation and treatment of meniscal tears in children, adolescents, and college-aged patients in the United States. Orthop J Sports Med 2019;7(10). 2325967119875079.
39. Olson M, Pandya N. Public insurance status negatively affects access to care in pediatric patients with meniscal injury. Orthop J Sports Med 2021;9(1). 2325967120979989.
40. Sood A, Gonzalez-Lomas G, Gehrmann R. Influence of health insurance status on the timing of surgery and treatment of bucket-handle meniscus tears. Orthop J Sports Med 2015;3(5). 2325967115584883.
41. Smith HE, Lyons MM, Patel NM. Epidemiology of Meniscal Allograft Transplantation at Children's Hospitals in the United States. Orthop J Sports Med 2021;9(9). 23259671211034877.

42. De Smet AA, Ilahi OA, Graf BK. Untreated osteochondritis dissecans of the femoral condyles: prediction of patient outcome using radiographic and MR findings. Skeletal Radiol 1997;26(8):463–7.
43. Linden B. Osteochondritis dissecans of the femoral condyles: a long-term follow-up study. J Bone Joint Surg Am 1977;59(6):769–76.
44. Twyman RS, Desai K, Aichroth PM. Osteochondritis dissecans of the knee. A long-term study. J Bone Joint Surg Br 1991;73(3):461–4.
45. Kessler JI, Nikizad H, Shea KG, et al. The demographics and epidemiology of osteochondritis dissecans of the knee in children and adolescents. Am J Sports Med 2014;42(2):320–6.
46. Patel NM, Helber AR, Gandhi JS, et al. Race Predicts unsuccessful healing of osteochondritis dissecans in the pediatric knee. Orthopedics 2021;44(3):e378–84.
47. Wall EJ, Vourazeris J, Myer GD, et al. The healing potential of stable juvenile osteochondritis dissecans knee lesions. J Bone Joint Surg Am 2008;90(12):2655–64.
48. Krause M, Hapfelmeier A, Möller M, et al. Healing predictors of stable juvenile osteochondritis dissecans knee lesions after 6 and 12 months of nonoperative treatment. Am J Sports Med 2013;41(10):2384–91.
49. Adams AJ, Talathi NS, Gandhi JS, et al. Tibial spine fractures in children: evaluation, management, and future directions. J Knee Surg 2018;31(5):374–81.
50. Leeberg V, Sonne-Holm S, Krogh Christoffersen J, et al. Fractures of the knee in children-what can go wrong? A case file study of closed claims in The Patient Compensation Association covering 16 years. J Child Orthop 2015;9(5):391–6.
51. Smith HE, Mistovich RJ, Cruz AI Jr, et al. Does insurance status affect treatment of children with tibial spine fractures? Am J Sports Med 2021;49(14).
52. Skaggs DL, Clemens SM, Vitale MG, et al. Access to orthopedic care for children with medicaid versus private insurance in California. Pediatrics 2001;107(6):1405–8.
53. Skaggs DL, Lehmann CL, Rice C, et al. Access to orthopaedic care for children with medicaid versus private insurance: results of a national survey. J Pediatr Orthop 2006;26(3):400–4.
54. Beck JJ, West N, Shaw KG, et al. Delays in Obtaining Knee MRI in Pediatric Sports Medicine: Impact of Insurance Type. J Pediatr Orthop 2020;40(10):e952–7.
55. Wiznia DH, Schneble CA, O'Connor MI, et al. Musculoskeletal urgent care centers in connecticut restrict patients with medicaid insurance based on policy and location. Clin Orthop Relat Res 2020;478(7):1443–9.
56. Patterson BM, Draeger RW, Olsson EC, et al. A regional assessment of medicaid access to outpatient orthopaedic care: the influence of population density and proximity to academic medical centers on patient access. J Bone Joint Surg Am 2014;96(18):e156.
57. Rabah NM, Knusel KD, Khan HA, et al. Are There Nationwide Socioeconomic and Demographic Disparities in the Use of Outpatient Orthopaedic Services? Clin Orthop Relat Res 2020;478(5):979–89.
58. Wallace J, Covassin T, Moran R. Racial disparities in concussion knowledge and symptom recognition in american adolescent athletes. J Racial Ethn Health Disparities 2018;5(1):221–8.
59. Post EG, Roos KG, Rivas S, et al. Access to Athletic Trainer Services in California Secondary Schools. J Athl Train 2019;54(12):1229–36.
60. Boulware LE, Cooper LA, Ratner LE, et al. Race and trust in the health care system. Public Health Rep 2003;118(4):358–65.

61. Adegbembo AO, Tomar SL, Logan HL. Perception of racism explains the difference between Blacks' and Whites' level of healthcare trust. Ethn Dis 2006; 16(4):792–8.
62. Brandon DT, Isaac LA, LaVeist TA. The legacy of Tuskegee and trust in medical care: is Tuskegee responsible for race differences in mistrust of medical care? J Natl Med Assoc 2005;97(7):951–6.
63. Druckman JN, Trawalter S, Montes I, et al. Racial bias in sport medical staff's perceptions of others' pain. J Soc Psychol 2018;158(6):721–9.
64. Todd KH, Deaton C, D'Adamo AP, et al. Ethnicity and analgesic practice. Ann Emerg Med 2000;35(1):11–6.
65. DelPizzo K, Fiasconaro M, Wilson LA, et al. The utilization of regional anesthesia among pediatric patients: a Retrospective Study. HSS J 2020;16(Suppl 2): 425–35.

Pediatric and Adolescent Knee Injuries

Risk Factors and Preventive Strategies

Lauren S. Butler, PT, DPT, SCS[a], Joseph J. Janosky, DrPHc, MSc, PT, ATC[b], Dai Sugimoto, PhD, ATC[c,d],*

KEYWORDS

- Injury risk factors • Injury prevention • Primary prevention • Secondary prevention
- Tertiary prevention • Neuromuscular training • ACL

KEY POINTS

- There are several non-modifiable and modifiable risk factors that contribute to sports-related injury among young athletes. Modifiable risk factors should be targeted with injury prevention interventions.
- There are three distinct types of injury prevention interventions: primary, secondary, and tertiary.
- There are empirical studies supporting the protective effect of neuromuscular training against knee injury, including anterior cruciate ligament tears, in young athletes.
- Future directions include improving the translation of research evidence to clinical practices and increasing the use of evidence-based health promotion strategies to protect young athletes from preventable injury.

 Video content accompanies this article at http://www.sportsmed.theclinics.com.

INTRODUCTION

An estimated 60 million children participate in organized sports each year in the United States.[1] Sports participation is a major cause of musculoskeletal injuries in children,

Disclosure of Funding Source: None.
Financial Disclosure: All authors have no financial relationships relevant to this study to disclose.
Conflict of Interest: All authors have no conflict of interest to disclose.
[a] Nicklaus Children's Hospital, 3100 SW 62nd Ave, Miami, FL 33155, USA; [b] Sports Medicine Institute, Hospital for Special Surgery, 535 East 70th Street, New York, NY 10021, USA; [c] TheMicheli Center for Sports Injury Prevention, Waltham, MA, USA; [d] Faculty of Sport Sciences, Waseda University, 2-7-5, Higashifushimi, Nishi-Tokyo City, Tokyo 202-0021, Japan
* Corresponding author.
E-mail address: dai.sugimoto.007@gmail.com
Twitter: @LaurenSchlacht (L.S.B.); @joejanosky (J.J.J.); @Dai_Sugimoto (D.S.)

which can create a significant public health burden.[2] The knee has been cited as one of the most commonly injured body parts, with an estimated 2.5 million sports-related knee injuries occurring in adolescents annually in the United States.[3,4] Sports-related knee injuries result in significant time loss from physical activity and sport and often require surgical treatment.[5,6]

Sports-related knee injuries are classified as overuse or traumatic, with overuse injuries being more common.[7,8] A study evaluating knee injury patterns in high-school sports found knee injuries to be more prevalent in competition than in practice, with the highest injury rates occurring in football and girls soccer.[9] Another study reported the greatest rates of adolescent knee injuries in soccer and basketball.[10] The most frequent traumatic injuries reported involve the cruciate and collateral ligaments (medial collateral ligament [MCL], posterior cruciate ligament [PCL], anterior cruciate ligament [ACL], and lateral collateral ligament [LCL]), menisci, and patella. The most frequent overuse injuries reported include Osgood–Schlatter disease, Sinding–Larsen–Johansson syndrome, patellofemoral pain syndrome, and tendonitis.[8,9,11,12] Overall, females are reported to have a higher risk of sustaining a knee injury than males.[10] Ligament injuries, specifically ACL injuries, are among the most devastating knee injuries for young athletes. Female athletes have two to eight times greater risk of sustaining an ACL injury as compared with male athletes.[13–15] After ACL injury, there is a significant risk of developing osteoarthritis regardless of the treatment intervention, such as ACL reconstruction surgery.[16] Given the significant physical burden of ACL and other sports-related knee injuries, especially in females, it is imperative that injury prevention interventions are developed to effectively address modifiable injury risk factors. The use of appropriate clinical screening tools and targeted injury prevention strategies has the potential to considerably reduce the incidence of knee and ACL injuries in young athletes.[15]

RISK FACTORS

To implement effective injury prevention interventions, it is vital to understand the factors that increase the risk of suffering a sports-related knee injury. Injury risk factors can be categorized as non-modifiable and modifiable factors.

Non-modifiable Risk Factors

Athlete age, gender, injury history, sports history, and anatomical factors have been identified as non-modifiable risk factors for athletic knee injuries in children and adolescents.[3,10,12–15,17–37]

Age and gender
Female athletes have been found to have a higher risk of sustaining a knee injury, specifically an ACL injury when compared with male athletes.[10,13–15] It seems that this increase occurs during puberty in females.[15,17] During puberty, children experience a variety of anthropomorphic and hormonal adaptations that result in changes to body mass and body dimensions.[20] In male athletes, increases in power, strength, and coordination occur at proportionate rates to these changes.[18–20] However, it seems that females experience a neuromuscular lag during which increases in power, strength, and coordination do not occur with the same synchronicity as male athletes. It is hypothesized that this neuromuscular lag in the growth spurt may be a contributing factor to knee injury risk.[15,18,19]

The growth and development process may also increase susceptibility to overuse injuries to the epiphyseal plate or apophysis.[23] In the growing child, the physis is the weakest part of the bone; thus, the physis is often susceptible to injury as a result of excessive stress. Similarly, overuse apophyseal injuries occur as a result of excessive stress to the areas with major tendon insertions.[3,12,24,25]

Injury history

Several studies have identified a history of the previous injury as a significant risk factor for any sports-related injury and specifically for sustaining an overuse injury to the knee.[8,24,26,27] In addition, a history of a previous ACL injury has been found to increase the risk of sustaining a subsequent ACL injury, particularly in young athletes.[15,28] ACL reinjury rates are reported as high as 33% in athletes younger than age 25 who return to sports.[29] Screening for injury history may be an important component of injury prevention. A study by Engebretsen and colleagues[30] found that a simple questionnaire asking about injury history was able to predict those who went on to suffer an in-season injury in youth soccer players. Those who were flagged as high risk with the questionnaire were twice as likely to sustain an injury.[30] This is an important finding from both an injury prevention and a screening standpoint.

Anatomical factors

Generalized ligamentous laxity has been reported as a risk factor for both patellofemoral pain syndrome and ACL injuries.[31,32] Similarly, a large Q angle has been reported as a risk factor for patellofemoral pain syndrome, patellar instability, and ACL injury.[31,38] Several additional anatomical risk factors have been reported for ACL injury, including decreased intercondylar femoral notch size, decreased depth of concavity of the medial tibial plateau, increased slope of the tibial plateaus, and increased anterior-posterior knee laxity.[34–36,39] In one study, the identification of a narrow intercondylar notch inlet was associated with a positive predictive value of 70% in identifying those who suffered an ACL injury.[37]

Modifiable Risk Factors

Biomechanical and neuromuscular risk factors, training loads, and body mass index (BMI) have been identified as modifiable risk factors for sports-related knee injuries.

Biomechanical and neuromuscular control

There is an abundance of evidence suggesting that poor neuromuscular control of lower extremity biomechanics, specifically as it pertains to knee joint loading, is a significant contributor to knee injury risk.[21,40] Identifying athletes who are unable to adequately use muscular strength, power, and recruitment (those with poor neuromuscular control) to limit high knee joint loads can be very effective when implementing injury prevention interventions.[40] It must be acknowledged that there are unique differences between male and female individuals in the evaluation of biomechanical and neuromuscular risk factors. A systematic review by Hewett and colleagues[15] found that male and female individuals have different trunk and hip neuromuscular control and biomechanics, with female individuals demonstrating greater lateral trunk displacement, altered trunk and hip flexion angles, and greater ranges of trunk motion compared with male individuals. These same movement pattern dysfunctions have also been associated with patellofemoral pain in female athletes.[41] Post pubertal female individuals also demonstrate greater landing forces, altered quadriceps and hamstring activation strategies, and altered hip recruitment strategies compared with male individuals.[15,18,42] These altered hip strategies contribute to higher knee to hip moment ratios, decreased gluteal activation, increased rectus femoris activation, and greater hip adduction angles and moments, which were theorized to have injury risk implications.[15,43] In female athletes, knee abduction loads predict ACL injury and trunk displacement predicts both knee and ACL injury with high sensitivity and specificity.[40,44] However, in male athletes, trunk displacement has not been found to be predictive of knee or ACL injury.[44] Poor frontal plane knee control has also been cited as a contributing factor to the increased risk of suffering an overuse injury to the knee.[11]

Video evaluation of actual ACL injuries revealed four common motor performance components, including lateral trunk deviation, knee abduction motion, flatfoot position, and increased hip flexion.[45,46] These movement patterns have been further classified into four neuromuscular imbalances known as dominance categories to help guide injury prevention interventions. The four dominance categories consist of ligament dominance, trunk dominance, leg dominance, and quadriceps dominance.

Ligament dominance. Ligament dominance is characterized by a frontal plane collapse of the hip and knee, with the athlete relying on static stabilizers (ligaments) to absorb ground reaction forces rather than lower extremity musculature.[47] As previously mentioned, female athletes adopt hip strategies during athletic movements that result in increased knee abduction moments and thus increase ACL injury risk.[15,42,45] Carefully observing the way an athlete lands from a jump can help identify if a ligament dominance movement pattern is present. When observing an athlete land from a jump, he or she will likely demonstrate a dynamic valgus collapse of the lower extremity. This may include thigh adduction or internal rotation, knee abduction, tibia external rotation, and/or foot pronation. **Fig. 1** illustrates an athlete with a ligament dominance landing strategy. The muscles of the posterior chain (gluteals, hamstrings, and gastrocsoleus muscles) are critically important in mitigating this frontal plane collapse and should be targeted with injury prevention interventions.[47] Exercises such as single-leg deadlifts, banded squats, and lateral step downs are effective for the rehabilitation of athletes with ligament dominance (Videos 1–3). In addition, implementing motor control strategies and biofeedback are important components of improving athletes' landing strategies. Performing double-and single-leg plyometric exercises while providing various types of feedback, aimed to improve the athlete's landing posture, are recommended. For example, visual feedback from a mirror or video playback, can be used to highlight suboptimal valgus landing postures to facilitate movement pattern correction. Tactile cues, such as placing a resistance band around the athlete's knees, can also be used to facilitate hip abduction and external rotation, allowing for more favorable landing strategies.

Trunk dominance. Decreased ability to control trunk displacement is a sensitive predictor of the knee, ligament, and ACL injury.[15] An athlete's inability to sense the position of their trunk in space, or so-called trunk proprioception, can lead to excessive trunk displacement. When excessive trunk lateral displacement occurs over the stance limb, there is an observed lateral shift of the center of mass. This lateral center of mass shift can result in valgus collapse at the knee, thus increasing injury risk.[47] Athletes with trunk dominance may present with sagittal or frontal plane trunk deviations during athletic tasks. They may also have difficulty maintaining lower limb placement underneath their center of mass. **Fig. 2** shows an athlete with a trunk dominant landing strategy. Postural control exercises that challenge the athlete's ability to maintain their center of mass over their base of support can be used to address trunk dominance. Exercises such as single-limb kneeling on an unstable surface and single-leg squats with trunk perturbation are examples of effective exercises to address postural control deficits (Videos 4 and 5).

Leg dominance. The muscular imbalance between limbs with regard to strength and muscle recruitment has been described as leg dominance, with greater asymmetry

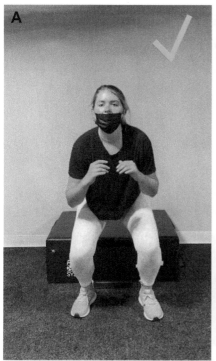 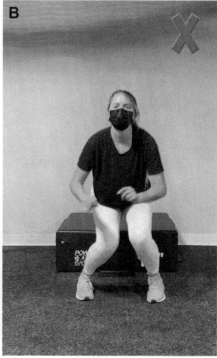

Fig. 1. An athlete landing from a drop vertical jump demonstrating good technique as shown with good frontal plane knee control (*A*) and poor technique with ligament dominance as shown with frontal plan collapse of the lower extremities into a dynamic valgus position (*B*).

resulting in a greater risk of future injury.[47] Women demonstrate greater differences in strength, flexibility, and muscle recruitment patterns between limbs compared with males.[47–50] These differences may lead to more significant asymmetrical lower extremity loading in female athletes. In addition, asymmetries in lower extremity loading are not uncommon after sports-related injuries.[51] Athletes with greater asymmetry in double-leg landing demonstrate a greater risk of injury.[40,47] Anecdotally, leg dominant movement strategies may be observed as a preferential loading of one limb over the other during bilateral tasks such as squatting and jumping. During single-limb tasks, differences in hop distances, vertical displacement, and quality of landings may be observed. **Fig. 3** highlights an athlete with a leg dominant movement strategy during an overhead squat. Single-leg training addressing strength and power and single-leg hopping drills addressing power and landing stability can effectively target a leg dominant movement strategy (Videos 6–8).

Quadriceps dominance. Quadriceps dominance describes a strategy used to stabilize the knee joint by primarily activating the quadriceps muscles.[47] In the clinic, this activation pattern may be present as stiff knee posturing on the jump and hop landings, loud landing contact sounds, and increased knee extension on the plant leg during a cutting maneuver. This extended knee posture can result in increased external knee extension moments, which, in the absence of adequate posterior chain muscle recruitment, increases stress on the knee joint and contributes to a higher injury risk.[47]

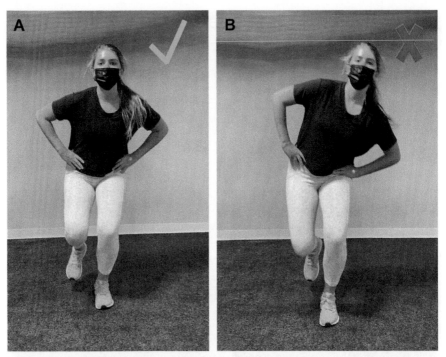

Fig. 2. An athlete landing from a single-leg hop demonstrating good technique as shown with the trunk maintained over the hips (*A*) and poor technique with trunk dominance as shown with an excessive ipsilateral trunk lean (*B*).

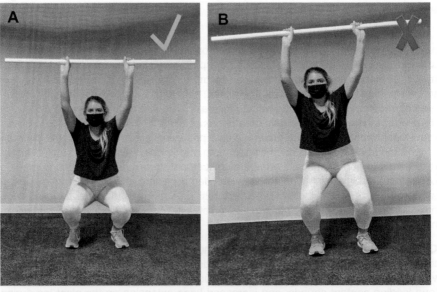

Fig. 3. An athlete performing an overhead squat demonstrating good technique as shown with symmetrical loading of the right and left lower extremity (*A*) and poor technique with leg dominance as shown with the athlete asymmetrically loading the right lower extremity greater than the left lower extremity (*B*).

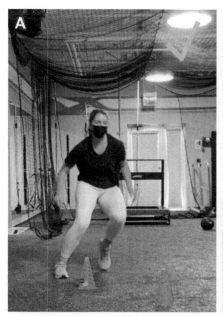
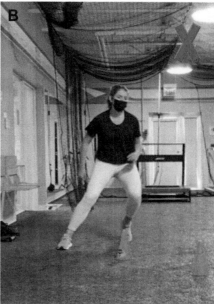

Fig. 4. An athlete performing a 45-degree side-step cut with good technique as shown with appropriate knee flexion during the loading phase (*A*) and poor technique with quadriceps dominance as shown with an excessively stiff and extended knee position during the loading phase (*B*).

Fig. 4 shows an athlete with a quadriceps dominant cutting strategy. Plyometric training is effective in addressing quadriceps dominance through the use of biofeedback aimed at increasing knee flexion and decreasing contact noise at landing. Neuromuscular reeducation focused on increasing knee flexion excursion during squatting, jumping, and cutting tasks is also recommended as shown in Video 9.

Training loads

Several studies have identified an association between high training volumes and increased risks of sustaining an overuse injury.[8,24,26] In a 2009 study examining sports injury risk factors in junior high-school athletes, the average weekly hours spent playing sports and the number of sports played were identified as the most significant risk factors for all sports-related injuries.[26] Specific to knee injuries, participation in sports greater than two times per week was identified as a significant risk factor for both traumatic and overuse knee injuries.[8]

Body mass index

Pediatric obesity is a major public health concern and increases a child's risk of developing orthopedic disorders of the knee joint.[52] In 2018, the prevalence of childhood obesity in the United States was 19.3%, affecting more than 14 million children.[53] In 2017, less than one-quarter (24%) of children aged 6 to 17 in the United States participated in the recommended 60-min of daily physical activity, whereas only 51% of high-school students participated in muscle-strengthening activities on at least 3 days per week.[54] Furthermore, according to a report by Ling and colleagues[55] (2020), less than 24% of children aged 8 to 17 years demonstrated the ability to complete fundamental movement skills and common neuromuscular training (NMT) exercises with proper technique. Considered collectively, high levels of obesity, low levels of physical activity, and poor overall movement quality among children contribute to widespread injury susceptibility. In a study of high-school athletes, obese athletes were found to sustain a larger proportion of knee injuries compared with normal-weight peers.[56] It was also found that underweight athletes sustained a larger proportion of overuse injuries.[56] Furthermore, having a greater BMI has been identified as a risk factor for noncontact ACL injuries in female athletes.[57] Higher BMI has been associated with increased anterior-posterior knee laxity and increased knee joint compression forces, which may lead to an increased risk of ACL injuries in young athletes.[58] Given the association between BMI and injury risk, it may be advantageous for sports medicine clinicians to educate young athletes on the importance of healthy eating and routine physical activity habits.

Summary

Numerous modifiable and non-modifiable risk factors are associated with athletic knee injuries in children and adolescents. Clinicians should aim to identify modifiable risk factors that can be targeted with specific interventions with the overall goal of reducing injury risk.

INJURY PREVENTION
Types of Prevention Strategies

The natural history of many knee injuries in the pediatric population, most notably ACL rupture, is associated with a plethora of physiological and biomechanical dysfunction. Secondary injury to knee cartilage, premature loss of joint surface integrity, and recurrent joint instability are common among active individuals who receive conservative (nonsurgical) treatment.[59] In addition, it has been reported that when ACL rupture is left untreated, it can lead to long-term osteoarthritic changes caused by joint laxity and rotatory instability.[60] The natural history of knee injuries mirrors that of the natural history of the disease that includes five fundamental phases underlying, susceptible, subclinical, clinical, and outcome.[61]

Strategies designed to prevent pediatric knee injuries and protect individuals from undesirable long-term sequelae typically consist of activities designed to reduce the risk of the injury and minimize the impact of injury on health. The US Centers for Disease Control and Prevention (CDC) presented a conceptual framework that categorized three types of injury prevention activities, commonly referred to as interventions, according to the phases of the natural history of injury.[62] The first category of preventive interventions corresponds to the underlying and susceptible phases of the natural history of injury and is referred to as primary preventive interventions. CDC described primary interventions as those designed to prevent injury among entire populations by maximizing the effects of protective factors and eliminating exposure to risk factors.[57]

The second category of preventive interventions corresponds to the subclinical phase and is referred to as secondary preventive interventions. Secondary interventions emphasize the early detection of injury risk factors and are typically implemented as screenings.[57] The third category of preventive interventions corresponds to the clinical and outcomes phases and is referred to as tertiary preventive interventions. CDC reported that tertiary interventions focus on reducing the severity of an existing injury and preventing the recurrence of an injury through the delivery of medical treatment and/or rehabilitative services.[57]

Primary preventive interventions

Primary preventive interventions targeting the youth population include public health-based education programs designed to promote health and decrease injury risk by increasing physical activity rates and promoting high-quality movement patterns. For example, a comprehensive guide to design and conduct school-based physical activity programs for teachers and school administrators was introduced,[63] whereas the Comprehensive School Physical Activity Program (CSPAP) was developed by CDC in collaboration with SHAPE America to develop new or improve existing school-based physical activity programs.[64] In addition, a curriculum designed specifically for middle- and high-school physical education teachers was released in 2021 to foster the delivery of movement training for school students.[65]

Young athletes constitute a segment of the broader youth population that is more susceptible to a knee injury, requiring more specific primary preventive interventions. Collectively, sports coaches are often prioritized as one of the most important groups to consider when designing and delivering interventions that ultimately benefit young athletes, but outcomes associated with the adoption and implementation through coach education are largely unknown. One study identified that training coaches helped to enhance adoption and implementation of an injury prevention program regardless of their perceptions of the injury prevention program.[66] Similarly, it has been reported that a coach education intervention improved adherence to recommendations for implementing an NMT program designed to serve as a protective factor against lower extremity musculoskeletal injury, whereas feedback cues can improve the alignment and technique of children performing ACL injury prevention exercises.[55] Contrastingly, several researchers have reported low compliance with the implementation of NMT by sports coaches, with many noting associations between low rates of compliance with injury prevention interventions and high rates of ACL injury.[13,67–69]

Secondary preventive interventions

The second category of preventive interventions is referred to as secondary preventive interventions. This category of interventions emphasizes the early detection of injury risk factors and is typically developed and implemented as screenings.[62] Screening tools capable of targeting those at high risk for a knee injury can help identify those who will benefit the most from injury prevention interventions.[15] Several screening tools are recommended to assess movement pattern dysfunction related to knee and ACL injury risk.

Anterior cruciate ligament nomogram. The ACL Nomogram is a clinic-based algorithm that assesses five biomechanical factors that have been shown to accurately identify high knee abduction moments during landings.[47,49,70] The algorithm captures tibia length, knee valgus displacement, knee flexion ROM during a drop vertical jump, body mass, and quadriceps: hamstring strength ratio.[47,49,70] The algorithm has been found to predict high knee abduction moments during a drop vertical jump with 84% sensitivity and 67% specificity in young female athletes.[49] The ACL Nomogram serves as a practical tool for clinicians to identify athletes who may demonstrate high knee abduction moments and a higher ACL injury risk.

Tuck jump assessment. The tuck jump assessment tool was developed to identify high-risk landing mechanics during a high-intensity plyometric task. It involves real-time or video-based scoring of a 10-s repeated tuck jump task and specifically evaluates the athlete's symmetry, trunk control, and landing quality. The tuck jump assessment tool has been found to have good to excellent inter- and intra-rater reliability when evaluating performance in male and female adolescent athletes.[71] Specific movement pattern dysfunctions identified with the tuck jump assessment tool can be targeted with injury prevention interventions.

Landing Error Scoring System. The Landing Error Scoring System (LESS) is a field-based assessment tool to identify high-risk movement patterns during a drop vertical jump.[33,72] The LESS involves scoring suboptimal movement patterns in both the frontal and sagittal planes, with higher scores indicating poorer landing technique. The LESS has demonstrated good inter- rater and intra-rater reliability and concurrent validity with three-dimensional (3D) motion analysis.[33,66] The predictive validity of the LESS has also been explored with conflicting results. One study found the LESS total score to have a positive predictive value of 1.6% in predicting ACL injury in youth soccer players (age = 13.9 ± 1.8 years; 25% from 11 to 12 years of age).[73] A similar study in multisport high-school and collegiate athletes found no relationship between the ACL injury risk and the LESS scores.[33]

Although more work is needed to establish its predictive validity in identifying those at high risk for ACL injury, the LESS is a valuable tool for assessing jump landing techniques.

Qualitative analysis of single-leg loading. The qualitative analysis of single leg loading (QASLS) involves dichotomous scoring of inappropriate movement strategies occurring in specific body regions (arm, trunk, pelvis, thigh, knee, and foot) during single-leg loading tasks.[74] The tool has been shown to have excellent validity compared to 3D motion capture kinematics during single-leg squatting and landing tasks.[74] It has also been found to have good to excellent intra- and interraterreliability.[75] Higher scores on the QASLS indicate poorer movement quality. Given the relationship between neuromuscular deficits and ACL and knee injury risk, screening tools that can aid in the identification of movement pattern dysfunction during single-leg squatting and landings are an important component of knee injury risk screening and prevention interventions.

Assessment of cutting technique. Knee injury often occurs with cutting or change of direction tasks in sport.[76] Specifically, lateral trunk motion with the body shifted over the stance limb, knee valgus, wide foot plant, knee extension, and decreased plantar flexion have been found to be related to high knee joint loads during the performance of a cutting task.[77,78] Cutting techniques and movement patterns are modifiable; therefore, screening tools capable of identifying risky movement patterns during a cutting task may aid in targeted injury prevention interventions. Furthermore, interventions aimed to modify suboptimal cutting techniques have been shown to be effective in reducing the occurrence of high-risk movement faults.[79] The Cutting Movement Assessment Score (CMAS), a qualitative scoring system to evaluate a 90-degree cutting maneuver, is a reliable and valid tool to assess risky movement patterns during a 90-degree cutting task.[73] The CMAS involves a visual assessment of eight movement variables observed in the frontal, sagittal, and 45-degree planes derived from 2D video recordings. Subjects with higher CMAS scores have been found to demonstrate higher knee joint loading, suggesting its efficacy in knee injury risk assessment.[73] Similarly, the Cutting Alignment Scoring Tool (CAST), a qualitative scoring system to evaluate at a 45-degree side-step cut, has also been found to be a reliable tool in assessing risky movement patterns. The CAST involves dichotomous scoring of four frontal plane movement variables observed from 2D video during a planned 45-degree side step cut.[80]

Tertiary preventive interventions

The third category of preventive interventions is referred to as tertiary preventive interventions. CDC reported that tertiary interventions focus on reducing the severity of an existing injury and/or preventing the recurrence of injury through the delivery of medical treatment and/or rehabilitative services.[62]

Tertiary preventive interventions targeting children and adolescents include health care services designed to promote recovery from injury and reduce the risk of subsequent injury.

Surgical treatment of sports-related knee injury is an increasingly common intervention among this population in the United States. According to a report, the rate of ACL reconstruction procedures among individuals aged 3 to 20 years increased from 17.6 per 100,000 in 1990 to 50.9 per 100,000 in 2009.[81] Similarly, another study queried the Pediatric Health Information System (PHIS) database and reported that the number of ACL reconstruction surgeries performed on individuals aged 18 years or younger increased 5.7-fold between 2004 and 2014, whereas all orthopedic surgeries in this population increased 1.7-fold.[82] It has been reported that although pediatric patients with ACL injury were most often evaluated objectively by a degree of knee joint laxity and subjectively with the International Knee Documentation Committee (IKDC) Subjective Knee Form, a standardized set of outcome measures is currently lacking.[83]

Physical rehabilitation is another widely used tertiary intervention that promotes recovery from a knee injury and helps to reduce the risk of recurrent injury. Standing in stark contrast to historical time-based standards, most current rehabilitation protocols use functional benchmarks to evaluate recovery status. Widespread support for supervised rehabilitation programs supported by evidence-based clinical reasoning and achievement of function-based milestones has been described.[84]

Injury Prevention Evidence

Concepts of primary, secondary, and tertiary preventions were highlighted in the recent ACL research retreat VIII summary statement.[85] Along with the three layers of preventive concepts, the effectiveness of NMT on ACL injury reduction was discussed, highlighting recent meta-analysis studies.[86] There have been several meta-analytic studies to determine the effectiveness of preventive NMT as a whole.[87] All documented studies suggested an approximately 50% reduction of ACL injury risk if NMT is performed.[87,88] In addition to ACL injury prevention, the prevention initiative using NMT extended to a groin injury in football/soccer field players,[89] a shoulder injury in football/soccer goalkeepers,[90] and an elbow injury in baseball throwers.[91]

Preventive NMT has various benefits beyond preventing musculoskeletal injuries in physically active individuals. According to Swart and colleagues,[92] if NMT is applied to all athletes as a "universal" training program, significant medical cost reduction along with ACL injury decline is estimated. Recent studies found reinjury rates can be as high as 33% following ACL reconstruction surgery.[29] In addition, substantial future osteoarthritis risk following ACL injury and reconstruction was well documented.[93,94] If ACL injury incidence is reduced by NMT, the risk of ACL reinjury and future osteoarthritis cases will also be reduced. Therefore, the objective of this section is to review previous NMT-based injury prevention programs and discuss key aspects to enhance prophylactic effectiveness.

Exercise recommendations for prevention

Numerous ACL injury prevention programs, such as PEP,[95] the "11",[96] HarmoKnee,[97] and HIP[98] have been cited in the last two decades. A few studies analyzed the effect of the NMT on neuromuscular and biomechanical variables in laboratory settings.[70,99] On the other hand, there were approximately 20 prospective studies that used ACL injury as an outcome variable to examine the effectiveness of NMT.[87] The NMT-based ACL injury prevention programs used in those prospective studies were diverse. However, two studies analyzed which type of exercises should be included in NMT to enhance prophylactic effectiveness.[87,100] One study identified that the NMT-based program needs to include multiple exercises instead of a single exercise type.[100] In addition, another study suggested to include muscular strength and proximal control exercises in NMT.[100] In this study, proximal control was defined as exercise that involved segments proximal to the knee joint.[101] There was one commonly used exercise that included both muscular strength and proximal control—the Nordic/Russian hamstring curl. Several NMT-based programs that used the Nordic/Russian hamstring curl exercise demonstrated notable ACL injury reduction.[95,96,102] Another investigation reported that studies that included both muscular strength and landing stabilization are the most effective.[87] The lead author of this study, Petushek, referenced a drop-landing maneuver and jump/hop and held as examples of landing stabilization exercises.[89] Lunges, hamstring exercises (Nordic/Russian hamstring curl), and heel/calf raises were also suggested as a part of ACL prevention best practices.[89]

Other key components for prevention

Along with the type of exercise, a few key components that enhance the prophylactic effectiveness of NMT are reported.[100,103] Two studies suggested that athletes younger than 18 years old showed greater ACL injury reduction than athletes over 19 years old if they performed NMT.[100,104] The two studies suggested that early teens or even younger ages are ideal to begin NMT. In addition to athlete age, NMT volume and dosage appear to be a vital aspect. One study investigated the amount of NMT that would need to be performed to effectively reduce ACL injury risk.[88] This study suggested an NMT volume of at least 30 min per week during in-season to show meaningful ACL injury risk reduction.[88] The authors suggested that performing NMT multiple times per week with a duration of 10–15 min per session may be a more practical approach instead of a single 30-min NMT session per week.[88] Another vital element of NMT that needs to be applied is verbal feedback. One study identified that high knee abduction during a jump-landing maneuver is the most sensitive and specific risk factor for noncontact ACL injury.[40] To reduce high knee abduction, an NMT program was implemented in a group of young athletes.[105] In this study, verbal feedback on movement quality during the session was given to one group, but not the other group.[105] After 8 weeks, young athletes in the verbal feedback group demonstrated a mean reduction of 6.7 degrees of knee abduction.[105] However, athletes who did not receive verbal feedback only saw a mean knee abduction angle reduction of 2.8 degrees.[105] Furthermore, elevated ground reaction force (GRF) was also identified in young athletes who sustained noncontact ACL injury compared with young athletes who did not.[43] Three laboratory studies that used plyometric exercises measured GRF between pre-training and post-training.[106–108] Two studies that provided verbal feedback in their training showed 22.0% and 26.4% of GRF reduction,[106] whereas the GRF reduction of the one study that did not give verbal feedback was 7.4%.[108] In short, there are several key components to enhance prophylactics of NMT, including athlete's age, dosage/volume of NMT, and status of verbal feedback. If 30 min of NMT with verbal feedback is performed on a weekly basis during the in-season among early teenage athletes, ACL injury risk can be considerably reduced.

Summary

Concepts of primary, secondary, and tertiary prevention strategies were summarized, and the efficaciousness of NMT on ACL injury reduction was presented. Moreover, parameters that enhance prophylactic effectiveness were highlighted.

FUTURE DIRECTIONS

Although the efficacy of some injury prevention programs has been documented in scientific journals, translating the research evidence to routine practice is challenging. One article highlighted that the complexity of translating injury prevention research evidence into handball training was well highlighted.[109] In this study, reduced ACL injury incidence rates were recorded as a knee injury prevention program was implemented with Norwegian female handball players over a 2-year period.[109] However, after program implementation ended, ACL injury incidence rates returned to pre-study levels.[109] Concerningly, the ACL injury incidence rate 2 years later was worse than baseline levels.[109] According to the authors, the increase in ACL injury incidence rates occurred because the handball coaches involved in the study did not continue to implement knee injury prevention programming with their players because they thought it was just a research study and did not realize the potential health benefits for their players. Subsequently, the research team recorded their knee injury prevention program exercises in digital video disc (DVD) format and provided it to the handball coaches. After the DVD distribution, ACL injury incidence rate showed an immediate decline.[109] This study highlighted the important role that researchers play in translating research evidence into practice.

Some researchers have examined adherence/compliance with recommendations for implementing ACL injury prevention programs.[110,111,112] Both high[98,112] and low adherence/compliance rates of ACL injury prevention programs were reported.[69,96,108] instead of sugimoto critical component In response to these conflicting findings, Joy and colleagues[113] asked football/soccer coaches for the reasons why prevention programs are not well used. The top reported barrier to program implementation by a sample of more than 700 coaches was a lack of knowledge about injury prevention.[112] Therefore, developing effective coach education programs and deploying education specialists to collaborate with sports coaches may be key factors for translating evidence to practice.

The translating research into injury prevention practice (TRIPP) theory was developed based on the four pillars of the injury prevention model developed by Van Mechelen.[114] In addition to the four pillars, two additional components were added to the model, which are (1) describing the intervention context and (2) implementing it in the real world and assessing its effectiveness.[113] Furthermore, one study introduced seven specific steps to implement a prevention program, which include (1) establishing administrative support, (2) developing an interdisciplinary team, (3) identifying logistical barriers and solutions, (4) developing an evidence-based prevention training program, (5) trainning the trainers and users, (6) managing progam fidelity (adherence/compliance), and (7) processing an exist strategy. Taking these steps may help facilitatethe successful adoption of injury prevention programs as routine practices.[115])

CDC usses a scientific method to develop injury prevention programs known as the public health approach to injury prevention. This process includes four unique steps: defining the problem, identifying risk and protective factors, developing and testing prevention strategies, and assuring widespread adoption of effective injury prevention principles and strategies.[116] Few knee injury prevention researchers have published studies that follow a public health approach to program development, implementation, and evaluation, contributing to the limited real-world effectiveness that has spanned at least 2 decades.

Effective injury prevention and health promotion programs share several common characteristics, including:

1. The application of behavior science during program development,
2. The use of evidence-based interventions during program implementation, and
3. The integration of formative, process, outcome, and impact evaluations during all stages of the program's lifespan.

Unfortunately, there is an alarming paucity of knee injury prevention programming and research that share all of these crucial attributes.

Meaningful reductions in rates of injury incidence and prevalence cannot be expected without a change in human behavior. Behavioral science can be leveraged to explain factors that contribute to injury and develop interventions to change behaviors that contribute to injury.[117] Despite the limited application of behavioral science in sports injury prevention research, many successful injury prevention programs have been developed with one or more behavior change theories as to their foundation. For example, the Theory of Planned Behavior, the Health Belief Model, the Integrated Behavior Model, Social Cognitive Theory, and the Transtheoretical Model have all been used to develop effective injury prevention programs.[118–121] Unfortunately, a few knee injury prevention programs incorporate behavior change theory during program development.

Similarly, most knee injury prevention programs focus on the implementation and evaluation of exercise-based preventive interventions (eg, NMT). The implementation and evaluation of education-based preventive interventions are notably underrepresented in the literature, whereas most programs lack comprehensive approaches to evaluation. Most knee injury prevention programs provide valuable summative evaluation data (eg, injury incidence rates) but fail to include formative evaluation data. Collaboration between sports medicine and public health practitioners may help to improve program design, implementation, and evaluation and positively impact the health of young athletes in the future.

SUMMARY

Given the high prevalence of sports-related knee injuries in the pediatric population, the identification and implementation of appropriate screening tools and injury prevention strategies is imperative. To develop successful injury prevention strategies, risk factor identification is an important first step. There are two types of risk factors: non-modifiable (age, gender, injury/sport history, and anatomical) and modifiable risk factors (biomechanical, neuromuscular control, training loads, and BMI). Three types of preventive interventions, primary, secondary, and tertiary, can address these risk factors. To enhance the efficaciousness of NMT for knee injury prevention, athlete's age, training dosage, exercise mode, and verbal feedback are critical components. Furthermore, to translate study evidence to clinical practices and routine training, awareness of injury prevention and health promotion needs to be further strengthened.

CLINICS CARE POINTS

- There are non-modifiable and modifiable risk factors. To develop injury prevention strategies, the focus should be on modifiable risk factors.
- Injury prevention strategies consist of multiple layers including primary, secondary, and tertiary interventions in the current public health promotion model.
- To enhance the efficaciousness of neuromuscular training for knee injury prevention, including ACL injuries, athlete's age, training dosage, exercise mode, and verbal feedback are critical components.

- Increasing the use of health promotion strategies when developing injury prevention interventions is necessary to improve effectiveness.

DISCLOSURE

The authors have nothing to disclose.

SUPPLEMENTARY DATA

Supplementary data related to this article can be found online at https://doi.org/10.1016/j.csm.2022.05.011.

REFERENCES

1. Calmbach WL, Hutchens M. Evaluation of patients presenting with knee pain: part I. history, physical examination, radiographs, and laboratory tests. Am Fam Physician 2003;68(5):907–12.
2. Goldberg A, Moroz L, Smith A, et al. Injury surveillance in young athletes: a clinician's guide to sports injury literature. Sports Med 2007;37(3):265–78.
3. Caine D, Maffulli N, Caine C. Epidemiology of injury in child and adolescent sports: injury rates, risk factors, and prevention. Clin Sports Med 2008;27(1): 19–50.
4. Gage BE, McIlvain NM, Collins CL, et al. Epidemiology of 6.6 million knee injuries presenting to United States emergency departments from 1999 through 2008. Acad Emerg Med 2012;19(4):378–85.
5. Fernandez WG, Yard EE, Comstock RD. Epidemiology of lower extremity injuries among US high school athletes. Acad Emerg Med 2007;14(7):641–5.
6. Rechel JA, Collins CL, Comstock RD. Epidemiology of injuries requiring surgery among high school athletes in the united states, 2005 to 2010. J Trauma Acute Care Surg 2011;71(4):982–9.
7. Jespersen E, Rexen C, Franz C, et al. Musculoskeletal extremity injuries in a cohort of schoolchildren aged 6–12: a 2.5-year prospective study. Scand J Med Sci Sports 2015;25(2):251–8.
8. Junge T, Runge L, Juul-Kristensen B, et al. Risk factors for knee injuries in children 8-15 years: the CHAMPS-study DK. Med Sci Sports Exerc 2016;48(4): 655–62.
9. Swenson DM, Collins CL, Best TM, et al. Epidemiology of knee injuries among U.S. high school athletes, 2005/2006-2010/2011. Med Sci Sports Exerc 2013; 45(3):462–9.
10. Louw QA, Manilall J, Grimmer KA. Epidemiology of knee injuries among adolescents: a systematic review. Br J Sports Med 2008;42(1):2–10.
11. O'Kane JW, Neradilek M, Polissar N, et al. Risk factors for lower extremity overuse injuries in female youth soccer players. Orthopaedic J Sports Med 2017; 5(10). 2325967117733963.
12. Arnold A, Thigpen CA, Beattie PF, et al. Overuse physeal injuries in youth athletes: risk factors, prevention, and treatment strategies. Sports health 2017; 9(2):139–47.
13. Hewett TE, Lindenfeld TN, Riccobene JV, et al. The effect of neuromuscular training on the incidence of knee injury in female athletes. Am J Sports Med 1999;27(6):699–706.

14. Arendt E, Dick R. Knee injury patterns among men and women in collegiate basketball and soccer: NCAA data and review of literature. Am J Sports Med 1995;23(6):694–701.

15. Hewett TE, Myer GD, Ford KR, et al. Mechanisms, prediction, and prevention of ACL injuries: Cut risk with three sharpened and validated tools. J Orthop Res 2016;34(11):1843–55.

16. Lohmander L, Östenberg A, Englund M, et al. High prevalence of knee osteoarthritis, pain, and functional limitations in female soccer players twelve years after anterior cruciate ligament injury. Arthritis Rheum 2004;50(10):3145–52.

17. Andrish JT. Anterior cruciate ligament injuries in the skeletally immature patient. Am J Orthop (Belle Mead NJ) 2001;30(2):103–10.

18. Quatman CE, Ford KR, Myer GD, et al. Maturation leads to gender differences in landing force and vertical jump performance: a longitudinal study. Am J Sports Med 2006;34(5):806–13.

19. Hewett TE, Myer GD, Ford KR. Decrease in neuromuscular control about the knee with maturation in female athletes. JBJS 2004;86(8):1601–8.

20. Lloyd RS, Oliver JL, Faigenbaum AD, et al. Chronological age vs. biological maturation: Implications for exercise programming in youth. J Strength Cond Res 2014;28(5):1454–64.

21. Hewett TE. Neuromuscular and hormonal factors associated with knee injuries in female athletes. Sports Med 2000;29(5):313–27.

22. Hewett TE, Zazulak BT, Myer GD. Effects of the menstrual cycle on anterior cruciate ligament injury risk: a systematic review. Am J Sports Med 2007;35(4):659–68.

23. Valovich McLeod TC, Decoster LC, Loud KJ, et al. National athletic trainers' association position statement: Prevention of pediatric overuse injuries. J Athletic Train 2011;46(2):206–20.

24. Caine D, Caine C, Maffulli N. Incidence and distribution of pediatric sport-related injuries. Clin J Sport Med 2006;16(6):500–13.

25. DiFiori JP, Benjamin HJ, Brenner JS, et al. Overuse injuries and burnout in youth sports: a position statement from the american medical society for sports medicine. Br J Sports Med 2014;48(4):287–8.

26. Emery C, Tyreman H. Sport participation, sport injury, risk factors and sport safety practices in calgary and area junior high schools. Paediatrics Child Health 2009;14(7):439–44.

27. Emery CA. Risk factors for injury in child and adolescent sport: a systematic review of the literature. Clin J Sport Med 2003;13(4):256–68.

28. Paterno MV, Rauh MJ, Schmitt LC, et al. Incidence of contralateral and ipsilateral anterior cruciate ligament (ACL) injury after primary ACL reconstruction and return to sport. Clin J Sport Med 2012;22(2):116.

29. Dekker TJ, Godin JA, Dale KM, et al. Return to sport after pediatric anterior cruciate ligament reconstruction and its effect on subsequent anterior cruciate ligament injury. JBJS 2017;99(11):897–904.

30. Engebretsen AH, Myklebust G, Holme I, et al. Prevention of injuries among male soccer players: a prospective, randomized intervention study targeting players with previous injuries or reduced function. Am J Sports Med 2008;36(6):1052–60.

31. Waryasz GR, McDermott AY. Patellofemoral pain syndrome (PFPS): a systematic review of anatomy and potential risk factors. Dynamic Med 2008;7(1):1–14.

32. Kramer L, Denegar C, Buckley WE, et al. Factors associated with anterior cruciate ligament injury: history in female athletes. J Sports Med Phys Fitness 2007;47(4):446.
33. Smith HC, Johnson RJ, Shultz SJ, et al. A prospective evaluation of the landing error scoring system (LESS) as a screening tool for anterior cruciate ligament injury risk. Am J Sports Med 2012;40(3):521–6.
34. LaPrade RF, Burnett QM. Femoral intercondylar notch stenosis and correlation to anterior cruciate ligament injuries: a prospective study. Am J Sports Med 1994;22(2):198–203.
35. Xiao W, Yang T, Cui Y, et al. Risk factors for noncontact anterior cruciate ligament injury: analysis of parameters in proximal tibia using anteroposterior radiography. J Int Med Res 2016;44(1):157–63.
36. Sturnick DR, Vacek PM, DeSarno MJ, et al. Combined anatomic factors predicting risk of anterior cruciate ligament injury for males and females. Am J Sports Med 2015;43(4):839–47.
37. Simon R, Everhart J, Nagaraja H, et al. A case-control study of anterior cruciate ligament volume, tibial plateau slopes and intercondylar notch dimensions in ACL-injured knees. J Biomech 2010;43(9):1702–7.
38. Clark D, Metcalfe A, Wogan C, et al. Adolescent patellar instability: current concepts review. Bone Joint J 2017;99(2):159–70.
39. Smith HC, Vacek P, Johnson RJ, et al. Risk factors for anterior cruciate ligament injury: a review of the literature—part 1: Neuromuscular and anatomic risk. Sports health 2012;4(1):69–78.
40. Hewett TE, Myer GD, Ford KR, et al. Biomechanical measures of neuromuscular control and valgus loading of the knee predict anterior cruciate ligament injury risk in female athletes: a prospective study. Am J Sports Med 2005;33(4):492–501.
41. Myer GD, Ford KR, Di Stasi SL, et al. High knee abduction moments are common risk factors for patellofemoral pain (PFP) and anterior cruciate ligament (ACL) injury in girls: Is PFP itself a predictor for subsequent ACL injury? Br J Sports Med 2015;49(2):118–22.
42. Ford KR, Shapiro R, Myer GD, et al. Longitudinal sex differences during landing in knee abduction in young athletes. Med Sci Sports Exerc 2010;42(10):1923–31.
43. Ford KR, Myer GD, Hewett TE. Longitudinal effects of maturation on lower extremity joint stiffness in adolescent athletes. Am J Sports Med 2010;38(9):1829–37.
44. Zazulak BT, Hewett TE, Reeves NP, et al. The effects of core proprioception on knee injury: a prospective biomechanical-epidemiological study. Am J Sports Med 2007;35(3):368–73.
45. Krosshaug T, Nakamae A, Boden BP, et al. Mechanisms of anterior cruciate ligament injury in basketball: video analysis of 39 cases. Am J Sports Med 2007;35(3):359–67.
46. Boden BP, Torg JS, Knowles SB, et al. Video analysis of anterior cruciate ligament injury: abnormalities in hip and ankle kinematics. Am J Sports Med 2009;37(2):252–9.
47. Hewett TE, Ford KR, Hoogenboom BJ, et al. Understanding and preventing acl injuries: current biomechanical and epidemiologic considerations-update 2010. North Am J Sports Phys Ther 2010;5(4):234.
48. Paterno MV, Schmitt LC, Ford KR, et al. Biomechanical measures during landing and postural stability predict second anterior cruciate ligament injury after

anterior cruciate ligament reconstruction and return to sport. Am J Sports Med 2010;38(10):1968–78.

49. Myer GD, Ford KR, Khoury J, et al. Development and validation of a clinic-based prediction tool to identify female athletes at high risk for anterior cruciate ligament injury. Am J Sports Med 2010;38(10):2025–33.

50. Ford KR, Myer GD, Hewett TE. Valgus knee motion during landing in high school female and male basketball players. Med Sci Sports Exerc 2003;35(10):1745–50.

51. Paterno MV, Ford KR, Myer GD, et al. Limb asymmetries in landing and jumping 2 years following anterior cruciate ligament reconstruction. Clin J Sport Med 2007;17(4):258–62.

52. Macfarlane GJ, de Silva V, Jones GT. The relationship between body mass index across the life course and knee pain in adulthood: Results from the 1958 birth cohort study. Rheumatology 2011;50(12):2251–6.

53. Centers for Disease Control and Prevention. Childhood obesity facts. 2021. Avaiable at: https://www.cdc.gov/obesity/data/childhood.html. Accessed November/9.

54. Centers for Disease Control and Prevention. Physical activity facts. 2020. Available at: https://www.cdc.gov/healthyschools/physicalactivity/facts.htm. Accessed May 15, 2021.

55. Ling DI, Boyle C, Janosky J, et al. Feedback cues improve the alignment and technique of children performing ACL injury prevention exercises. J ISAKOS 2021;6(1):3–7.

56. Yard E, Comstock D. Injury patterns by body mass index in US high school athletes. J Phys Activity Health 2011;8(2):182–91.

57. Shimozaki K, Nakase J, Takata Y, et al. Greater body mass index and hip abduction muscle strength predict noncontact anterior cruciate ligament injury in female japanese high school basketball players. Knee Surg Sports Traumatol Arthrosc 2018;26(10):3004–11.

58. Hashemi J, Breighner R, Chandrashekar N, et al. Hip extension, knee flexion paradox: a new mechanism for non-contact ACL injury. J Biomech 2011;44(4):577–85.

59. Dingel A, Aoyama J, Ganley T, et al. Pediatric ACL tears: natural history. J Pediatr Orthop 2019;39(Issue 6, Supplement 1 Suppl 1):S47–9.

60. Wheeless C. Natural history of the ACL-deficient knee. In: Wheeless CR, editor. Wheeless' textbook of orthopaedics. Towson, MD: Digital Trace Publishing; 2019.

61. Kisling LA, Das J. Prevention strategies. In: StatPearls [internet]. Treasure Island, FL: StatPearls Publishing; 2022. Available at: https://www.ncbi.nlm.nih.gov/books/NBK537222/.

62. Teutsch SM. A framework for assessing the effectiveness of disease and injury prevention. MMWR Recomm Rep 1992;41(RR-3):1–12.

63. Rink J, Hall TJ, Williams LH. Schoolwide physical activity: a comprehensive guide to designing and conducting programs. Human Kinetics; 2010.

64. Centers for Disease Control and Prevention. Physical education and physical activity 2021. Avaiable at: https://www.cdc.gov/healthyschools/physicalactivity/index.htm. Accessed November/10.

65. MOVE BETTER physical education workshop. Avaiable at: https://sports-safety.hss.edu/p/move-better-pe-curriculum-workshop. Accessed November/9.

66. Barden C, Stokes KA, McKay CD. Utilising a behaviour change model to improve implementation of the activate injury prevention exercise programme in schoolboy rugby union. Int J Environ Res Public Health 2021;18(11):5681.
67. Heidt RS, Sweeterman LM, Carlonas RL, et al. Avoidance of soccer injuries with preseason conditioning. Am J Sports Med 2000;28(5):659–62.
68. Myklebust G, Engebretsen L, Brækken IH, et al. Prevention of anterior cruciate ligament injuries in female team handball players: a prospective intervention study over three seasons. Clin J Sport Med 2003;13(2):71–8.
69. Söderman K, Werner S, Pietilä T, et al. Balance board training: prevention of traumatic injuries of the lower extremities in female soccer players? Knee Surg Sports Traumatol Arthrosc 2000;8(6):356–63.
70. Myer GD, Ford KR, Khoury J, et al. Biomechanics laboratory-based prediction algorithm to identify female athletes with high knee loads that increase risk of ACL injury. Br J Sports Med 2011;45(4):245–52.
71. Herrington L, Myer GD, Munro A. Intra and inter-tester reliability of the tuck jump assessment. Phys Ther Sport 2013;14(3):152–5.
72. Padua DA, Marshall SW, Boling MC, et al. The landing error scoring system (LESS) is a valid and reliable clinical assessment tool of jump-landing biomechanics: the JUMP-ACL study. Am J Sports Med 2009;37(10):1996–2002.
73. Padua DA, DiStefano LJ, Beutler AI, et al. The landing error scoring system as a screening tool for an anterior cruciate ligament injury–prevention program in elite-youth soccer athletes. J Athletic Train 2015;50(6):589–95.
74. Herrington L, Munro A. A preliminary investigation to establish the criterion validity of a qualitative scoring system of limb alignment during single-leg squat and landing. J Exerc Sports Orthop 2014;1(2):1–6.
75. Almangoush A, Herrington L, Jones R. A preliminary reliability study of a qualitative scoring system of limb alignment during single leg squat. Phys Ther Rehabil 2014;1(1):2.
76. Takahashi S, Nagano Y, Ito W, et al. A retrospective study of mechanisms of anterior cruciate ligament injuries in high school basketball, handball, judo, soccer, and volleyball. Medicine (Baltimore) 2019;98(26):e16030.
77. Donelon TA, Dos'Santos T, Pitchers G, et al. Biomechanical determinants of knee joint loads associated with increased anterior cruciate ligament loading during cutting: a systematic review and technical framework. Sports Medicine-Open 2020;6(1):1–21.
78. Kristianslund E, Faul O, Bahr R, et al. Sidestep cutting technique and knee abduction loading: Implications for ACL prevention exercises. Br J Sports Med 2014;48(9):779–83.
79. Dos'Santos T, McBurnie A, Comfort P, et al. The effects of six-weeks change of direction speed and technique modification training on cutting performance and movement quality in male youth soccer players. Sports 2019;7(9):205.
80. Butler LS, Milian EK, DeVerna A, et al. Reliability of the cutting alignment scoring tool (CAST) to assess trunk and limb alignment during a 45-degree side-step cut. Int J Sports Phys Ther 2021;16(2):312.
81. Dodwell ER, LaMont LE, Green DW, et al. 20 years of pediatric anterior cruciate ligament reconstruction in new york state. Am J Sports Med 2014;42(3):675–80.
82. Tepolt FA, Feldman L, Kocher MS. Trends in pediatric ACL reconstruction from the PHIS database. J Pediatr Orthop 2018;38(9):e490–4.
83. Zebis MK, Warming S, Pedersen MB, et al. Outcome measures after ACL injury in pediatric patients: a scoping review. Orthopaedic J Sports Med 2019;7(7). 2325967119861803.

84. Moksnes H, Grindem H. Prevention and rehabilitation of paediatric anterior cruciate ligament injuries. Knee Surg Sports Traumatol Arthrosc 2016;24(3):730–6.

85. Shultz SJ, Schmitz RJ, Cameron KL, et al. Anterior cruciate ligament research retreat VIII summary statement: an update on injury risk identification and prevention across the anterior cruciate ligament injury continuum, march 14–16, 2019, greensboro, NC. J Athletic Train 2019;54(9):970–84.

86. Nyland J, Greene J, Carter S, et al. Return to sports bridge program improves outcomes, decreases ipsilateral knee re-injury and contralateral knee injury rates post-ACL reconstruction. Knee Surg Sports Traumatol Arthrosc 2020; 28(11):3676–85.

87. Petushek EJ, Sugimoto D, Stoolmiller M, et al. Evidence-based best-practice guidelines for preventing anterior cruciate ligament injuries in young female athletes: A systematic review and meta-analysis. Am J Sports Med 2019;47(7): 1744–53.

88. Sugimoto D, Myer GD, Foss KDB, et al. Dosage effects of neuromuscular training intervention to reduce anterior cruciate ligament injuries in female athletes: meta-and sub-group analyses. Sports Med 2014;44(4):551–62.

89. Harøy J, Thorborg K, Serner A, et al. Including the copenhagen adduction exercise in the FIFA 11 provides missing eccentric hip adduction strength effect in male soccer players: a randomized controlled trial. Am J Sports Med 2017; 45(13):3052–9.

90. Al Attar WSA, Faude O, Bizzini M, et al. The FIFA 11 shoulder injury prevention program was effective in reducing upper extremity injuries among soccer goalkeepers: a randomized controlled trial. Am J Sports Med 2021;49(9):2293–300.

91. Sakata J, Nakamura E, Suzuki T, et al. Throwing injuries in youth baseball players: Can a prevention program help? A randomized controlled trial. Am J Sports Med 2019;47(11):2709–16.

92. Swart E, Redler L, Fabricant PD, et al. Prevention and screening programs for anterior cruciate ligament injuries in young athletes: a cost-effectiveness analysis. J Bone Joint Surg Am 2014;96(9):705–11.

93. Webster KE, Hewett TE. Anterior cruciate ligament injury and knee osteoarthritis: an umbrella systematic review and meta-analysis. Clin J Sport Med 2022;32(2): 145–52.

94. Poulsen E, Goncalves GH, Bricca A, et al. Knee osteoarthritis risk is increased 4-6 fold after knee injury–a systematic review and meta-analysis. Br J Sports Med 2019;53(23):1454–63.

95. Mandelbaum BR, Silvers HJ, Watanabe DS, et al. Effectiveness of a neuromuscular and proprioceptive training program in preventing anterior cruciate ligament injuries in female athletes: 2-year follow-up. Am J Sports Med 2005; 33(7):1003–10.

96. Steffen K, Myklebust G, Olsen OE, et al. Preventing injuries in female youth football–a cluster-randomized controlled trial. Scand J Med Sci Sports 2008; 18(5):605–14.

97. Kiani A, Hellquist E, Ahlqvist K, et al. Prevention of soccer-related knee injuries in teenaged girls. Arch Intern Med 2010;170(1):43–9.

98. Omi Y, Sugimoto D, Kuriyama S, et al. Effect of hip-focused injury prevention training for anterior cruciate ligament injury reduction in female basketball players: a 12-year prospective intervention study. Am J Sports Med 2018; 46(4):852–61.

99. Imwalle LE, Myer GD, Ford KR, et al. Relationship between hip and knee kinematics in athletic women during cutting maneuvers: a possible link to

noncontact anterior cruciate ligament injury and prevention. J Strength Cond Res 2009;23(8):2223–30.

100. Sugimoto D, Myer GD, Foss KDB, et al. Specific exercise effects of preventive neuromuscular training intervention on anterior cruciate ligament injury risk reduction in young females: meta-analysis and subgroup analysis. Br J Sports Med 2015;49(5):282–9.

101. Sugimoto D, Myer GD, Barber Foss KD, et al. Critical components of neuromuscular training to reduce ACL injury risk in female athletes: meta-regression analysis. Br J Sports Med 2016;50(20):1259–66.

102. Myer GD, Sugimoto D, Thomas S, et al. The influence of age on the effectiveness of neuromuscular training to reduce anterior cruciate ligament injury in female athletes: a meta-analysis. Am J Sports Med 2013;41(1):203–15.

103. Gilchrist J, Mandelbaum BR, Melancon H, et al. A randomized controlled trial to prevent noncontact anterior cruciate ligament injury in female collegiate soccer players. Am J Sports Med 2008;36(8):1476–83.

104. Myer GD, Stroube BW, DiCesare CA, et al. Augmented feedback supports skill transfer and reduces high-risk injury landing mechanics: a double-blind, randomized controlled laboratory study. Am J Sports Med 2013;41(3):669–77.

105. Hewett TE, Stroupe AL, Nance TA, et al. Plyometric training in female athletes: decreased impact forces and increased hamstring torques. Am J Sports Med 1996;24(6):765–73.

106. Irmischer BS, Harris C, Pfeiffer RP, et al. Effects of a knee ligament injury prevention exercise program on impact forces in women. J Strength Cond Res 2004; 18(4):703–7.

107. Vescovi JD, Canavan PK, Hasson S. Effects of a plyometric program on vertical landing force and jumping performance in college women. Phys Ther Sport 2008;9(4):185–92.

108. Sugimoto D, Myer GD, Bush HM, et al. Compliance with neuromuscular training and anterior cruciate ligament injury risk reduction in female athletes: a meta-analysis. J athletic Train 2012;47(6):714–23.

109. Myklebust G, Skjolberg A, Bahr R. ACL injury incidence in female handball 10 years after the norwegian ACL prevention study: important lessons learned. Br J Sports Med 2013;47(8):476–9.

110. Åkerlund I, Waldén M, Sonesson S, et al. High compliance with the injury prevention exercise programme knee control is associated with a greater injury preventive effect in male, but not in female, youth floorball players. Knee Surg Sports Traumatol Arthrosc 2022;30(4):1480–90.

111. Steffen K, Emery CA, Romiti M, et al. High adherence to a neuromuscular injury prevention programme (FIFA 11+) improves functional balance and reduces injury risk in canadian youth female football players: a cluster randomised trial. Br J Sports Med 2013;47(12):794–802.

112. Joy EA, Taylor JR, Novak MA, et al. Factors influencing the implementation of anterior cruciate ligament injury prevention strategies by girls soccer coaches. J Strength Cond Res 2013;27(8):2263–9.

113. Padua DA, Frank B, Donaldson A, et al. Seven steps for developing and implementing a preventive training program: Lessons learned from JUMP-ACL and beyond. Clin Sports Med 2014;33(4):615–32.

114. Van Mechelen W, Hlobil H, Kemper HC. Incidence, severity, aetiology and prevention of sports injuries. Sports Med 1992;14(2):82–99.

115. Finch C. A new framework for research leading to sports injury prevention. J Sci Med Sport 2006;9(1–2):3–9.

116. Centers for Disease Control and Prevention. Our approach 2020. Available at: https://www.cdc.gov/injury/about/approach.html. Accessed November/10.
117. Gielen AC, Sleet D. Application of behavior-change theories and methods to injury prevention. Epidemiol Rev 2003;25(1):65–76.
118. Gabriel EH, Hoch MC, Cramer RJ. Health belief model scale and theory of planned behavior scale to assess attitudes and perceptions of injury prevention program participation: an exploratory factor analysis. J Sci Med Sport 2019; 22(5):544–9.
119. Barros PM, Vallio CS, de Oliveira GM, et al. Cost-effectiveness and implementation process of a running-related injury prevention program (RunIn3): Protocol of a randomized controlled trial. Contemp Clin Trials Commun 2021;21:100726.
120. Simons-Morton B, Nansel T. The application of social cognitive theory to injury prevention. In: Gielen A, Sleet D, DiClemente R, editors. Injury and violence prevention: behavioral science theories, methods, and applications. Jossey-Bass/Wiley; 2006. p. 41–64.
121. Village J, Ostry A. Assessing attitudes, beliefs and readiness for musculoskeletal injury prevention in the construction industry. Appl Ergon 2010;41(6):771–8.

UNITED STATES POSTAL SERVICE ® Statement of Ownership, Management, and Circulation (All Periodicals Publications Except Requester Publications)

1. Publication Title	2. Publication Number	3. Filing Date
CLINICS IN SPORTS MEDICINE	000 – 702	9/18/2022

4. Issue Frequency	5. Number of Issues Published Annually	6. Annual Subscription Price
JAN, APR, JUL, OCT	4	$368.00

7. Complete Mailing Address of Known Office of Publication (Not printer) (Street, city, county, state, and ZIP+4®)

ELSEVIER INC.
230 Park Avenue, Suite 800
New York, NY 10169

Contact Person
Malathi Samayan

Telephone (Include area code)
91-44-4299-4507

8. Complete Mailing Address of Headquarters or General Business Office of Publisher (Not printer)

ELSEVIER INC.
230 Park Avenue, Suite 800
New York, NY 10169

9. Full Names and Complete Mailing Addresses of Publisher, Editor, and Managing Editor (Do not leave blank)

Publisher (Name and complete mailing address)

Megan Ashdown, ELSEVIER INC.
1600 JOHN F KENNEDY BLVD. SUITE 1800
PHILADELPHIA, PA 19103-2899

Editor (Name and complete mailing address)

Megan Ashdown, ELSEVIER INC.
1600 JOHN F KENNEDY BLVD. SUITE 1800
PHILADELPHIA, PA 19103-2899

Managing Editor (Name and complete mailing address)

PATRICK MANLEY, ELSEVIER INC.
1600 JOHN F KENNEDY BLVD. SUITE 1800
PHILADELPHIA, PA 19103-2899

10. Owner (Do not leave blank. If the publication is owned by a corporation, give the name and address of the corporation immediately followed by the names and addresses of all stockholders owning or holding 1 percent or more of the total amount of stock. If not owned by a corporation, give the names and addresses of the individual owners. If owned by a partnership or other unincorporated firm, give its name and address as well as those of each individual owner. If the publication is published by a nonprofit organization, give its name and address.)

Full Name	Complete Mailing Address
WHOLLY OWNED SUBSIDIARY OF REED/ELSEVIER, US HOLDINGS	1600 JOHN F KENNEDY BLVD. SUITE 1800 PHILADELPHIA, PA 19103-2899

11. Known Bondholders, Mortgagees, and Other Security Holders Owning or Holding 1 Percent or More of Total Amount of Bonds, Mortgages, or Other Securities. If none, check box ▶ ☐ None

Full Name	Complete Mailing Address
N/A	

12. Tax Status (For completion by nonprofit organizations authorized to mail at nonprofit rates) (Check one)
The purpose, function, and nonprofit status of this organization and the exempt status for federal income tax purposes:
☒ Has Not Changed During Preceding 12 Months
☐ Has Changed During Preceding 12 Months (Publisher must submit explanation of change with this statement)

PS Form **3526**, July 2014 [Page 1 of 4 (see instructions page 4)] PSN 7530-01-000-9931 PRIVACY NOTICE: See our privacy policy on www.usps.com.

13. Publication Title	14. Issue Date for Circulation Data Below
CLINICS IN SPORTS MEDICINE	JULY 2022

15. Extent and Nature of Circulation		Average No. Copies Each Issue During Preceding 12 Months	No. Copies of Single Issue Published Nearest to Filing Date
a. Total Number of Copies (Net press run)		179	171
b. Paid Circulation (By Mail and Outside the Mail)	(1) Mailed Outside-County Paid Subscriptions Stated on PS Form 3541 (Include paid distribution above nominal rate, advertiser's proof copies, and exchange copies)	111	99
	(2) Mailed In-County Paid Subscriptions Stated on PS Form 3541 (Include paid distribution above nominal rate, advertiser's proof copies, and exchange copies)	0	0
	(3) Paid Distribution Outside the Mails Including Sales Through Dealers and Carriers, Street Vendors, Counter Sales, and Other Paid Distribution Outside USPS®	34	38
	(4) Paid Distribution by Other Classes of Mail Through the USPS (e.g. First-Class Mail®)	0	0
c. Total Paid Distribution (Sum of 15b (1), (2), (3), and (4))	▶	145	137
d. Free or Nominal Rate Distribution (By Mail and Outside the Mail)	(1) Free or Nominal Rate Outside-County Copies included on PS Form 3541	20	18
	(2) Free or Nominal Rate In-County Copies Included on PS Form 3541	0	0
	(3) Free or Nominal Rate Copies Mailed at Other Classes Through the USPS (e.g. First-Class Mail)	0	0
	(4) Free or Nominal Rate Distribution Outside the Mail (Carriers or other means)	0	0
e. Total Free or Nominal Rate Distribution (Sum of 15d (1), (2), (3) and (4))	▶	20	18
f. Total Distribution (Sum of 15c and 15e)	▶	165	155
g. Copies not Distributed (See Instructions to Publishers #4 (page 83))	▶	14	16
h. Total (Sum of 15f and g)	▶	179	171
i. Percent Paid (15c divided by 15f times 100)	▶	87.87%	88.38%

* If you are claiming electronic copies, go to line 16 on page 3. If you are not claiming electronic copies, skip to line 17 on page 3.

PS Form **3526**, July 2014 (Page 2 of 4)

16. Electronic Copy Circulation		Average No. Copies Each Issue During Preceding 12 Months	No. Copies of Single Issue Published Nearest to Filing Date
a. Paid Electronic Copies	▶		
b. Total Paid Print Copies (Line 15c) + Paid Electronic Copies (Line 16a)	▶		
c. Total Print Distribution (Line 15f) + Paid Electronic Copies (Line 16a)	▶		
d. Percent Paid (Both Print & Electronic Copies) (16b divided by 16c × 100)	▶		

☒ I certify that 50% of all my distributed copies (electronic and print) are paid above a nominal price.

17. Publication of Statement of Ownership

☒ If the publication is a general publication, publication of this statement is required. Will be printed in the OCTOBER 2022 issue of this publication.
☐ Publication not required.

18. Signature and Title of Editor, Publisher, Business Manager, or Owner

Malathi Samayan — Distribution Controller

Malathi Samayan

Date 9/18/2022

I certify that all information furnished on this form is true and complete. I understand that anyone who furnishes false or misleading information on this form or who omits material or information requested on the form may be subject to criminal sanctions (including fines and imprisonment) and/or civil sanctions (including civil penalties).

PS Form **3526**, July 2014 (Page 3 of 4) PRIVACY NOTICE: See our privacy policy on www.usps.com

Moving?

Make sure your subscription moves with you!

To notify us of your new address, find your **Clinics Account Number** (located on your mailing label above your name), and contact customer service at:

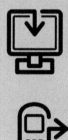

Email: **journalscustomerservice-usa@elsevier.com**

800-654-2452 (subscribers in the U.S. & Canada)
314-447-8871 (subscribers outside of the U.S. & Canada)

Fax number: **314-447-8029**

Elsevier Health Sciences Division
Subscription Customer Service
3251 Riverport Lane
Maryland Heights, MO 63043

*To ensure uninterrupted delivery of your subscription, please notify us at least 4 weeks in advance of move.

Moving?

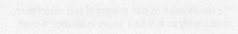

Printed and bound by CPI Group (UK) Ltd, Croydon, CR0 4YY

08/05/2025

01864704-0002